Dr. Bodo Otto

and

The Medical Background of the American Revolution

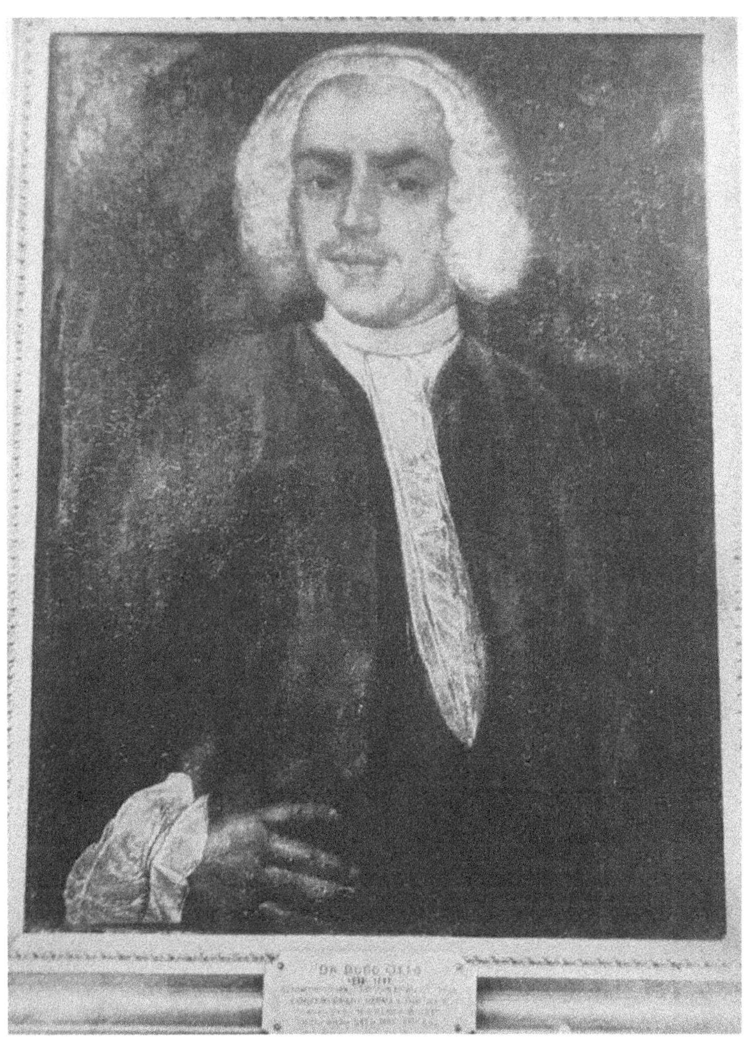

Dr. BODO OTTO

Born Hanover, Germany, 1711. Died Reading, Pennsylvania, 1787.

DR. BODO OTTO

and the Medical Background of the American Revolution

By

JAMES E. GIBSON

AUTHOR'S NOTE

THE WRITINGS of our colonial people were often involved. Sentences frequently became so lengthy as to cover several sheets of paper, resulting in complicated grammatical construction. Such conditions having been encountered in many of the letters and articles herein reproduced, the author has taken the liberty of doing some editing of them for the purpose of clarity.

TABLE OF CONTENTS

CHAPTER ONE

BODO OTTO'S ANCESTORS • Early Training • Apprenticeship • The Guilds • "The Dragoons" and the Army

IT IS A FAIR ASSUMPTION, though based on circumstantial evidence, that Bodo Otto's ancestors originally came from Saxony, having migrated in the seventeenth century to the neighboring province of Hanover. It is also believed that these forebears were foresters by profession, and it is known that an existing German branch of the family has continued in that profession these many centuries. A repetition of family Christian names over a long period of time on official government papers furnishes corroborative proof of the forestry connection far back into German history.

During the Thirty Years' War, Lauterberg, where the Ottos settled, was frequently raided and often devastated by marauding troops; once, the town was almost entirely destroyed, and its people were either killed or driven away. After the Peace of Westphalia in 1648, many Saxons from Southern Germany moved into the Harz section of Hanover, attracted by the vast mineral deposits and forestry wealth of the neighborhood.

It was in the year 1650 that there came into the Lauterberg district a "Saxon Mounted Forester" by the name of Michael Otto, who settled on the Oderfield. This Michael had several brothers, but only one, Hans Claus, likewise recorded as a "Chief Forester," is mentioned by name in Lauterberg Otto family records. Michael's oldest son, Hans Valentine, who was born in 1658, began a genealogical chart, and his descendants have continued it to the present generation. A German genealogist and Harz historian has expressed an opinion that Christopher Otto, Bodo's father, was the son of one of Michael's brothers, possibly Hans Claus and that ancestors of the American branch of the family settled in the Lauterberg neighborhood some time later. A search among the old church books of the Scharzfels parishes might clear up many uncertain points and establish definite dates, but the opportunity for an examination does not at present exist.

It is quite possible that Christopher Otto and his father before him were Chief Foresters for the estate of the Counts of Oberg, for the Oberg family likewise originated in Saxony. A bit of circumstantial evidence to support this probability is that when Christopher Otto required an affidavit to confirm his marriage claim and the birth of his son that Bodo might be legally apprenticed, he obtained two foresters for witnesses who testified they were all three in the service of Baron Bodo von Oberg at the time of the wedding.

Christopher's birth date was 1667, but unfortunately, we have no positive knowledge of where he was born or in what place he spent his youth and early manhood. Our first official record of him is that of his marriage in 1710 when he was forty-three years of age. The period between his birth and 1710 was full of important historical events, and one is curious as to whether Christopher took any active part in them and if they influenced his life. The Peace of Ryswick of 1697 brought to a close the prolonged war in the Low Countries between Louis XIV of France and the German Emperor. Christopher was between twenty and thirty years of age while this conflict raged and old enough to have entered it had he been so inclined. He was thirty-five when William, King of England, expired, and Sophia, Dowager Electress of Hanover, was elected to succeed to the English throne should Queen Anne die without issue.

It was but two years later that the Duke of Marlborough fought and won the brilliant battle of Blenheim, in which Hanoverian troops participated. Did Christopher Otto take part in these late seventeenth and early eighteenth century wars, and does it account for an official statement that the marriage of 1710 with Maria Magdalena Menechen was his first, or was this record an error on the part of the scribe? It does seem strange that a German of that period would remain single until arriving at the age of forty-three unless perhaps wars and absence from home had denied him the opportunity for a domestic life.

A certified abstract from the marriage register of St. John's Church in Hanover reads:

"On the 10th of June, 1710, the Licentiate Erythropel united in the bonds of matrimony, Christopher Otto and Maria Magdalena Menechen (in Krantz)."

What is the significance of the ending of this record reading "in Krantz?" Can it mean that she was adorned with a wreath, which was used to symbolize the bride as a maiden, or does it indicate the origin of the bride or possibly the residence of her family, and if so, is it the town "Kranz" located on the Baltic Sea? True, this is a long distance from the Hanover capital, but there was a related family of the Ottos, likewise foresters, living in that part of Germany, and this may explain Christopher's contact with that distant town.

Judge William T. Otto, President Lincoln's Assistant Secretary of the Interior, a great-grandson of Dr. Bodo Otto, learned of this Prussian branch of the family in 1884 and was referred to them in his efforts to trace the early Otto history. Again, within the past year, a correspondent in Lauterberg wrote of calling upon two old ladies of the Otto blood, who reported that some of the early archives were believed to be in the possession of a branch of the family located in East Prussia.

The history of St. John's Church, where Christopher was married, is interwoven with that of the Royal Chapel in the Elector's Castle.

The various reigning Dukes of Hanover for many generations had professed the Evangelical Lutheran faith and the Chapel had been so maintained until the accession of Duke Johann Friedrich, a Roman Catholic. The service then being that of the Church of Rome, the Duke's Protestant relatives and courtiers were deprived of their religious home and so they laid the foundation of a church in Neustadt. The Duke graciously issued a decree that the new building should be erected at the expense of the State, but before it was consecrated on April 10, 1670, Duke Johann Friederich passed away, and Ernest Augustus, a Protestant, succeeded. The Lutheran service was then resumed in the Castle, and from that time on, the records of the new church known as St. John's, as well as "Hof und Stadtkirche" and the Royal Chapel, have been combined. One year after Christopher's wedding, a son was born to him, and the archives of the Court record the christening in the Royal Chapel:

"Otto:-On July the 20th (1711), the Licentiate Erythropel baptized the son of Christopher with the name of Bodo. The godfather was the Privy Councillor, Von Oberg."

Whether the absence of Bodo's mother's name from the baptismal record was then customary or signified her death previous to that time, is not known. Not many years afterward, Christopher referred to this wife as "the late mother of the boy," and the same document indicated he had again married.

The Elector's Castle at Hanover containing the Chapel, was originally a monastery but had been so changed and rebuilt by the many succeeding generations of the ducal family that but little of the original structure existed. A member of an English Commission sent by Queen Anne to Hanover in 1702 has left an interesting description of the Royal Chapel. He wrote that it contained an unusually beautiful altarpiece, and the walls were wonderfully decorated with frescoes representing the crucifixion, while most of the needlework had been executed by the Dowager Electress Sophia with her own hands.

Baron von Oberg not only stood as godfather to Christopher Otto's son but conferred on Bodo his own Christian name.

There are many incidents in the lives of both Christopher and Bodo that suggest the existence of a close bond and even relationship between the Oberg and Otto families.

The Counts of Oberg were of a very noble house. They possessed numerous estates located in Hanover, Brunswick, and Magdeburg, though Obergen was their principal place of residence. They also had landed possessions in Hildesheim, Hoya, and Lüneburg. The first public account of them appears in a document dated 1103, and from that time down to the middle of the nineteenth century, they played important parts in affairs of war and peace as Commanders of fortresses and armies, Counsellors to the reigning Dukes and Ambassadors for the Electors as well as Bishops of the Church at Hildesheim.

Baron Bodo von Oberg was a man of great prominence in the Hanoverian Government. He was born in 1657 and, from 1683 until 1707, served as the Elector as Ambassador in the Courts of Berlin, Dresden, Stockholm, Vienna, Sweden, Saxony, and

Poland. During his presence in Berlin in 1684, he negotiated the marriage of the Elector's daughter, Sophia Charlotte, with the Crown Prince Frederick of Brandenburg, who in 1701 became the first King of Prussia. She was the grandmother of Frederick the Great and is said to have had beauty, charm, and unusual intellect. Baron Bodo von Oberg became a member of the Privy Council of Hanover, and in 1710 or 1711, the Financial Ministry of the State was conferred upon him.

It was from Baron Bodo von Oberg that Christopher Otto received his appointment as Controller or Tax Collector for the District of Scharzfels, but it is doubtful whether Christopher held that office at the time of his marriage or of Bodo's birth. This conclusion is based on the absence of any official title in the parish or Royal Court Records, for it has always been a German custom to include government honors in all public or church documents. So there comes the suggestion that Christopher Otto's presence in Hanover in the years 1710 and 1711 was connected with some private or estate business of Baron Bodo von Oberg. It is probable that Christopher received his appointment sometime between 1711 and 1713 and immediately left for his Scharzfels post, for later events indicate that Bodo was then too young to have any recollection of a time spent in Hanover. Young Bodo Otto's godfather died in 1713, just three years after his elevation to the Financial Ministry. Baron von Oberg's death, when his godson was but two years old, precludes any possibility that he was personally responsible for the appointments and honors that later came to Bodo, and again comes the thought of some strong bond between the two families, for the influence of the Obergs was present in matters affecting the State of Hanover for several succeeding generations.

The next account of Christopher Otto is obtained from a very ornate parchment record issued in 1724 by the Royal Court at

Uslar. It was a document made necessary by the absence of marriage and baptismal certificates that Bodo might be apprenticed to a surgeon. It has been translated twice by German scholars and reads:

"The highly esteemed Christopher Otto, having been appointed Controller by the Elector of Brunswick-Lüneburg for the County of Sharzfels, appeared in Court on the date given below and declared on oath that he had a son by his first marriage by the name of Bodo who desired to acquire a knowledge of surgery. Therefore, he made an application to a well-experienced surgeon by the name of Augustus Daniel Meier in the town of Harzburg near the Harz (mountains). A contract had to be made in order to acquire knowledge of the profession and a creditable testimony, or at least a baptismal certificate of his legitimate birth.

"Christopher Otto did then declare on oath in Court that he had married Maria Magdalena Neinekin, the late mother of the boy in A.D. 1708, while in the service of Baron Bodo von Oberg, a nobleman in Hanover. The above mentioned marriage took place in the Neustädter (St. John) Church of Hanover by the Court Chaplain, Rev. Wahrendorff, and in the next year Bodo was born. In due time, he was baptized, and the above-mentioned nobleman, Bodo von Oberg, became his sponsor. After a time, the preacher was promoted and sent to Dresden, but there were now two Royal Officers here, named Johan Friedrich Rischman and Johan Friedrich Bürgen, who would testify that the marriage was consummated according to the laws of the land.

"These two witnesses appeared in Court in order to be heard. They then testified that while they, too, were in the service of Baron von Oberg, Christopher Otto had been married to Maria Magdalena Neinekin by the Court Chaplain in Hanover and that she had worn a bridal wreath when united in church with Christopher Otto. They declared they knew no more except that the child of this marriage was born a year later and, shortly after his birth, received in Holy Baptism the name of Bodo. To this, these two witnesses testified on oath.

"Therefore, in accordance with my office and the duty devolving upon me, I have issued this certificate because I am fully convinced that the above testimony is correct and fully sustained.

"Hence, I herewith sign and corroborate the affirmation of the above-named persons and allow the seal of my office to be attached to the official document.

"So written at Uslar, March the fifteenth, in the year A.D., One thousand seven hundred and twenty-four."

–Friedrich Martin Hartlorff

(Seal)

Several mistakes appear in this old document; first, the spelling of the name of Christopher's wife, which is of no great importance, but the incorrect dates of his marriage and Bodo's birth have caused confusion in American records ever since. The pen and ink ornamentation on the certificate is of such an elaborate nature that it must have required a long time in the making and it is quite probable that the scribe is responsible for the errors. Dr. Bodo Otto brought this document with him to Pennsylvania in 1755, and in the absence of a birth attestation it has apparently been the authority used for his age. The certification of his marriage and regularity of his son's birth were what Christopher really sought, and the mistakes of time incorporated therein were of no great importance to him, but had Bodo's own mother been living, the wrong dates would probably have been corrected.

The wording of the Uslar attestation leads one to believe that Christopher had again married, and though no American family record mentions other children than Bodo, there was at least a daughter, for in 1756, Bodo Otto advertised in a Philadelphia newspaper asking for information of his brother-in-law, Maurice Zinche, who had emigrated from Lauterberg three years before.

Bodo Otto was only thirteen years of age when his father arranged an apprenticeship for him with a master surgeon. This, of a certainty, seems young for so serious an undertaking, but early contracts for training were the custom of those days. "Barber-Surgeons" schooling was a matter of only three years' application, and though its completion permitted a restricted practice, the attainment of that title never satisfied the more ambitious student, for it was the lowest rung on the professional ladder. The plan for Bodo's future was the beginning of a twelve-year preparation with travel, study, and hospital experience before settling down to private practice.

An apprentice, when starting training, lived in the house of his preceptor and obtained academic instruction while pursuing the rudiments of his professional studies. The duties of the boy included grinding powders, mixing medicines, accompanying the doctor on his visits, holding the basin when the patient was bled, helping to adjust bandages, besides many domestic chores about the house.

Bodo Otto's first apprenticeship was not served under August Daniel Meier as expected, for about one month after the arrangements were consummated, Dr. Meier died, and the parochial book at Harzburg of 1724 records his death with the notation that:

"On the 14th of (April, Mr. August Daniel Meyer was buried in the evening."

A second contract was then made with a surgeon of the College of Hildesheim by the name of Albrecht Henrick Klarig.

Among the records of the "Barber and Chirurgeon Guild" on file in the Hildesheim City Hall is the notice:

"June 26: In the year 1724, Johanni (Fall), I have registered my in Lauterberg, apprentice boy, Bodo Otto, born in Lauterberg, in the presence of all the co-masters, to study with me for three years. His birth certificate is on file.

"MASTER ALBRECHT HENRICK KLARIG "JOSBST FRIEDRICH WILCKEN ("Past Master") "HENNIG PERLE "JOHANN KLARE."

Then appears a list of the graduates, stating:

"In the year 1727, on April 1st, I have taken the name of my apprentice boy Bodo Otto off the roll of apprentices in the presence of all my co-masters.

"CONRAD FRIEDRICH FEGEBARICH (Past Master)

"HENNING PERLE, Sen. "I. H. GOSSLING

"ALBRECHT HENRICK KLARIG, Master."

Hildsheim, April 1st, 1927.

Another entry in the old guild book is in Bodo Otto's own handwriting and reads:

"I, Bodo Otto, born in Lauterberg, have studied in Hildesheim with H. Klarig of the new city and am now in that very place in Hildesheim.

"May 5th, 1727" An interesting error is contained in these Hildesheim archives, which may have some significance. It will be noticed that Lauterberg is credited with being Bodo's birthplace, both by his "master" and in Bodo's own statement, but the Archivist of Hildesheim has written that the birth certificate correctly records it as "Hanover." Does this not prove that Bodo

Otto left Hanover when so young that he had no recollection of that city and, knowing only Lauterberg as his home, considered it his birthplace?

To understand the importance of the "Barber and Chirurgeon Guilds" in which Doctor Otto began his training and its relation to the tuition of professional men of the times, will require a brief review of medical history. Even less than 200 years ago, graduates of the Barber and Chirurgeon Guilds were doing most of the surgery in Europe. Early Roman records present barber surgeons as men of great notoriety and their shops as resorts of the better class. Horace credits them with being most accurately informed, and stated much news could be obtained through them. The "Barber Surgeons," however, were of the lowest order in medical attainments, but most of those who aspired to the highest classification began as such. The famous Ambroise Paré was the son of one, as well as having had the same initial training. In early times, a social as well as professional distinction existed between "physicians, the surgeons of the Long Robe," who served under the physicians, and the "surgeons of the Short Robe," which included "barbers" and "apothecaries." Many "Barber-Surgeons" attended and gave baths, besides bleeding, cupping, leeching, giving enemas, and extracting teeth.

In Germany, they were required to pass examinations given by the four oldest Guild masters and the City physician, as well as to present evidence of legitimate birth. They were also required to travel for three years to gain additional experience from professional contacts. Among the better surgeons, apprentices were called "assistants" and paid as much as 300 marks. The "Barber-Surgeons" were a real power in France, Germany, and England, for they were the doctors of the common people and, consequently, the most valuable of all the professions.

As late as the eighteenth century, German surgeons were quite separated from physicians and not esteemed of equal importance, either socially or professionally, though special attention had always been given to surgical training in German institutions. Conditions of professional respect were just the reverse in the American Colonies, where surgeons were scarce, and their technical skill was highly honored. During the American Revolution, men who could qualify as surgeons were eagerly sought out and given hospital positions of great importance.

The German professional fees charged at the end of the seventeenth century may not have prevailed at the time when Bodo Otto practiced in Hanover, but they were recorded then as being:

40 pfennigs for office visits
1.35 marks for house visits
1.70 " " night calls
and one gulden for consultation.

A surgeon received 10½ marks for setting a broken arm, 20½ if two bones were broken, and 30.85 marks for a dislocated elbow or knee joint; 31 marks were paid for amputating an arm and 41 for a leg, but a surgeon could claim only half pay if his patient died.

Pest House physicians received salaries of 2,000 marks, while army surgeons were only paid 15 to 52 monthly, varying with different branches of the service. "Official District Surgeons" exercised all the functions and authority of "State Physicians."

These last few records are of special interest to us, for Bodo Otto served in the Hamburg Pest House as surgeon to the Duke of Celle's "Dragoons" and as chief of the District of Scharzfels.

Hildesheim, where Bodo began his professional training, was a medieval town not far from his home. It was the seat of the Bishopric, a hereditary office of the Oberg family, and this fact may have had some influence on Christopher's sending his son to that place. The old section of the city is most interesting, for it comprises many timbered buildings, with excellent examples of Romanesque and Renaissance architecture. The streets are narrow and crooked and the wall of the town has been converted into a promenade. Against the façade of the ancient cathedral stands a rose bush 25 feet high, reputed to be 1,000 years old.

Just when Bodo Otto left Hildesheim and began the period of travel to extend his training is not known, but in a document issued by him in Philadelphia in 1766, he wrote:

"After the expiration of mine apprenticeship (at Hildesheim), I served as a surgeons' man (assistant) under several masters at Hamburg and attended the Lazaretto where there is a conflux of both internal and external ailments."

This statement registers an advancement from the "Barber Surgeon" classification, in which he was restricted to the treatment of wounds and external diseases.

The selection of Hamburg for advanced study and experience was a wise choice. It was then the largest city in all of Germany, but its water supply was obtained from the badly polluted river Elbe, resulting in frequent epidemics of cholera, etc., so Bodo Otto said truly when he claimed the Lazaretto or Pest House, brought him experience in many ailments. It was a rare opportunity for observation and practice in different diseases, especially in the early part of the eighteenth century, when hospitals were not numerous.

Hamburg is believed to have been founded by Charlemagne in 805 when he built a castle as a defense against the heathen Slavs. It became the center of Northern European civilization and was repeatedly plundered and burned by the Danes and Norsemen. By the Treaty of 1240-49, it entered the Hanseatic League, and from that time on, the wealth and commercial importance of the town greatly increased. Hamburg officially adopted the reformed religion very early and received many foreign refugees.

Bodo Otto's army service with the Duke of Celle's "Dragoons" may have predated his Hamburg training, for the Lüneburg certificate, which mentions it states he enrolled under General Bottmar, who, it has been ascertained, commanded the regiment between 1690 and 1729.

The chronicles of the "Dragoons," later known as the "Sixth Cavalry Regiment of Kur-Hanover," would undoubtedly furnish information on its activities during the period Bodo Otto served as its surgeon. All this might be found in Werche's "History of the Army of Hanover" if the opportunity existed to examine the book.

The Duke of Celle was an uncle of the Elector, and as one of the reigning family, his regiment may have then been attached to the Court. Hanover was not involved in war during the period of Bodo's connection with the army, and peace-time medical duties were not arduous or such as required constant presence, so they need not have interfered with other study and training. Bodo Otto's service was at a time when Spain threatened the peace of Europe through a treaty with Charles VI of Austria, which brought France, Prussia, and England into a strong alliance. It was then that Spain attacked Gibraltar, and Charles threatened to invade Holland. The dual obligations of the Georges as Kings of England and Electors of Hanover involved the German Province in every European peril that threatened, and it is known that the

Elector frequently marshaled his subjects when war clouds gathered. The English Minister Walpole was largely responsible for averting many serious European conflicts during the reigns of both George I and George II, and his efforts at this time prevented a war that would have involved the regiment in which Bodo Otto served.

The record of the Duke of Celle's "Dragoons" is one of glory and honor extending as far back as the Thirty Years' War. In 1702, the regiment was with the Army of the Reich on the upper Danube opposing the French, and on August 13, 1704, it fought under the English Duke of Marlborough and Prince Eugene of Austria in the battle of Blenheim. Here, it is related: "The Dragoons of Celle's regiment, under von Bottmar, rode into the enemy at full speed with swords in fists and without stopping as usual to first discharge their pistols."

On July 6, 1711, the "Dragoons" were in the attack at Douay and in 1712 at Le Quesnoy, France, while later they took part in the war of the Austrian Succession and engaged in the battle of Dettigen. The regimental uniform was light blue with silver ornaments. Its staff included one field surgeon with two helpers. A sword, now in the Berks County Historical Society, presented by one of the Otto family, bears a notation that it was carried by Bodo Otto at Valley Forge. This cannot be correct, for American surgeons did not wear side arms or uniforms until after 1800. It is possible the sword was brought from Germany and had been worn by Bodo when in the Hanoverian Army, but it is also probable it was given to him by a grateful wounded Hessian officer who was a patient in Dr. Otto's Trenton hospital in the summer of 1777. This, in fact, is the family tradition, and it is further believed that the donor was the same Lieutenant who inscribed and presented a German songbook to Bodo's son and assistant, Dr. John A. Otto.

CHAPTER TWO

LÜNEBERG • Medieval Traditions • The City Hall and Salt Feasts • Otto's Second Marriage • Kalkberg Fortress

IT IS IN LÜNEBURG, situated on a tributary of the Elbe River, about thirty miles southeast of Hamburg, where we pick up Bodo Otto's history from official records. Just when he transferred his activities from Hamburg, or the army, to the town of Lüneburg is not known, but the certification of his admission to practice recites that Bodo had previously served under Lüneburg master surgeons. The city taxpayers' list also includes his name as a citizen prior to the date of his professional examination, so he may have resided and studied in Lüneburg for some time before presenting himself for a final examination on June 13, 1736.

The city of Lüneburg, founded by Henry the Lion, is medieval in appearance, with narrow streets and ancient buildings. It was originally a fortress town and part of the aged walls still stand. The old city possesses many fine examples of wood carving, paintings and murals. It was once an influential member of the Hanseatic League and, at the time of the Reformation, was one of the richest towns in Northern Germany. The population of Lüneburg in the Middle Ages is believed to have been 14,000 and the town to have contained 2,000 houses. Every taxpayer was required to personally convey the amount of his assessment to the City Hall, and it was against the law to delegate even a member of one's own family. Taxation was based on self-appraisement, and honesty in such matters seemed to have been expected and assured by the citizen oath. Custom required that every taxpayer be treated with refreshments by the city officials, and there still exist the old silver beakers from which wine was served to those who paid large amounts, while the citizens contributing small dues were content with beer served in zinc mugs. Councilmen served the city without salaries but received honor gifts of several casks of wine and, at Lenten time, an additional honorarium of a barrel of herring. In the City Hall are kept the bones of a pig in honor of a tradition that in the twelfth century, it acted as a messenger of the gods and accidentally made known the vast salt deposit on the outskirts of the town when it appeared with brine upon its bristles.

The Lüneburg City archives, which are very numerous, began with documents dated 1514, and many writings of Martin Luther are included in the collection; among them is the letter in which he wrote: "In all, I hate nobody more than those who convert liberty into oppression."

The oldest document among these papers is a communication from a Lüneburg citizen, Johann Funke, who complained he had been exiled from home because he had read the writings of Dr. Martin Luther and sung the German Psalms at church.

At the beginning of the sixteenth century, the Lüneburg City Council was opposed to the Lutheran movement and warned the citizens against the dangers of supporting the sect. They also obtained several priests from the nearby monastery of St. Mary's in an effort to counteract the movement by preaching the old faith to the people.

Lüneberg's Protestantism developed quickly in spite of official opposition. At an Evangelical meeting held in the large assembly room of the City Hall, the rope supporting the heavy stone weight of the tower clock was cut, resulting in a ruined ceiling but fortunately without serious casualty. It was in the City Hall of this ancient town that Bodo Otto reported on June 13, 1736, to undergo an examination after twelve years of preparation. The City records contain the following certificate, which qualified him to practice among the physicians and surgeons of Germany:

"WHEREAS, BODO OTTO, a Native of Hanover, who according to his Indenture produced before us, has served a regular apprenticeship of three years to Mr. John Albrecht Klarchen, Member of the College of Surgeons at Hildesheim, concerning which he has also shown a proper testimony; and has afterwards been Surgeon to a company of Cavalry in the Regiment of Lieutenant General BOTTMAR, in which Service he behaved to everyone's satisfaction, as his Discharge witnesseth; and has likewise with several Masters here at Lüneburg, at Hamburg, etc., practised the Art of Surgery: And being now desirous to be received a Member of the College of Surgeons in this city; therefore we the physicians whose Names are hereunto subscribed, with the Assistance of three Surgeons of the College, viz. Mr. FRANCIS JULIUS PFEIFFER, Mr. J. BUNCKE, and Mr. PHILIP GERHARD DOPKING undertaking, according to the King's Order, his Examination on the 13th day of June 1736, the said Candidate, having previously declared his Intention to remain by the Art of Surgery, and to improve himself therein, have questioned him on the Osteology, Splanchnology, the Circulation of the Blood, Bleeding, and the necessary Precautions with regard to it, as well concerning the Cure of an Artery accidentally touched, as also the knowledge about the Gangraena and the Sphacelus and the proper Remedies for their Cure; likewise concerning Wounds and their accidents; and lastly about the Instruments and the external Remedies to be applied by Surgeons; all according to the Tenour of the original Writings thereof, kept in our Office of Records: Leaving, for the present, the rest of the Examination, respecting Luxations, Fractures, etc., to the College of Surgeons here.

Now, the above-mentioned Candidate BODO OTTO, having honourably answered his Examinations, we, together, have in Witness of the Truth, granted him this authentic Attestation, corroborated by our Hands and Seals, to the End, that thereupon (performing well the rest of His Art) he may be received a Member of the College of Surgeons at this Place, and be entrusted with a Surgeon's Office.

Done at Luneburg in the Lesser Secretary's Office, at the City Hall, on the 13th day of June, 1736.

B. A. NOTTELMANN, Dr. H. C. CRUGER, M.D.
Civit. Luneb. Proto-Physic & Civ. Luneb. Phys. Ord. (L.S.)
(L.S.) FRANCIS JULIUS PFEIFFER
Surgeon to the Regency of the City (L.S.) JACOB BUNCKE,
Provincial Surgeon
(L.S.) PHILIP GERHARD DOPKING, Surgeon"

These so-called "College of Surgeons," maintained in all large German cities, were not professional educational institutions but might be compared with American medical examining boards before which a newly arrived physician and surgeon or recently graduated apprentice was required to appear and prove his qualifications for the classification to which he belonged.

Next to the churches of Lüneburg, the City Hall held the highest practice in rank among the important buildings of the city. Compared with other similar buildings in the Fatherland, the one in Lüneburg stands in first place. The structure itself is monumental, and in both exterior and interior appearance, it is claimed to be artistically perfect. The history of its erection is said to extend through seven centuries, for it reached its present size and perfection through the efforts of many generations of citizens.

Every year before deciding upon the seasonal sales price of salt, a great feast was held in the City Hall to which were invited the City Scribe, the official physicians, the Superintendent of the Mint, the leaseholder of the City Hall wine cellar, the caretaker of the Kalkberg, the Ducal Tax Collector, the Guest Master of the Holy Ghost, the Church Lord and Sexton of St. Lamberti, and the entire clergy. The festivities lasted three full days, and all entertainment was free to the guests, but if anyone wished to continue the celebration beyond that time, pay was demanded for the meat and drink consumed.

Bodo Otto's marriage to his first wife, Elizabeth Sauchen, probably occurred about the time of his examination in Lüneburg, for on May 1, 1737, a daughter was born and christened Mary Elizabeth. She later accompanied her father and his family, by a second wife, on their emigration to America and died in New Jersey in 1768. She was married, as recorded in her father's will, to George Marx. If he were George Wilhelm Marx registered as landing in Philadelphia on August 31, 1750, it would seem that the wedding occurred in America after the Ottos' arrival. Bodo's wife, Elizabeth Sauchen, died in 1738 and is buried in Lüneburg.

Four years later, the Parochial Book of St. Lamberti's Church of Lüneburg, for the month of April in 1742, records the marriage of "Bodo Otto, chirurgicus of this place and the virgin Catharina Dorothea Dahncken, daughter of the late Johann Dahncken of Schwerdfigers, legitimately born."

An interesting portrait of Catharina Dorothea (Dahncken) Otto remains in possession of the family. A tradition handed down is that she was of noble birth, but of this there is no proof, though the poise and beauty of the painting suggests that the subject was a patrician.

Bodo's and Catharina's first child was born on the 22nd of August, 1743, and christened Frederick Christopher after his grandfather; the next, Dorothea Sophia, born November 16, 1744, lived only until February 28, 1748, and she too was buried in Lüneburg. A second son arrived on September 14, 1748, and was baptized Bodo, Jr., in honor of his father. The birth date of the youngest, John Augustus, was July 30, 1751, several years after the family had moved to the Scharzfels district.

St. Lamberti's Church, where Bodo Otto's marriage to his second wife occurred, was located in the parish of the same name and dates from 1209. It was closely related and dependent upon the salt deposits and, according to the custom of the Middle Ages, the church served not only in its religious capacity but as the meeting place for the officials of the saline organizations. Here new officers were appointed and old ones dismissed; questions pertaining to the management of salt production, such as wages of workers and even the social affairs of the families of the employed, were subjects of discussion and decision. The church was materially interested in the financial success of the salt mines, for the salaries of the Lamberti church lord, priests, clock setter, and all others were obtained from the sale of the product.

In 1511 there existed a charitable society in Lamberti to attend the poor of the congregation and care for the Eternal Light maintained in the church.

Celebrations and feast days were observed by the church attendance of the City Council and other high civic and religious officials, and after services they were served with claret wine and

Einbecker beer. During the Reformation, St. Lamberti was fully in agreement with the new teachings and in 1531, Martin Luther spent Palm Sunday in Lüneburg, holding service in the church during Easter Week.

Early in 1703, structural weakness appeared in the old building, and though repairs were frequently made and reinforcing members were later introduced, the deterioration of ages became too great to be overcome, so in 1861, after 552 years of service, this ancient church was condemned as unsafe. Today it exists only on old city maps but remains a glorious memory in the religious history of Lüneburg. The church contained many beautiful and artistic paintings, which, with the famous high altar erected about 1460, were transferred to honor places in the Lüneburg Church of St. Nicklai. In November of 1747, Bodo Otto requested and received an attestation of his skill and fidelity from Dr. Henry Christian Kruger, the official physician of Lüneburg, and this possibly was sought in anticipation of his leaving that city for the Harz, for about a year later he asked for a similar document from Lt. Col. P. A. de Rion, the commanding officer of the Kalkberg Fortress. The two documents follow:

MR. BODO OTTO, Surgeon of the College of this City, having requested of me an Attestation about his Skill and Experience in Surgery, I think it incumbent on me to testify by these Presents that he did not only well answer to his Examination before the late Mr. Nottelmann, the first physician to the City, and me, in 1736, and that thereupon he was received a Member of the College of Surgeons and permitted to keep 2 Surgeon's Office; but that also, since that time to this day he has sufficiently shown his ability in Surgery, in many particular and difficult Cases; having but lately made a successful amputation of a Leg, and happily and well cured the wound.

In Witness of the above attestation, I have hereunto set my Hand and Seal.

Done at Lüneburg, the 25th day of November, 1747.

(L.S.) DR. HENRY CHRISTIAN KRUGER,

physician to the city.

WHEREAS BODO OTTO, of the College of Surgeons of this City, has intimated to me that he has lately sold his Office and consequently can no longer attend or cure the Invalids quartered in this Place, being obliged to prepare for his Removal to his new Post on the Hartz; and has therefore requested an attestation respecting his good Behavior and assiduous attendance to his Duty. NOW, the said BODO OTTO, having, at all times, and by all accidents that have occurred, shown himself as an honest, experienced and faithful surgeon, both to the Prisoners in the Fortress Kalkberg at this Place as also to the Invalids quartered here; I, readily complying with his request, do by these Presents attest his above said Qualifications, and recommend him in the best manner to everyone's Favour. Lüneburg, November the First, in the year 1748.

(L.S.) P. A. DE RION

Lieutenant Colonel of a Company of Invalids belonging to His Majesty the King of Great Britain and Electors of Brunswick-Lüneburg.

What tales Bodo Otto might have told of his twelve years' contact and service as Chief Surgeon in this ancient Fortress of Kalkberg! It is claimed that its history extends back 6,000 years before the birth of Christ, and the evidence to support such a belief is found buried in the soil within the boundaries rather than in documents, for excavations and old graves furnish the proof through stone and bronze implements uncovered. The commanding site of the Kalkberg readily suggested a defensive use. Steep cliffs, hardly accessible, were supplemented by artificial fortifications that were easily defended by a handful of brave men. As a fortress, the Kalkberg was never conquered. Its garrison was not allowed to leave the walled enclosure between sunset and sunrise, and vicious dogs supplemented the soldiers on guard duty. A watch was constantly maintained on the Kalkberg towers, and the surrounding country was continuously under observation for suspicious movements indicating the presence of an enemy or robber band. Arms, armor, rifles, powder, and even crossbows were always kept in readiness for attack or defense, and the area within the fortress was sufficiently large to take thousands of people under its protection. A fortified castle, eventually erected within the Kalkberg walls, became the seat of the local reigning Duke. Long before that time, tradition has it that an ancient pagan shrine was located on the site and a slender Italian column of marble now reposing in the museum is believed to have supported the idol. On this spot of heathen worship, the Benedictine cloister of St. Michael's was established, and from that place, the Christian faith was forced upon the pagan inhabitants of Lüneburg. Many a Saxon was forcibly converted to Christianity, for until the year 959 all properties of those refusing to renounce their pagan gods were confiscated and given to the Church.

Under the reign of Emperor Otto the Great, bitter wars were fought between the German and the Wendish nations and throughout centuries of conflicts that followed, the Wendish Army never penetrated beyond the Ilmenau River because of the unconquerable Kalkberg.

In 1071, a Swabian King attempted to obtain possession of the Fortress through trickery, but the seventy warriors he smuggled into the Kalkberg to overthrow the garrison were quickly starved into submission. Until the fourteenth century, the Lords of the Kalkberg castle had always been protectors of the Lüneburg people, but under the then-reigning Duke Magnus, they were so oppressed that the natives rose in rebellion. A group of brave young men, adopting women's dress, joined a procession of females attending worship in the Kalkberg Chapel and, at a signal from their leader, threw off their disguise and, overpowering the garrison, made the entire ducal family their prisoners. Denouncing all allegiance to the Duke, they destroyed the menacing castle with the exception of the Watch Towers. Sometime later, the Lüneburg citizens rebuilt this castle, but thereafter, they retained physical possession of both castle and fortress.

The name Kalkberg is incorrectly applied to this natural stronghold, for it is not composed of Kalk or lime, as the term might indicate, but is, in fact, a massive formation of gypsum. Much of this deposit was carried away during the recent World War for use in the manufacture of sulphuric acid and sulphur, so greatly needed in explosives for the German Army.

The Kalkberg was also employed a hundred years ago to establish trigonometric points when the German Government developed the metric system. Efforts are now being made to obtain the necessary funds to restore the ancient fortress to its condition of the Middle Ages. Its glorious history and the scenic grandeur surrounding its site certainly warrant the efforts. It has been said that if one wishes to enjoy a beautiful view of Lüneburg and the surrounding country, he should visit the Kalkberg in May or June when the evening sun dips toward the horizon, and the magnificent beauty of the scene will remain in the memory forever...

CHAPTER THREE

THE DISTRICT OF SCHARZFE-LS • Hunting Ground of Emperors • Religious Cloisters Local Superstition

IT WAS SOMETIME between the end of the year 1748 and the beginning of 1750 that Bodo Otto, with his second wife and two sons, together with a daughter by his first marriage, moved from Lüneburg to their new home in the Harz mountains.

Lauterberg, Scharzfeld and the Castle of Scharzfels lie adjacent to each other, and it was in this immediate neighborhood that Bodo settled a district steeped in such splendid history, traditions, and folklore that it must have quickened the heartbeat and stirred the imagination of Bodo's young family.

The District of Scharzfels obtained its name under the reign of Emperor Charles the Great when he introduced the Frankish Constitution and form of government. The early history and traditions of this section tell of many different groups of people who governed the territory or were subject tribes as the fortunes of war decided. Conflicts with Rome had taught the Germans they could conquer their enemies if they would only act together when mutual interests made it necessary. Even when they united in a common cause, each tribe retained its own laws and leaders.

Very often they elected a supreme commander from the strongest group, even adopting his tribal name for all of them, and it was under such circumstances that the Saxons became the dominant people in the Harz mountains. One part of this tribe had drifted to England and there strongly established themselves very early in history. It was in their native territory that the Germans came in contact with the Franks," and this was the beginning of wars and hatreds that seem likely to continue as long as the two nations exist. This small section of the Harz, especially Scharzfels, Harzburg and Pöhlde, became a favorite hunting ground of the Saxon Emperors who often visited these parts. There, beautiful views delighted the eye while fertile valleys and meadows provided food for the cattle and men. Then came religious monasteries into the neighborhood with their followers and culture. Ilfeld, Walkenried and Pöhlde were established, and the Saxon Emperors provided the monks and everybody connected with the religious orders and golden opportunities for peace and plenty; wherever these retreats were located, far from the tumult and activities of the world, villages sprang up because of the need of laborers to work the fields and craftsmen to supply their wants. And thus came into being the town of Lauterberg in which the Otto family settled and to which Bodo was returning with a physician-and-surgeon qualification and with honors conferred on him by his sovereign.

The village of Scharzfeld was built near Pöhlde Abbey, and it is first noted in an official document dated 952 issued by Emperor Otto I. He was the son of Queen Mathilda, who founded the monastery between 947 and 951 in honor of John the Baptist and the martyr Servatius.

Until the end of the eighth century, the old Saxons steadfastly clung to their pagan deities, made sacrifices and resisted the teaching of Christianity, but after this neighborhood came under the influence of the Pöhlde Abbey, fields were cultivated, houses built, and a church erected in which the converted Saxons worshipped.

Bodo Otto's youngest son, John Augustus, wrote in his Bible that he was born in Lauterberg and again that it was from that place they began their journey to Philadelphia, so it is assumed that the village of Lauterberg, centrally located in the district to which Bodo was officially credited, served as his family residence.

The property erected or acquired by the first of the Ottos, who settled in Lauterberg about 1650, has remained in the possession of the family down to the present time, although the house has been twice rebuilt in the intervening centuries. It is located adjacent to the Evangelical Lutheran Church in which both Christopher and Bodo worshipped, and its present owners are two sisters of seventy-five and eighty-five years of age; one, still a Miss Otto, and the other a widow. From them it was learned the house had always been maintained by the family even when its master was required to live elsewhere because of public duties. Here, the Ottos returned after they retired from official life, and spent their last days.

During some extended repair and replacement work on the old house in 1863, a family document dated 1788 was found in the wall. It, too, told of reconstruction work executed in that year and reported evidence found that the building had been on fire at some previous time—possibly during the Thirty Years' War—and that silver coins of early dates were recovered from under the stairs. It also described a cannonball and some rifle bullets found among débris under the floor and recorded the belief they had been fired during the War of 1618-48. This document of 1788, signed by the City Scribe, also described the ceremony of installing the "House Door." It is believed the original paper is in the possession of a branch of the family living in Lehnsan, Holstein, Prussia, which descended from Chief Forester Wilhelm Otto, born in 1796.

A strange and interesting tale comes to us from a historian of the Harz about Dr. Christian Barnhardt, who was a predecessor of Bodo Otto as chief surgeon of the Scharzfels. The story, as told by the old people of the neighborhood, relates that Dr. Barnhardt was a great traveler, and on one of his extended trips that carried him over the sea, he met and married a mermaid whom he brought to his home. The upper part of this wife was formed quite like a woman, but the lower half of her resembled a fish, and she lived in a large spring of cold water. The Doctor's neighbors greatly feared and disliked this misshapen creature though her hair was said to have been like spun gold and her complexion as beautiful as apple blossoms. One day, when the Doctor had gone to a distant village to attend to a sick patient, the people sat in judgment on this unnatural female and decreed that she be poisoned unto her death; the good Doctor was grief-stricken in his loss and with the money his mermaid had brought him from the bottom of the sea, said to have been a leather sack full of gold, he established a fund for the benefit of the needy of the district. Like most folklore tales, this story is built upon certain proven facts. It is true there was a Scharzfels physician by the name mentioned who, like Bodo Otto, was Chief Surgeon of the district, and he was a bachelor and a great traveler. On one of his travels, he acquired a seal, which he brought home and kept in a subterranean stream flowing through his cellar. The ignorant and superstitious people of the neighborhood considered it a monster cursed by God and made away with it. On the Doctor's death it was found he had left his estate to the district authorities under a provision that the interest be distributed among the poor. Unfortunately, the value of the investments held in the trust disappeared in the recent German inflation, and this wonderful charity, which kept alive a fantastic tale, ceased to function. Very recently the cold stream in which the seal lived was uncovered when extending a cellar in the Doctor's old house and traced to its source in the depths of a hillside mine.

In the year 1131, the Castle of Scharzfels was built on a lofty site that towered above the village of Scharzfeld. Situated on a steep barren rock, it dominated and protected the surrounding country. It was in this castle on January 31, 1750, that Bodo Otto was administered an interesting oath of fidelity as "Chief Surgeon of the District of Scharzfels," and among his cherished papers brought to America is the original subscribed and attested document which reads:

"His Britannic Majesty's Privy Councillors for the Regency of the Electorate of Brunswick-Lüneburg, having appointed BODO OTTO, after due inquiry into his ability and skill, Chief Surgeon of this Bailiwick, and he having first heard the Warning against Perjury, the following Oath was administered unto him: 'You shall vow and swear on Oath unto GOD and by His holy Word, that you will always, in undertaking Chirurgical Cures, as also in sections and Inspections, make known and indicate the true Circumstances, to the best of your Knowledge and Understanding, and that you will not fail so to do, for the sake of any Reward, Favour, Hatred, Friendship or Enmity, or for anything else that might be devised by the Senses of Man. So help you, GOD and His holy Word."

The early history of the Scharzfels Castle is wrapped in deep mystery but even the first known records of it are surrounded with romance. Nature dictated the design of the defense with its steep cliffs and deep ravines that only needed a roof to make the beginning of an unconquerable fortress. A drawbridge gave ingress to the court which was enclosed in a half circle of gigantic rocks, and long stone stairs led to a second hanging bridge that furnished an entrance to the large-domed hall. From this point, wide passageways cut through solid stone gave access to the abode of the Castle Lord. An engraving of the Scharzfels Fortress and Castle made in 1650 shows it in all its medieval grandeur, and though it has since been destroyed, it is said the surrounding woods and fields appear very like they did two hundred and eighty-five years ago. On the main road at the foot of the hill, along which the gentry and peasantry traveled, was the Customs House and Tax Collector's residence and both structures are shown. These two buildings are of special interest to the Otto family, for it was here that Christopher Otto performed his duties as "Controller" and maintained his official residence.

It is not known when people first realized the value and importance of the natural fortress of Scharzfels, but according to traditions it had been a retreat of the early Saxons. The first document relating to the Scharzfels were those ceding it to Pöhlde Abbey, but it remained in possession of that order only for a short time and soon became the property of the Count of Lauterberg. When old Count Werner von Lauterberg died in 969, his estate was divided among four sons, the third of whom, Bodo by name, obtained the "House of Scharzfels," as it was called. The family of Lauterberg eventually lost the title, and in 1130, Scharzfels became a Castle of the German Reich and later by gift from the Emperor it changed hands many times. One of the owners erected a high watch tower on a commanding spot from which the entire country could be observed. Whenever merchants' caravans were seen approaching, a trumpet sounded, and the Count and his men in armor would mount their horses and gallop away to waylay and rob the traveler whom they also held for ransom.

It was in the year 1525 that the peasants revolted and made their twelve demands in an effort to correct both religious and economic ills. Their grievances were very real, and the solutions suggested were equally just, but the peasants were badly advised and poorly led. Mobs became active throughout the land and directed their attacks against castles and

monasteries, and though the Scharzfels Fortress was too strong to be captured, they destroyed the nearby Pöhlde buildings, leaving only the bare walls of the church and twenty-four chairs from the choir.

In 1617 Scharzfels Castle came into possession of a Duke of Celle of the ranking family of the State. It was from a later generation of the blood that the Elector of Hanover and a King of England was chosen and it was said the mining and forestry properties attached to the Scharzfels furnished them a private income of £300,000 annually.

Scharzfels survived the Thirty Years' War though suffering at the hands of uncontrolled bands of soldiers that plundered the country. On September 12, 1641, the nearby town of Lauterberg was ruthlessly looted and set on fire by the Emperor's troops.

Many traditions and folklore tales are still related to the old castle, but the story called "The Ghost of the Scharzfels" is perhaps the most interesting. It is told that in the eleventh century, during the reign of Emperor Henry IV, there lived in the fortress a noble Count and his beautiful wife whom the Emperor greatly desired. There also dwelt in the Scharzfels a little elf or gnome who, for many generations, was frequently seen in the shape of an old man, clad in the clothes of a miner. His abode was in a lookout tower, and whenever a joyous happening for the inmates was in store he appeared before the event in a lively and jolly mood and danced out of sheer joy in the courtyard and on castle walls.

He was, however, very sad when a calamity approached, and once upon a time, when the Count and his beautiful wife returned to the Scharzfels after attending a Court festivity, they espied the elf sitting upon the terrace with every appearance of great grief; his eyes were full of tears which overflowed and wetted his long white beard that reached to the ground. The Count and his wife were greatly disturbed for fear that some dreadful disaster was about to happen. Not long afterwards, a renegade monk, the private chaplain of the Emperor, appeared at the Castle with a command from his Master for the Count to leave immediately on a state mission of importance. Soon after his departure and apparently quite accidentally, the Emperor and his Chaplain arrived at Scharzfels seeking shelter from a threatening storm. With the help of the infamous monk, the Emperor imposed his will on the defenseless Countess. Then there resounded throughout the Castle a terrible noise! The elf had hurled down the roofs of the many towers and, from the walls, loudly announced to all the wicked deed that the Emperor, assisted by the monk, had wrought upon the Countess. Tradition claims that the elf so persistently and terribly pursued the monk that he threw himself over the cliffs into the Harz River, and today, the spot is called the "Rock of Disgrace," while the Emperor was afflicted with remorse all through the remainder of his life. This tradition, like most folklore tales, has some foundation of truth. The facts are that Emperor Henry had a Knight, Albrecht von de Helm, who, as Chief of Mines throughout the entire Harz Mountains, maintained his residence in the Scharzfels Castle. The Emperor, who, with Archbishop Adelbert von Brener, lived a life of great dissipation in the nearby Castle of Harzburg, forced his attention on the beautiful wife of the Count while her husband was absent. On Albrecht von de Helm's return, the Countess informed him what had happened in his absence, and Albrecht demanded satisfaction but was laughed at for his presumption. Crazed with anger, the Count planned vengeance upon the

Emperor and set fire to every government-owned mine and smelter in the district; he fled with his wife beyond the boundaries of the kingdom, aided in his escape by the Archbishop of Cologne.

With altered methods of warfare and vehicles of attack, the old fortress of Scharzfels lost its reputation and the confidence of the people as the unconquerable defense of the Harz. The beginning of the eighteenth century found it reduced to a garrison of invalids and retired soldiers.

Here, they lived in peace and quiet, spending the remaining days of their lives exchanging reminiscences of wars and experiences with the satisfaction of years honorably spent in service to the State. For their sustenance they cultivated gardens and brewed beer to supplement the "bread of Grace" they daily received. These were the men who came under the professional care of Bodo Otto when he became Chief Surgeon of the district. For five years, he attended their ills in an atmosphere of happiness and peace, but at the beginning of 1756, one year after Bodo Otto's departure for America, their quiet and contentment were disturbed by the sound of marching feet and the tumult of battle.

Three times was the Scharzfels captured during the Seven Years' War, as the enemy advanced and retreated across Brunswick-Hanover, and twice was it recovered without great damage being done to the Fortress. The third attack in September 1761, made by an army of 11,000 Frenchmen, met with such stubborn resistance from a handful of old German soldiers that the enemy, in revenge, reduced the Fortress to utter ruins. When the French began their assault on September 16th, bringing heavy artillery into action, the Scharzfels were garrisoned by only 250 invalids, 40 artillerists and 100 local sharpshooters. From the time of the Thirty Years' War until the present day, the men of the Harz Mountains have been celebrated for their marksmanship. Beginning in 1652, they held an annual

Schützenfest, the winner of which was crowned king of the sharpshooters and given a sum of money and a silver plaque. Of such were the soldiers who helped defend the Castle in 1761 and gave their enemy an impression of a large and aggressive defending garrison. The return fire from the Fortress was most effective, and the fighting and bombardment continued day and night. During the siege of Scharzfels, neighborhood people were compelled to supply the assaulting French army with food and were forced to erect protective fortifications for the enemy.

The batteries and sharpshooters in the Castle did heavy damage to the besieging army, and seven days passed with the old Fortress maintaining its previous reputation of being unconquerable when properly defended. The French were about ready to abandon the attack and withdraw when a traitorous inhabitant divulged a secret path to a nearby mountain where batteries were placed and executed great damage. Further resistance was then impossible, and the fate of the Scharzfels was sealed, so on September 25, 1761, after seven days of continuous fighting, the Fortress surrendered. The 100 sharpshooters, who knew every path and ravine in the country, escaped down vine-covered cliffs, and by densely wooded passes, they reached the safety of their Harz forests. Even before the French could occupy the Castle, a courier was dispatched to Paris with news of the difficult capture of the strong Scharzfels and a claim that it had been defended by a large army supported by many guns.

Perhaps it was the humiliation of finding the captured garrison composed of only 290 men, of whom 250 were incapacitated retired soldiers, and the many guns to be but a few cannons that decided the fate of the Fortress. On September 29 and 30, 1761, while Paris was celebrating the French victory with artillery fire and a Te Deum service in the Church of Notre Dame, the commanding officer at Scharzfels requisitioned miners from nearby Lauterberg to blast down the walls that had stood for five hundred and thirty years. The French, in their blind rage and fury, because of a seven-day resistance of 390 men against 11,000, even tried to destroy the rock upon which the Castle stood. The approach of Duke Ferdinand of Brunswick with a force of Hanoverian troops caused the enemy to hastily withdraw and saved the neighborhood from further acts of vengeance.

The destruction of the Scharzfels Castle and Fortress was almost complete, and they have never been rebuilt. All that remains are picturesque and interesting ruins. Here, the fall winds blow through the forest, brushing dying foliage from the trees, while overhead dark clouds float across the sky and cover the moon; ghostly bats and owls rush through the air, while on the ground, small animals glide through the underbrush like fairies or spirits of men who throughout the centuries had lost their lives in the Castle's defense. Deserted now is the old Fortress where, many ages ago, knights in shining accouterments gathered for pleasure and tournaments or assembled for war—where tilting was done for the smile and favor of fair maidens or men summoned to fulfill feudal obligations to their chief.

Today, the ruin of the Scharzfels is a place of amusement for neighborhood people. The view from the top of the rock embraces the charming valley of the River Oder and the peaceful villages of Barbis, Bailolfeld and Scharzfeld. The old Castle of Harzburg, now used as a Law Court and State Prison, is within the range of vision, and when the weather is clear, the monument of the Kyffhauser, the tower of Possen and the Hills of Gottingen can be seen.

It was sometime after 1748, while living in the neighborhood, that Bodo Otto "frequented the physical, anatomical and botanical lectures of two eminent professors" at the newly established University of Gottingen, situated within the Scharzfels district.

The registry of the university does not include his name, but this is readily explained. Dr. Otto was then a practicing physician and not a medical student in preparation for a degree, so he was never entered on the college rolls.

The faculty of the German universities, though receiving salaries from the State, obtained the greater part of their income from fees paid directly to them by students who attended lectures. The relations between teacher and pupil were then quite personal and not a matter of official notice until the scholar appeared for an examination and a university diploma. The lecture charges for academic courses were sixteen shillings, sixpence, but for the "Art of Healing," as medical lectures were called, they were two and even three times as much.

The Evangelical Lutheran Parish Book of Lauterberg contains the final story of Christopher Otto and closes the German church records of the family, for his son Bodo left his native land not long afterwards, never to return.

"The Licent Controller, Christopher Otto of the District of Scharzfels, died at Lauterberg on August 21, 1752, in his eighty-fifth year. He was publicly buried, with great honor, on August 25, in the Evangelical Cemetery."

This burial ground on the outskirts of the town is shown in an old engraving made in 1650, but the cemetery no longer exists, for the village encroached upon its site, and a school building and playground now cover it.

CHAPTER FOUR

ENROUTE TO AMERICA • Change of Residence • International Dissension • The Trials of Traveling • Sickness

LONG AFTER THE DEATH of Christopher Otto, his grandson John Augustus wrote in his journal: "Grandfather being dead, Father decided to emigrate to America," so Bodo Otto evidently considered a change in his residence sometime prior to 1752 and possibly deferred action during the lifetime of his old father. Neither family records nor traditions explain why Dr. Otto, who enjoyed an enviable position in his native land as well as holding an official appointment from the King, was willing to forego these advantages and assume the uncertainties of life in a new country among strangers. Several published sketches of his life claim the underlying reasons were political dissensions and revolutions, but history fails to record any such disturbing conditions. Religious peace was universally enjoyed in Hanover in the eighteenth century and the Evangelical Lutheran Church, to which Bodo Otto belonged, was the one officially recognized by the State. The country was perfectly content under the Regency, for the absent Elector and the people were happily governed, so it could not have been any of the accredited reasons. Was it, then, a love of adventure? Bodo Otto had many of the characteristics and the spirit of a pioneer, but he was forty-four years old, an age when most men are well settled and not easily fired by tales of excitement; besides, he was the head of a young family and therefore less likely to take chances just for the thrill of them. Could it have been a desire for economic betterment with greater opportunities for his three growing sons? This may have had a great influence, for despite Bodo Otto's established position, there was uncertainty about the future caused by widespread unemployment in the Harz between 1750 and 1755, with corresponding local economic disturbance. In addition, as a contributing cause of the depression, there had been a succession of poor harvests and a conflagration that ruined 199 mines in the Scharzfels district. The distress of the people was further increased by an epidemic of plagues and pests that swept through the countryside and caused the shutting down of the remaining mines and smelters. Truly this combination of circumstances might have inclined any man to consider a possible chance of improving his condition. If these problems disturbed Bodo Otto's peace of mind, perhaps the war clouds that were gathering over Europe in the apprehension of the Seven Years' War caused the important decision for a change and the beginning of a new life in the Colony of William Penn. Surely the mustering of troops in France, Austria, Prussia, and England had a significance not to be ignored. Did Bodo Otto realize that a war between France and Austria, as allies against Prussia and England, would necessarily draw Hanover into the conflict and that the Scharzfels district, situated between the contending countries, would become a battleground of the pending European War?

Contrary to an agreement with England, the French had built a line of American forts along Lakes Erie and Ontario and were extending them to the Mississippi River. The English Government took no steps to retaliate until early in 1755 when France attempted to reinforce its Canadian army and fleet. British men of war then pursued the French squadron and an engagement took place off Newfoundland, with two French ships striking their colors. The French Ambassador in London requested his passports and returned to Paris, but his Government delayed a declaration of war for two reasons; first, they were anxious that England should take the war initiative so that they might claim the benefit of their treaty with Spain, stipulating an offensive alliance if France were attacked in Europe; and, second, the French Navy was composed of only 113 vessels, against 213 possessed by the British. Both nations began increasing the number of their ships of war and building privateers. Recruiting stations were established in Hanover, and French troops moved into the Low Countries on the German border. Sea raids on each other's commerce immediately started. The danger of a passage to America was reflected in the withdrawal of emigrant ships from the trade and an eight percent increase in insurance rates. Frederick the Great had said early in 1754 that war between France and England was inevitable. He was at that time under a treaty of offense and defense with France which would expire early in 1756. France, anxious to renew the agreement, requested the Prussian Ambassador in Paris to write his sovereign suggesting that Frederick attack Hanover, saying:

"He will find there fine pillage, for the treasury of the King of England is well furnished, and he has but to siege."

The King of Prussia reasoned that if he renewed the Treaty with France, the French would surely attack Hanover, and this would bring Austria and Russia, presumably English allies, down upon him, while a compact with England might prevent the war being carried into Germany. King George of England was well informed of the situation and first appealed to Frederick through the Duke of Brunswick and later by a personal request for an alliance. A decision depended upon the attitude of Russia, which had not been friendly to Prussia, and the English sovereign informed Frederick of a Russian agreement to support him with troops, which later proved otherwise, so Prussia signed an English offensive and defensive treaty. Louis XV was very resentful of Frederick the Great for this change of "Allies," so they sought a compact with Austria, Prussia's hereditary enemy. Thus, Europe's powers aligned when open warfare began in 1756, and for seven years, there was continuous fighting in the Scharzfels district of Bodo Otto's old home. The London newspapers of April 26, 1755, carried an item that:

"His Majesty went to Leicester House this day to take leave of his family before visiting his German Dominion."

This, in reality, was for the purpose of contacting the King of Prussia, and on May 10th, the day the Ottos began their long journey to America, it was published:

"The King has left orders that if during his absence the lords of the Regency should find it expedient to declare war, the yacht should be dispatched for his return." Even if Bodo Otto had all these facts before him it must have been difficult to reach a decision on so momentous a matter of whether to stay at home or emigrate. If he remained in Lauterberg, he was confronted with the certainty of active participation in a war in which he had no patriotic interest, leaving his wife and young children to contend with hostile troops. On the other hand, should he leave the Scharzfels, he faced the uncertainty of finding a ship sailing from Rotterdam to America, and if successful in this first step, what were the chances that the vessel would ever reach its destination? A decision not only involved his own future and that of the family but might even become a matter of life or death. That he was fortunate in discovering a vessel destined for Pennsylvania is confirmed by the fact that only two ships carrying Germans sailed for Philadelphia in the year 1755, for the impending danger of war had resulted in their withdrawal from the American trade. Even before Bodo Otto's ship left England for Pennsylvania, London newspapers reported that many owners thought it prudent to hold their vessels in port even though most of them were fitted out with guns and British men of war well spread out over the seas. John Augustus Otto's journal records the important decision in his entry:

"On May 10, 1755, father moved with his family from Lauterberg to Philadelphia in America," and so Bodo Otto began his journey to the Pennsylvania Colony in a period of official peace but was obliged to pass through thoroughly alarmed countries with many of the incidental dangers and discomforts of actual warfare.

Dr. Otto's emigrating family consisted of his second wife; a daughter, Mary Elizabeth, aged 18 (by his first marriage); Frederick Christopher, a boy of twelve; Bodo, Junior, seven years old; and John Augustus, a boy approaching four.

It is regretted that no account or tradition exists of their trip to Rotterdam, of their passage to and delay in England, or their voyage to America. However, other emigrants have written much of the discomforts, suffering and privations of the German pioneer, from which some impression may be gained of what Bodo Otto and family may have in part experienced. Most of these accounts, however, deal with the water route down the Rhine to the port of embarkation. It might reasonably be expected that at least this portion of the journey to America could have been made in comfort and with good dispatch, but such is not the record.

Gottlieb Mittleberger, who came to Philadelphia in 1750, bringing an organ for the St. Michael and Zion Lutheran Church, wrote that the hardships of attending the German river trips were impossible to describe. The main reason for the discomfort and vexation was the requirement that Rhine boats pass through thirty-six towns, all of which made custom examinations and assessed duties. The time consumed by these stops and inspections depended entirely upon the temper and convenience of Government officials and accounts for the fact that passage of the Rhine required from four to six weeks. Delays necessarily resulted in additional and often unexpected expenses which, with arbitrary assessments of duties on personal effects, ate into the emigrants' supply of accumulated money. Many who started with ample funds reached their destination in debt to the shipmaster for part or all of their passage.

Another route used by Germans living adjacent to rivers flowing into the Baltic Sea was through Hamburg, with sailing direct to the Colonies.

Lauterberg was not conveniently located for a river passage to Holland, and it appears likely that Bodo Otto reached Rotterdam, his port of embarkation, either by means of public stagecoach or, if his household effects were numerous enough to require it, by private conveyance.

An English diplomat has left an interesting account of the conveniences of the main traveled German stagecoach routes and told of well-marked roads with distances to and from the next village painted on the signpost. He complained bitterly, however, of the taverns' poor food, dirt, inconvenience, and high costs. Travelers, out of necessity, carried their own bedding, and sharing a room or even a bed with others was the universal rule. He mentioned the smoke and smell encountered, for he said the houses were not ventilated, and open doors were the only means of eliminating both offenses.

The Reverend Henry Melchior Mühlenberg, who lived in the neighborhood of Lauterberg, used the public coaches when setting out for America in 1742 and his diary gives many incidents of day-to-day travel. True, he first went to the city of Hanover, possibly fifty miles to the north, but the distance from that city to the Holland border is comparable with that from Lauterberg, and the routes are fairly parallel. Mühlenberg left Hanover on April 5, 1742, reached Osnabuck in western Germany on April 7th, crossed into Holland on the 10th and arrived at Amsterdam the next day. By scaling the map of Germany and Holland, this indicates an average daily travel of forty miles with but a week of elapsed time; surely a much better record with at least less time for discomfort than any river trip promised.

In the "Life and Times of Henry Melchior Mühlenberg," the details and incidents of this trip so briefly outlined may be found. It tells that he abandoned the coach at "Norden" on April 10th, boarding a boat propelled by horses. The name of the town must be a typographical error, for Norden is a German village some ninety miles due north of the direct route to Holland. Possibly "Nord horn," just over the Holland border, was the town really meant for it is situated on a river that empties into the Zuider Zee; but it probably was Naarden, a village located a few miles from Amsterdam, though it seems strange that Mühlenberg transferred from stagecoach to boat when so near his destination.

The arrival of the traveler at Rotterdam often marked the beginning of another period of uncertain and expensive waiting. Many of the ships carrying emigrants to America sent agents through Germany to solicit passengers for the Colonies. Very often, these representatives were unscrupulous rascals whose misrepresentations of conditions caused needless mental and physical suffering. With the congestion of people waiting for both the uncertain arrival and departure of the boat on which passage was expected, emigrants stormed the first ship available, regardless of her size and accommodation.

The prevailing fare from Europe to America varied from forty to fifty dollars, half payable on departure and the balance on arrival at the destination, but funds were often depleted and even exhausted before that time. The only recourse then left was a contract with the shipmaster permitting him to sell the passenger's services for a sufficient length of time to cover the amount due. Adults were bound for from three to six years, depending upon age, physical condition, and the nature of their trade. Children from ten to fifteen years old were required to serve their masters until they were twenty-one years old.

Many abuses and cruel injustices resulted from these contracts for passage, sometimes occasioned by the deliberate intent of the captains but more often the outcome of misunderstandings that naturally arose between people speaking different languages. It was for the purpose of protecting the German settler from imposition as well as his own mistakes that the Pennsylvania German Society was organized in 1764 by members of the Philadelphia Lutheran churches. Bodo Otto became an active member of this organization after his return to Philadelphia practice after six years of residence in New Jersey.

Vessels sailing from Holland were quite dependent upon freight to the Colonies for their expenses and profits, and frequent stops for the purpose of collecting cargo were made at different Channel ports. Consequently the relatively short sail from Holland to the last port of call consumed from three to four weeks. Then followed a final ship inspection and fitting out with more delays to further exhaust the emigrants' patience and funds. There is a record of boats carrying Palatinates from Plymouth to New York being held in the harbor from Christmas Day until Easter.

Bodo Otto's ship, the "Neptune," probably enjoyed favorable winds and weather en route to America, for she made the voyage in eight weeks' time, arriving in Philadelphia on October 7, 1755. This indicates the "Neptune" sailed from England about August

12th and leaves three full months to be accounted for after leaving Lauterberg in Hanover. Could war preparations in Germany have delayed Bodo Otto's reaching Holland, or was there a long wait in Rotterdam and many stops en route to England? Unfortunately neither family papers nor traditions supply the answer.

The Philadelphia port records inform us that the "Neptune" cleared from Gosport, England, and this fact permits one to build a story around this ship that has all the possibilities of romance. Gosport, opposite Plymouth, was originally called "Gods Port," for it was so christened by Bishop Henry de Blois in 1158 when it gave him a haven from a violent storm. It was a naval station, not a commercial port, and only two ships out of 324 were recorded as sailing from England to Philadelphia, with German emigrants cleared from this harbor. What, then, is the significance? Did the "Neptune" enter Gosport to be fitted out with guns for her own protection, or was she waiting there for the sailing of men of war to the Colonies in order that she might have a convoy for at least the beginning of her voyage?

English naval stations had been busy accumulating war supplies, conditioning and outfitting ships from early 1755, and 300 privateers were said to be under construction. The French were equally active in this respect, and a fleet of flat boats was assembled in Brittany for the contemplated use of a French army of 250,000 men to invade England. Paris news dispatches recited that France was only delaying a declaration of war until she had acquired the desired number of warships and privateers. The French fleet was assembled in the harbor of Brest, and the English squadron off Plymouth. Captured merchantmen were constantly being brought into English ports, and France retaliated by seizing all English ships and merchandise found in French harbors. George II was still in Germany on July 26, 1755, when a news dispatch was published in London that:

"It is currently reported that the King of Prussia has entered into an offensive and defensive treaty with his Majesty at Hanover."

A week later, it was further reported:

"The present state of affairs between England and France, requiring his Majesty's departure, is fixed for the 26th instant."

The methods of aligning European powers show little change today over those used in 1755. England and France were the only real enemies involved, destined to settle their differences by recourse to arms. The participation of Austria, Prussia, Poland, Sweden, and Russia was purely a matter of some possible advantage to be gained, so a subject of negotiation and barter without regard to any national grievance. Russia, presumably an ally of England, threw its strength, unexpectedly, to France, and on the death of the sovereign, Elizabeth, and succession of Peter III, switched to the English side because of Peter's admiration for Frederick of Prussia, but when that Czar was deposed by Catherine the Great she withdrew her troops from active participation in the conflict. War was nothing then but a State business and national pastime and had little appeal to the patriotism of individual citizens.

The following published dispatches furnish a reason for believing the "Neptune" had anchored in Gosport while waiting for the protection of British men of war:

"Gosport, July 10, 1755, His Majesty's Ships, Warwick, Greenwich, and Winchester have come into the harbor to be sheathed and fitted out with all expedition, being intended for the West Indies; the guns, stores, etc., are being taken out with great diligence."

"Gosport, Aug. 1, 1755, Commander Frankland has hoisted his pennant on His Majesty's ship 'Winchester' and Capt. Le Grosse is expected to sail with the squadron very soon."

"London, Aug. 9, 1755, We hear that six French men of war are cruising in the mouth of the Channel, but Admiral Hawke is sailing in quest of them."

"August 11, 1755, We hear that Commander Frankland sails next week with ten men of War of the Line for the West Indies."

Then there appeared the convincing dispatch that:

"The Lords of the Admiralty have informed merchants that some of His Majesty's ships are sailing for the Mediterranean and

West Indies and would take their ships under convoy if sent to Spithead."

The precaution of waiting for protection was apparently a wise one, for on August 12, 1755, the day the "Neptune" is believed to have sailed, the following dispatch was published at Cadiz:

"The French squadron, which has been at anchor some time in this Bay, sailed today bearing its course northeast. It was afterwards met by two Masters of Ships who saw the English fleet commanded by Admiral Hawke but a small distance apart, but that there did not appear any disposition to attack each other."

What stories might be told by the log of the "Neptune" were it available for examination! The record would probably reveal days of feverish outfitting with guns, reports and rumors of dangers lying off the coast, of prize crews bringing captured French merchantmen into Gosport and then the start to America, under the protection of the British Navy. What a contribution to Colonial history could have been made had the Pennsylvania Assembly required captains of emigrant ships to file copies of their logs as well as lists of their German passengers!

Unfortunately, no record of the voyage of the "Neptune" has been found to tell us whether the days were fair or stormy or if the trip was made in anxiety and fear or with a feeling of security and protection.

In the absence of a diary kept on the "Neptune," a reference to records of other voyages may be of some interest.

With the raising of the anchor at the English port of departure, the real misery of many an emigrant's trip began. The ships were small and often overcrowded, and sometimes, the sleeping allotment of space for a passenger was only two by six feet. Under such circumstances, with seasickness, fever, diarrhea and even smallpox present, deplorable conditions were experienced, and many a German regretted the day he left home. Large numbers died, and the mortality among children was almost unbelievable, for those between one and six years of age had a small chance of surviving serious illness on a rough and prolonged voyage.

In addition to sickness, many suffered the pangs of hunger and thirst, for provisions and water were often exhausted when storms and adverse winds retarded the ship.

Rain was frequently the only resource for drinking water, and many times, it was caught on spread canvas to save a desperate situation. The Reverend Doctor Mühlenberg wrote in his diary of resorting to this method of replenishing the supply and mentioned that in their great need the captain had remembered a quantity of vinegar that might in extremity be used to quench thirst. To their disappointment and surprise many of the bottles were found half empty. The mystery was solved when rats were observed gnawing off the corks and inserting their tails as a method of getting at the drink they, too, were seeking.

The "Neptune's" quick passage precludes the possibility of any tales of suffering from exhausted supplies, while the Philadelphia port physician's report indicates a voyage without serious sickness aboard, for he found:

"The passengers are all in good health except one man and woman, and they but very slightly ailing so that we can not report any infectious distemper being aboard the said vessel; therefore, there can be no objections to her being admitted to enter the port."

The two Philadelphia weekly papers announced on October 9th, 1755:

"Tuesday last (Oct. 7) arrived here the ship 'Neptune,' Capt. George Smith from Rotterdam but last from Cowes in eight weeks."

The time consumed on the "Neptune" voyage was much less than the average required, for most ships reported twelve weeks necessary to make the trip and often fifteen elapsed.

A second news item stated:

"By Captain Smith we have letters from London as late as August 5th, which say that they soon expect a declaration of war and that insurance from London to America was eight guineas and from West Indies to London 13%."

After the emigrants had been duly examined and passed by the port physicians, they were marched to the Philadelphia Court House, where they took the two required Oaths and signed their names. One was a declaration of allegiance, and the other of abjuration, denying the right of the Pope to depose rulers and referring to descendants of James II who still claimed the throne of Great Britain.

Ninety-three names appear on these old Pennsylvania documents, signifying there were that number of males over sixteen years of age on board the "Neptune" and that the balance of the 226 whole freights reported by the captain were women and children, each adult being considered one whole and every child a half freight.

Dr. Wm. J. Hinke, in his book on the Pennsylvania German Pioneers, has said that the order of the names appearing on the two Prescribed Oaths was of great importance and significance for the Peaders or, most important, of the emigrants, usually signed first. Both signed lists were headed by Reimer Landt and followed by Bodo Otto.

The second and last German emigrant ship to arrive at Philadelphia in the year 1755 was the "Pennsylvania," which entered port on November 1st with but thirty-four "whole freights." On November 10, 1756, the "Snow Chance" arrived with 109½ "whole freights," and then German immigration entirely ceased for five full years. On October 23, 1755, an advertisement appeared in a Philadelphia paper:

"FOR CHARLES-
TOWN SOUTH
CAROLINA, THE
SHIP 'NEPTUNE'
GEORGE SMITH
COMMANDER

> Will sail in fourteen days. For freight or passage agree with Benjamin and Samuel Shoemaker or said Commander on Board."

The November 13, 1755 newspaper contained the announcement in news of the port:

"OUTWARD
BOUND SHIP
'NEPTUNE'
GEORGE SMITH
FOR SOUTH
CAROLINA"

CHAPTER FIVE

THE COLONIAL PHYSICIAN • Epidemics • Importance of Colonial Physician • Colonial Medical School

THE DISEASES THAT ATTACKED the early American Pioneers in their new environment were similar to those they had experienced in Europe. Very few of the expeditions to America were accompanied by accredited physicians and surgeons, so the first colonists relied on the family's medical resources for remedies and on past experience for guidance in nursing. Medical men soon followed the early emigrants and the history of many of those who practiced in New England, the Middle and Southern Colonies, has been preserved.

Epidemics of various kinds appeared in a short time and, on several occasions, destroyed entire settlements. Smallpox was one of the scourges soon encountered, frequently devastating Indian villages as well as white settlements. The Pilgrims, while regretting the resulting mortality among the natives, often looked upon the Indian casualties as acts of Providence sent for the white man's protection. In 1690, Lieutenant John Hubbell, while marching his company of Connecticut soldiers to revenge an Indian massacre in New York, was stricken with smallpox and died. His remains were buried where he expired, and the Indians, disinterring his body to take his scalp and divide his clothes, spread the infection among their own people, and half the tribe succumbed to the malady. Other epidemics, including measles, influenza, diphtheria, dysentery, pleurisy and various kinds of fevers, were encountered, so the Colonial physician had many problems to solve and, at times, numerous patients to see.

It has been claimed that the professional men of those days were unusually well educated, and it was written:

"The doctor of the seventeenth and eighteenth century was a great personage; that no one questioned his authority on any point, and to his utterances the people paid great heed; while the power of his presence was only second to that of exalted church dignitaries."

Of his appearance, it was said:

"The European physicians wrote great wigs, a distinctive dress of black cloth almost clerical in effect, and carried gold-headed canes."

In the provinces, the medical profession did not follow these formal fashions to any great extent. Though wigs were sometimes worn, the American custom of wearing the hair long and tied back was found more convenient and much less expensive, while dark clothes and walking sticks were not serviceable for country practice.

Dr. Bodo Otto's portrait presents him arrayed in the conventional Continental mode with a wig and flounced shirt, but all the characteristics of the artist's technique indicate the picture to have been painted prior to Dr. Otto's emigration to America.

The Colonial physician, the judge, and the minister were the most important people in the community. He was his patients' beloved friend, confidant and counselor, sharing both their joys and sorrows. The frequency with which we find the doctor's name as witness to wills, executor of estates and guardian for children is evidence of deep affection and entire confidence. Neighbors committed their interest to him when selecting representatives for committees, conventions, assemblies and for such public positions as judges over the courts, with the firm conviction they would be faithfully served and well represented. Even the Quakers showed deference to the honor of his position and, ignoring their rule regarding the non-use of titles, addressed him respectfully as "Doctor."

The professional preparation of the Colonial physicians, compared to present-day requirements, seems woefully inadequate, for prior to 1762, when Dr. William Shippen, Jr., introduced public medical lectures for students and young practitioners, the only available method of learning "the art and science of physic and chirurgery," was through apprenticeship with some local medical man whose training, in the great majority of cases, had been similarly obtained. Proud was the physician who possessed an institutional medical degree or a technical library. Opportunities in the provinces to learn the intricacies of anatomy through dissection and operations were very rare, so the young apprentice acquired a knowledge of the location and relations of the organs of the body from rough pictures and charts rather than through clinics and lectures.

When Dr. Shippen, Jr., journeyed abroad to continue his studies after a three-year American apprenticeship, his father wrote an English friend that while his son had enjoyed all the professional advantages available in Philadelphia,

"For the want of that variety of operations and those frequent dissections which are common in older countries, I must send him to Europe."

Dr. Fothergill, a prominent Quaker physician of London and friend of Benjamin Franklin, had shown great interest in the professional problems of the Colonies as well as in the young American students in Europe, and writing in 1762 to James Pemberton of the Pennsylvania Hospital, said:

"I need not tell thee that the knowledge of anatomy is of exceeding great use to practitioners in physics and surgery and that the means of procuring subjects with you are not easy. Some pretty accurate anatomical drawings, about half as big as life, have fallen into my hands, which I propose to send to your hospital, to be under the care of the physicians and to be by them explained to the pupils who may attend the hospital.

"In the want of real subjects these will have their use, and I have recommended to Dr. Shippen to give a course of anatomical lectures to such as may attend. He is very well qualified for the subject and will soon be followed by an able assistant, Dr. Morgan, both of whom, I apprehend, will not only be useful to the province in their employments but, if suitably countenanced by the Legislature, will be able to erect a school of physic among you, that may draw students from various parts of America and the West Indies, and at least furnish them with a better idea of the rudiments of their profession than they have at present the means of acquiring, on your side of the water."

The Fothergill charts and drawings used in Dr. Shippen's lectures were kept under lock and key, but it was advertised they were subject to examination by the interested and curious for a fee of one dollar. These beautifully colored drawings, seventeen in number, are still preserved in the archives of the Pennsylvania Hospital, and they were recognized in John Adams' diary notation: I as a work of art is evident by

"Dr. Shippen carried us into his chamber where he showed a series of anatomical paintings of exquisite art. Here was a great variety of views of the human body, whole and in part. The Doctor entertained us with a clear, concise, comprehensive lecture upon all the parts of the human frame. The entertainment charmed me."

Shippen's newspaper announcement of a public lecture course read:

"Phila., Nov. 11, 1762

"Please to inform the public that a course of anatomical lectures will be opened this winter in Phila., for the advantage of young gentlemen now engaged in the study of physics in this and the neighboring province, whose circumstances and connections will not permit of their going abroad for improvement to the anatomical schools of Europe; and also for the entertainment of any gentleman who may have the curiosity to understand the anatomy of the human frame tickets for the course to be had of the doctor at five pistoles each and any gentleman who may be inclined to see the subjects prepared for the lectures and learn the art of dissecting, etc., is to pay five pistoles more."

The result of Dr. Shippen's initial effort was an enrollment of ten students. In 1774, twelve years after these lectures began and in the ninth year of the Philadelphia Medical College's existence, Dr. Chovet also offered a series of public lectures, illustrated with waxworks and mechanical apparatus, to explain the action of the different organs of the body. His newspaper advertisement read:

"At the anatomical museum, in Vider Alley 2nd St., on Wednesday, the 7th of December, at six in the evening.

—Dr. Chovet—

will begin his course of anatomical lectures, in which the several parts of the human body will be clearly demonstrated with their mechanism and action together with the Doctrines of Life, Health and the several effects resulting from the action of the parts, in a curious collection of anatomical waxworks and other natural preparations; to be continued the whole winter until the course is completed. As this course can be attended without the disagreeable sight and smell of recent diseased and putrid Carcasses, which often disgust even the student in physics as well as the curious, otherwise inclined to this useful and sublime part of natural philosophy, it is hoped the undertaking will meet with suitable encouragement."

John Adams, after inspecting this exhibit, wrote:

"Went in this morning to see Dr. Chovet and his skeleton and waxworks. This exhibit is much more exquisite than that of Dr. Shippen's at the hospital. The Doctor reads lectures for 21/2 joes* a course which takes up four months, the waxworks are all of the Doctor's own hands."

Of such were the means of studying anatomy in the latter half of the eighteenth century, for dissections of human bodies had so excited and angered the people that, in 1765, Shippen publicly denied a report he used corpses stolen from graveyards and, when the story was again circulated, in 1770, a mob attacked his home, compelling the doctor to leave his house by the back door to avoid personal violence. One source of Dr. Shippen's subjects were bodies of suicides and executed criminals, and these were few in number. Under such methods, with limited opportunities, the knowledge attained by an apprentice in his pursuit of a medical education depended mainly on an acumen of observation and a retentive memory. While admittedly far from perfect, much can be said for a system of teaching where the student is subject to constant personal instruction and direction from a successful preceptor. Intimate association with one who knows and the opportunity to try out new theories have produced many remarkable men in both science and art. One wonders, however, what misadventures occurred when the average youthful physician was first released for independent practice.

The period of colonial medical apprenticeships varied from three to seven years, depending often upon the student's capacity and the extent and opportunities afforded by the preceptor's practice. Many apprentices with an academic foundation, sufficient capital and necessary ambition supplemented their provincial preparation with further instruction from recognized authorities abroad, where they acquired a medical degree. John Morgan and Benjamin Rush, in addition to Wm. Shippen, Jr., were typical examples. Morgan had obtained a bachelor's degree from the College of Philadelphia before entering the Philadelphia office of Dr. John Redman. After a short period of service in the French and Indian Wars, he traveled to Edinburgh, acquiring his doctor's degree in 1763. Rush graduated at Princeton with the Class of 1760 and, after a six-year apprenticeship under the same Dr. Redman continued his medical studies for three years in Edinburgh, London and Paris.

It was due to Dr. Morgan and Dr. Shippen, later ably supported by Dr. Rush and others, that in 1765, the first colonial medical school in the College of Philadelphia was established.

The Colonial physician was necessarily an apothecary, for he prepared his own remedies and frequently maintained a public establishment for the purpose. Most provincial medical supplies originated abroad, and it is recorded that German contributions to the American Lutheran Church, as well as family remittances to Colonial settlers, were often in the form of drugs, for they found ready sale and were easily converted into cash.

Homeopathy and small doses were unknown in American practice. Large quantities of unpleasant-tasting and ill-smelling concoctions were the rule, with regular preventive dosings at stated intervals a national habit. In the Spring, the blood was purified, the kidneys excited, and the bowels purged, necessitating a daily regimen of effective drugs, and in many ailments, the patient was frequently bled.

Surgical skill, even measured by the standard of those days, was a rarity. With the exception of provincial apprenticed physicians who later obtained training in hospitals abroad or the experienced European surgeons who emigrated to the Colonies, the most successful American surgeons were those who had served in the French and Indian War. Much has properly been credited to those Colonial physicians who completed their preparation for practice in England and Scotland, for to them we are indebted for the establishment of higher standards of professional education and for the beginning of provincial medical schools, but comparatively little honor of recognition has been accorded those emigrant physicians and surgeons like Bodo Otto, who also made contributions to American Medical advancement, though admittedly in a different manner.

Apprentices who were privileged to study under their direction received something more than was possible from American-trained preceptors, including an appreciation of the advantages that might be gained by continuing their study in the Old World.

It would be interesting to reproduce a medical apprenticeship contract, but search among the Archives of the University of Pennsylvania, the College of Physicians, Ridgway Library and the Historical Society of Philadelphia has failed to discover any contractual agreement of that nature.

With the completion of an apprenticeship, signified by a written certification to that effect from his preceptor, the young physician was released to practice, with but few restrictions or conditions. A typical certificate indicating a student's discharge follows:

"Springfield, Essex Co., N.J.
April 13, 1773

"This is to certify, to whom it may concern, that the Bearer, Mr. James Davidson, has served an apprenticeship under me of two years six months in the study and practice of physics and surgery, during which time he was industrious and studious; therefore, I can with candor recommend him to the public, qualified to be useful in the above branches."

JAMES DAYTON

Massachusetts, New York and Virginia adopted a few laws relating to the practice of physics, but they had little influence on the qualifications or restrictions of practice. The Duke of York published a code for some of the Colonies as early as the seventeenth century and issued a license to practice in the following language:

"Greetings-being well informed of your knowledge, skill and judgment in the practice of chirurgery and physics, I do hereby license and authorize you to practice the said science of chirurgery and physics within His Majesty's Province of New Jersey for and during his pleasure."

William Smith wrote, in 1758, regarding the prevalence of medical quacks in the Colonies and of the many poorly prepared practitioners imposing on the public, saying:

"The profession is under no kind of regulation. Loud as the call is to our shame, be it remembered we have no law to protect the lives of the King's subjects from the malpractice of pretenders. No candidates are either examined, licensed or sworn to fair practice."

It may possibly have been a realization of this situation that prompted Bodo Otto to publish, in pamphlet form, the records of his German preparation and of his service and honors, as the explanation on the first page reads:

"CANDID READER

Counting myself the least of all practitioners in physics and surgery, it is not from ostentation or a vain endeavor to make myself valued above the rest of my brethren that I have had the following documents translated and printed.

In many English families where I have the honour to practice, I have not only been advised but urgently pressed to do so for the following two reasons:

First, in order to let the public know that I am no interloper who by chance has picked up a receipt on how to prepare a plaster or to serve some drops, let it be to some or no purpose, but that I have had the regular education of a surgeon. That, after the expiration of mine apprenticeship, I have served as surgeon's man under several masters abroad, and at Hamburg attended the Lazaretto, where there is a conflux of both internal and external ailments. And having afterwards, at the University of Göttingen, frequented the physical, anatomical and botanical lectures of two eminent professors, I was at Luneburg received a member of the College of Surgeons and had the care of the prisoners in the Fortress and the Invalids quartered in the town; people among whom a surgeon has abundant opportunities to become a proficient both in the theory and practice of his art.

Secondly, that since I am a stranger in this part of the world, magistrates may be convinced that I have enjoyed in Europe the protections of persons of dignity and that both my conduct and talents have been approved by them.

So consequently, I make bold in America, not to claim but to beg the favour of the public in general and the patronage of persons of distinction in particular, assuring every one of his stations that it shall be my unwearied endeavor to merit the name of

Their faithful and devoted humble servant

BODO OTTO"

The American physicians later adopted a pledge of fair practice as suggested by William Smith, but many years before that time, Bodo Otto had taken an oath of fidelity to his professional obligations in the old Scharzfels Castle in the Harz Mountains of Germany.

The introduction of medical lectures in the Colonies suggested the value of meetings of practicing physicians for the exchange of experiences and also led to the formation of the first medical society. In their organization meeting held in New Brunswick, N.J., in 1766, they adopted a schedule of professional fees which in part provided:

"Visits in town, whereby the physician and surgeon can be readily attending the patients without ridding, to be charged for, according to the duration of the ailment and degree of attendance.

Per week:

In other cases, requiring longer and daily care and attendance, in proportion for lesser or more time, exclusive of medicines—10 shillings.

Visits in the country:

Under half a mile to be charged for as in town.

Above half a mile and not more than one and one-half mile–1 shilling.

Above one and a half miles and not exceeding fifteen miles–1 shilling for each additional mile.

Every visit above fifteen miles and not exceeding twenty-five miles–1 shilling for each additional mile.

Above twenty-five miles–2 shillings per mile.

Consultation fees:

Every first visit and opinion of the consulting physician or surgeon–

15 shillings, exclusive of traveling fees.

Every succeeding visit and advice, by same 7 shillings, 6 pence."

Surgical fees for many operations were also listed but are too numerous to mention. Among them, however, is included the delivery of a child, which provides:

"Delivery of a woman, in natural cases, £1 10 shillings; in preternatural cases, including those requiring forceps, £3."

If it were the intention of the medical society to approve a schedule of professional fees in language the layman could not understand, the cited list might be considered a great success; but, if the agreement were made for the purpose of regulating competition between physicians and communities, it would seem they needed an arbitrator as part of their organization. The decade before the American Revolution marked the beginning of better medical education opportunities, but the change from private preceptors to public institutions, with greater expense and often with the necessity which the student was under of leaving home, was a slow process, and it is recorded that only fifty men received medical college degrees between 1765 and 1776. Many local apprentices and young practitioners, however, took advantage of opportunities to attend some of the special private or institutional lecture courses by paying a fee to the officiating instructor.

A great majority of the faculties of the early Colonial medical schools were Americans who had studied under the best masters and institutions abroad with the avowed intent of returning home to establish provincial colleges where all the advantages of

European methods, including anatomical lectures, dissections and hospital clinics, could be obtained.

This organizing ability, necessary to bring into being a system of medical education foreign to Colonial practice, involved qualifications so greatly needed when the medical department of the Continental Army was authorized. True, these same medical men undertook the work of organizing the medical department of the Continental Army. They then filled the higher positions of the organization, but the unity of purpose displayed in their earlier work was lacking. Had it not been so, a different history regarding the suffering and mortality of Revolutionary soldiers might have been written. The directing heads had the experience and the capacity to accomplish many seeming impossibilities, but to their great shame be it, said jealousy, ambition, greed, and revenge prevented the perfecting of an organization that would have reflected credit and honor on all and possibly have even saved the lives of many who needlessly died

CHAPTER SIX

PHILADELPHIA • Establishment of Practice • Germantown and Reading • The Beginning of the Revolution

GOTTLIEB MITTELBERGER, a German organist, has left a record of his impressions of Philadelphia, its people and customs, written in 1754, just one year before Bodo Otto and his family arrived. Mittelberger wrote that the city was large, regularly laid out and handsomely constructed, having broad streets and many cross alleys; that it was steadily growing with 300 houses yearly, and, it was believed, would become one of the largest cities in the world. He said the houses were built of brick or stone, were roofed with cedar shingles, and some of them were four stories high. The town, he commented, was so extensive that it required almost an entire day to explore it.

Ships were constantly arriving from all principal ports of the world, bringing the products of many nations, and local trade was active and increasing.

The German citizens of the city were highly respected and influential in business and public affairs, but they were inclined to be clannish and to find their amusements and social life closely associated with their Church.

Mittélberger commented on the trusting and generous characteristics of the people of the Colony and asserted that a perfect stranger could travel about the province for a whole year without its costing him a cent, for wherever he might stop, an invitation would be extended to remain. Houses faced the street or country road, with porches in front, where the family sat during summer evenings and greeted passing neighbors or travelers.

The liberties enjoyed by the people of Pennsylvania greatly surprised the German settlers. Freedom from molestation and low tax rates were new experiences. It also amazed them that no restrictions were placed on the choice of a vocation and that a citizen was permitted to change his business activity as often as he wished.

Mittelberger observed that the cost of living was extremely low, and most families in Philadelphia served meat and butter or cheese with bread at every meal; those greetings, when friends met, were accompanied by a handshake, a custom strange to him; he wrote that death and funerals were announced to near neighbors, who in turn informed others, until the entire countryside learned of the bereavement; one or more from each family then attended the interment, after which cake and wine or punch would be served to all. Mittelberger thought it odd that everyone rode horseback, even to do errands nearby. It surprised him there was so little music, and that the Germans were the only ones who had imported organs for their churches. Indians walking the streets, clad only in blankets, shocked him, as did also the luxury of the clothing worn by both the men and women of English extraction.

Pennsylvania boasted of having four printing establishments, and Philadelphia was proud of its College, where several languages were taught. Eight churches served possibly 2,500 families in the city, and Sabbath-breaking and swearing in public were punished with fines of five pounds.

Philadelphia was a city of approximately 15,000 inhabitants when Bodo Otto began a new professional life in the country of his adoption. Watchmen walked the streets at night, crying out the hour and announcing important news. Sidewalks were littered with refuse, and epidemics of disease were quite frequent. It was in the year 1755 that the cornerstone of the Pennsylvania Hospital was laid, that the people might be better served in their illnesses. This institution was then four years of age, and among the English physicians who fostered it were Doctors Thomas Bond, Sr., his brother Phineas, Cadwalader, Kearsley, Moore, Redman, and Dr. William Shippen, Sr.

It is very probable that a few of Bodo Otto's friends had preceded him to Philadelphia and that he brought letters of introduction to other Germans so his European medical experience may have been known. It was customary in Germany, and, therefore, not considered unprofessional, for members of the medical profession to publish the record of their training, qualifications and specialties in the public press. Therefore, two months after Bodo Otto arrived, The Pennsylvania *Berichte*, a German newspaper, contained the following announcement:

"Phila., Pa., December 16th, 1755.

"Reimer Land and Bodo Otto, who arrived from Germany are now living with Henry Hoffecker in Front Street, near Benjamin Shoemaker's. They give notice herewith that both of them have studied in German Universities as Doctors of Medicine and Surgery and have practiced in anatomical institutions and hospitals. They now offer their services, in company, for all manner of curable ailments, exterior wounds and injuries. Those suffering from gout and rheumatism–they promise relief from pain. Venereal diseases they will cure without torment. Fractures, dislocations, cancer, eruptions, old fistulas and all kinds of wounds will also be treated. They pledge themselves to give all, an intelligent explanation of their illness and the medicines used, and, above all, they wish to be differentiated from such doctors in the land who do not understand the nature of the illness or injury suffered by their patients, or the power of the drugs they use."

Truly, some remarkable claims are made here, but it must be remembered that the word "cure," as used in the Colonial medical vernacular, meant "treat." It should also be recalled that at the time this announcement was issued, the Colony contained many poorly prepared and ignorant physicians, for there were no laws requiring qualifications for practice.

It has been impossible to locate Dr. Otto's host, Henry Hoffecker definitely, or to learn anything regarding him, but as there were then over one hundred taverns in Philadelphia, it is probable he was an innkeeper, patronized by the German element of the city. His house was likely situated somewhere north of High Street, for Benjamin Shoemaker, an ex-Mayor of Philadelphia, maintained an office at his wharf in that neighborhood.

What, if any, blood relationship existed between Bodo Otto and Reimer Land or Landt, as he registered on his arrival, is not known. Partnerships in the medical profession were not infrequent, as an examination of early Philadelphia directories will prove. The association of these two, however, was not continued any length of time, for Dr. Land soon moved to Faulkner Swamp and, several years afterward, advertised his arrival in Germantown.

During the winter of 1755-56, an unusual amount of smallpox was present in Philadelphia. Many of the Indians who had accepted the Assembly's invitation to visit the city suffered from the infection and died. The Acadian refugees from Nova Scotia also lost fifty of their members. Later in the year, the malady became a dangerous epidemic, and the Surgeon of the English troops quartered in the town wrote his commanding officer:

"I am sorry to be obliged to inform you that the smallpox is increasing among the soldiers, and as their quarters are so scattered and the convenience of attending them so bad, I would venture to affirm that unless a proper hospital is soon provided, every house in this place will be infected within a fortnight. The safety of the town, the recovery of the sick soldiers, and the principles of humanity all show the necessity of a hospital being immediately provided."

It was under such conditions of unusual sickness that Bodo Otto quickly established a large practice among his compatriots. His long European medical and surgical experience brought him many patients, consultations and operations, resulting in the necessity of being better located near the center of the German population of the neighborhood counties, so the year following his settling in Philadelphia, a newspaper announced that:

"Doctors Reimer Land and Bodo Otto, because of their many patients in the surrounding neighborhood, have found it desirable that one should live in the City and the other in the Country. Therefore, Reimer Land will remain in the first-mentioned place, and Bodo Otto may be consulted in Germantown, in the house of Cornelius Engle. Whoever wishes to be served by one or both may follow his preference."

Germantown, in 1756, was a village of an unrecorded number of inhabitants but covered a considerable area, by reason of the fact that the early settlers had built their homes along the Main road for a distance of two miles. These first homes were quite small, one or one and a half stories in height, but as wealth increased and the people felt more confident in their own future, more pretentious houses were erected of stone or brick, with two stories and an attic.

Paul Engle was one of the early settlers and held title to several sections of land at the northern end of the original Germantown survey. Sometime about 1750, his son Cornelius erected a large two-story stone house, designed for two families, on Lot 21, facing the great road, and here Bodo Otto took residence and established his office. This old house stood for over one hundred and sixty years, passing through several alterations to meet the requirements of trade as business encroached upon the neighborhood until, in 1911, it was demolished that Tulpehocken Street might be extended to the eastward.

Germantown was a busy community when Bodo Otto settled in its midst. The people were successful, sociable, and kindly disposed, and the town was distinctly German in its character. Good living was universal, for besides the products of the garden, food of all kinds was plentiful, and bear, deer, wild turkey and other game could be found on the outskirts of the village. Indians, in considerable numbers, were frequent visitors and often remained for several months while they made and exchanged their native products for articles they needed. In addition to the various craft enterprises that distinguished Germantown, a large country trade had been developed with the people in the surrounding counties, for the neighborhood farmers were more inclined to do their trading here than carry their crops to a larger market, over the extremely bad roads that entered Philadelphia. Professor Kalm commented, in 1748, after a visit to Germantown, on the town's activity, and said that one might see dozens of county wagons in the village, and the people were so numerous that the street seemed always to be filled.

Few available records might tell of Bodo Otto's professional contemporaries in Germantown, but it is known that there still lived the renowned Dr. Christopher Witt, a man of many interests and attainments. He was not only a successful physician but a botanist of note and a great friend of John Bartram. Witt was a Pietist, an intimate of Kelpius, the hermit, and was credited with occult powers. As he, two, lived on the great road, not more than two city blocks beyond, it is probable that Bodo Otto and Christopher Witt exchanged many friendly visits. Not far away, on the other side of the street, stood the two-story brick house that Arent Klinchen had erected. Its completion had been celebrated with a dinner attended by the host's good friend, William Penn. Next to this was the home of Arent Klinchen's son Antony, a great hunter, of whom it was told that he tagged and dated his game so that it might be eaten in regular sequence. Other near neighbors were Justus Johnson, Dirk Keyser and Christian Warner, who fell heir to Dr. Witt's estate as a reward for kindnesses extended to the old man; Reuben Haines, who owned "Wick," where Lafayette was entertained when he returned to America in 1824. Not far away stood the Saddlers Tavern, established by Daniel Pastorius and his wife, Sarah Shoemaker, but then maintained by Pastorius' widow, who had married Daniel Macknett. The Inn was celebrated for its good food, and many were the Philadelphia sleighing parties that patronized it. Some years later, in 1775, Dr. William Shippen, Jr., acquired a country home in the neighborhood, and here, in the first three-story house of Germantown, which still stands, he eventually retired from active practice. Some distance to the north was the house built by John George Binsell in 1727, which was later known as the Billmeyer Mansion, in front of which Washington held a council of war during the battle of Germantown. At the same distance to the south stood the home of Melchoir Meng, which the British commandeered as an emergency hospital because of the many barrels of vinegar available to stanch the flow of blood. Below the Square or Market, which was located in the center of Germantown, lived Christian Lehman, a land surveyor who made many of the early maps of the village and with whom Bodo Otto maintained a friendship for many years. John Wister was another distant neighbor whose sister, Maria Barbara Hitner, was John Otto's wife's grandmother. Christopher Sauer, the printer of a German newspaper of great influence throughout the Colonies, also lived and had his shop in that section of the town.

The two religious sects, Mennonites and Quakers, that dominated Germantown, in the beginning, had restricted the use of the church graveyards to their own members, so in 1724, a piece of ground was set aside in the upper end of the settlement for the use of anyone having need of it. Among its records of 1758 was found an entry, in the German language, of the interment of a woman from the household of Dr. Bodo Otto, but the English translation of this old book has erroneously published it as "wife" instead of "woman" (servant).

The Lutheran Church, which served the Germantown people, was located a full mile and a half from the center of the town, toward Chestnut Hill, and here in a little stone building, which still exists, was the parish school which Bodo Otto's children probably attended. Educational facilities were found inadequate to the needs of the village in 1759, about the time Bodo Otto again changed his residence, so the Germantown Academy was organized, and to meet a similar situation in 1775, the Concord School was started not far from Dr. Otto's old home.

Available files of German newspapers for several years prior to 1760 are incomplete, or it might be possible to learn just when Bodo Otto responded to the need for a physician in Southern New

Jersey, where a serious epidemic of sickness had occurred. Cohansey was the name given to a large section of territory situated in Cumberland County, New Jersey, bordering a creek that had its headwaters in Salem County and emptied into the Delaware River. Bridge Town was the County seat, and somewhere in this Cohansey neighborhood, Bodo Otto established his residence before the year 1760. Many Germans, some of whom had been shipmates with Dr. Otto on his voyage to America, had settled in that section, influenced by the fertility of the land and the need for craftsmen in the manufacture of glass. The southern part of New Jersey was considered very unhealthful in Colonial times, for fever and ague were always present during the summer and fall. Very few of the inhabitants escaped attacks of the malady, and Ephraim Harris wrote in his journal a record:

"That fatal and never-to-be-forgotten year 1759, when the Lord sent His destroying angel to pass through this place and remove many of our friends into eternity in a short space of time."

It is now thought that the epidemic to which he referred was smallpox, an affliction which Bodo Otto well understood. What prompted Dr. Otto's move to the Cohansey district is not recorded. He was a man with an unusual sense of professional obligation, and it may be that a feeling of duty influenced him to make the change, for Jersey medical history does not record many physicians in that section of the State at that time. It is also possible that his friend, the Rev. Henry M. Mühlenberg, urged it, for there was a German Lutheran Church in the neighborhood, in which Mühlenberg was especially interested and which he often visited. In any event, the parish book at Freasberg, dated January 1760, informs us that Bodo Otto and wife, Catharina Dorothea, stood sponsors in baptism for the daughter of Marcus Kirmann and his wife, Maria Elizabeth, with several similar entries extending into the year 1766.

In 1762, it was recorded that:

"Frederick Christopher, a son of Dr. Bodo Otto, had in his nineteenth year, attended the church with ten others, and renewed his baptismal vows and promised fidelity."

Frederick was even then receiving his medical training in his father's office, for in 1768, we find a reference to him stating he had been practicing physics in the county for several years. The other children probably attended the parish school that was maintained on the church grounds by the Lutheran preacher. Though always identified as an active member and supporter of the Lutheran Church, Bodo Otto's help and purse were often available to other struggling denominations. It was six years after he left New Jersey that the remembrance of such aid caused the rector of the Trinity Episcopal Church at Swedesboro to write in his parish book:

"The two Doctors Otto, Senior and Junior, were exceedingly kind and generous toward me on all occasions."

Part of the time of Bodo Otto's residence in Southern Jersey coincided with that period of resistance to the Stamp Act, when citizens refused to comply with the law, and the transfer of property was not registered because of the legal necessity of recording the objectionable instrument. This condition may account for the fact that no tax or property record can be found that might give a clue about Bodo Otto's home.

Sons of Liberty Societies had been formed in every county of the State to encourage the people to ignore the Stamp Law, and at Elizabeth, a gallows was erected, and it was declared that the first person who complied with the Act would be hanged without a judge or jury. The King's agent, appointed to issue the stamps in New Jersey, was visited by a committee with a demand that he immediately resign, and this was accompanied by a written message saying:

"If, Sir, you refuse our very reasonable request, it will put us to the trouble of waiting upon you in such a way and manner as perhaps will be disagreeable both to yourself and to us."

Strong circumstantial evidence exists that two of Bodo Otto's sons were in some way involved in the activities of the local Sons of Liberty, for both Frederick and young John, who was then only fourteen years of age, were among a number summoned to appear as witnesses in the Cumberland County Court, by order of the King. Nothing was cited in the writ that gave information of the charges involved, but after several postponements the case was finally dropped about the same time the Stamp Act was repealed.

New Jersey historians have often credited the honors and experiences of Bodo Otto to his namesake son, who remained in Gloucester County after his father had left the State. Here, Bodo, Junior, gained a reputation and a place in Jersey's archives as a physician, patriot, Member of the Assembly, Judge, Surgeon in the Army, and Colonel of New Jersey troops. It was the Senior, however, who was meant when it was written that:

"Bodo Otto from Germany, known as the Prussian physician, was always called upon in difficult cases, not only in the neighborhood where he resided but throughout the surrounding counties."

Thomas Clark, one of the most prominent Colonial men in Gloucester County, wrote in his journal:

"During the time I lived in Vanneman's plantation, I had a bad spell of sickness, with a white swelling on my right thigh, and Dr. Bodo Otto, Senior, attended me. He wanted to amputate my leg above the swelling, but I would not suffer it. I, at last, consented to have it lanced deep to the bone, and there came out a whit scum, like unto a hickory nut with prongs; when that healed, I got well, and blessed be God for it."

A physician friend to whom this experience was read has described the trouble as "sequestrium," a bone growth that often interferes with circulation, resulting in gangrene and sloughing off of the limb. Amputation in such cases is frequently the only recourse, but in this instance, it appears that the growth had loosened from the leg bone and was, therefore, easily removed.

During the six or seven years Bodo Otto lived in New Jersey, he served as preceptor to at least three medical students who attained success and renown in both their professional and public life. Two of these were his sons, Frederick Christopher and Bodo Junior, and the third was Jonathan Elmer, who served his State and nation in many important positions. Both Bodo Otto, Jr., and Jonathan Elmer finished their medical education in the College of Philadelphia and were among the first graduates to receive professional degrees.

The burial book of the Evangelical Lutheran Church of the Cohansey district, under the date of August 11, 1765, tells of the death and interment of:

"Bodo Otto's wife Catharina," the mother of his three boys. Not long afterwards, either changed conditions in New Jersey or the restlessness which seemed to possess him caused Dr. Otto to turn over his practice to his son, Frederick, and again, the newspapers announced:

"Pennsylvania Staatsbote May 5th and 12th, 1766 Bodo Otto who for many years has, by the Blessings of God, been recognized for his successful treatment of disease, and who is able to produce credentials from authorities under whom he has practiced, takes the liberty of making known to the Public that he is now established in Philadelphia and ready to practice. He, therefore, seeks, by this means, those who may stand in need of him to ask that they honor him with their favor and goodwill.

A long description of the curing [treatment] of this or that disease and of operations performed, he thinks unnecessary to give; he promises those persons who will entrust themselves to him, in illness or other trouble, to serve them as an honorable and intelligent physician. Those who, because of poverty, are unable to place themselves under the care of a physician may apply to him, and he will supply medicine and treatment with the greatest consideration.

His address at present is the care of Herr Leonard Melchior, and his Apothecary Shop is nearby."

The family name of Bodo Otto's host is frequently found in Colonial and Revolutionary War archives, and in 1772, Leonard Melchior was listed as an Innkeeper in the Mulberry Ward, paying taxes on:

A dwelling, etc.

One servant	£96	– 0	–	0
Two horses and one cow	1	– 10	–	0
Stores in his possession	1	– 13	–	4
	10	– 0	–	0
	£110	– 7	–	4

The wording of Bodo Otto's announcement suggests that his residence with Leonard Melchior was only temporary, and he was probably seeking a house, for he was accompanied by his youngest son, John, then fifteen years old, and Bodo Junior, who came to attend the Medical College and the clinics at the Pennsylvania Hospital. Possibly, Dr. Otto may have been anticipating his third marriage, for the parish book of St. Michael's Lutheran Church, under the date of September 18, 1766, records:

"By authority of a license dated September 12th, 1766, Bodo Otto, Practitioner in Physics, and Maria Margaretta Paris, both of this City, are joined together in holy matrimony."

According to a Bible entry of John Otto, his stepmother was an English woman, and at the time of her marriage, forty-seven years old, a suitable age for her husband, who was then fifty-five.

The Philadelphia to which Bodo Otto had returned included 4,000 homes, containing between twenty-five and thirty thousand souls. Dr. Benjamin Franklin, on being examined by the House of Commons on conditions in the Colony, expressed the belief that Pennsylvania then totaled 160,000 inhabitants, of whom one-third were Germans, one-third Quakers, and the remaining third other nationals and sects. A few years later (1771), Philadelphia County and City listed 10,455 taxable citizens, of whom 3,751 resided in the town. The export trade of that year was conveyed in 361 square-rigged ships, 391 sloops and schooners, and their total tonnage was 46,654.

As the city increased in population, so did the number of Lutherans until St. Michael's Church could no longer contain them, so the construction of another still larger one, called Zion, was begun in June 1766, just one month after Bodo Otto had returned to Philadelphia.

Charges of fraud against the skippers of ships arriving with German immigrants became so frequent and violent that in 1764, members of the Lutheran congregation fostered the formation of the German Benevolent Society to protect their countrymen from imposition and to render aid and advice to them when in trouble. Bodo Otto became one of this organization in 1766, when residence in the city made it possible for him to participate in the work. Another special effort, to which he contributed money and gave his time, was the endowment and direction of the Lutheran Seminary, conceived to educate preachers for the Church and teachers for the parish schools. The Reverend Henry Melchior Mühlenberg, the patriarch of the Lutherans in America, always believed that church and school should be maintained side by side, and this combination of preaching and teaching was generally observed. Usually, the pastor served as an instructor to the children of the neighborhood, but frequently, when no regular ordained minister was installed, a schoolmaster was assigned, and on Sundays, he read prepared sermons submitted by the Synod. Much difficulty was encountered in the effort to obtain the necessary number of men to supply the scattered eighty-one congregations in the Colonies, and the Rev. Doctor Mühlenberg wrote to Halle University in Germany:

"The importation of well-educated and efficient preachers from Germany is connected with so many difficulties and great costs that it is impossible to send over as many as a general and sufficient supply would necessitate."

Mühlenberg had long foreseen that the American church would eventually have to educate and supply its own preachers and teachers but realized this would involve an expense that the Lutheran Synod was in no condition to assume. It was not until 1772 that a start was made to establish such a school. Its beginning was to be modest, but the ultimate expectation was to create an institution that would parallel all the activities of Halle University of Germany. Twenty-four of the most prominent Lutherans in Philadelphia then met, endowed and organized "The Society for the Propagation of Christianity and Useful Knowledge among the Germans in America," and among them was Bodo Otto. The resulting school opened its doors on February 15, 1773, and continued to function until the British occupied the city in 1777 when the German Academy closed. Whether the dream of Mühlenberg, visualizing an American Halle University, with its many departments and diversification, could have eventually been realized is an interesting speculation. The capacity to conceive, direct and teach undoubtedly existed in the Board of Directors and the faculty, but the seemingly insurmountable obstacle seems to have been the raising of the large sum of money which the scope of the work made necessary. Most of the Lutheran congregations were heavily in debt, and many were not even self-supporting, so it proved an impossible task to accumulate the requisite endowment fund. Another condition that made ultimate success doubtful was the existence of the College of Philadelphia, which received financial support from both the Provincial Assembly and the citizens at large. The result was that the University of Pennsylvania eventually absorbed the German school and faculty, and the Reverend Kunze received the appointment of "German Professor of Philology" and became one of the Governing Boards, where he continued his effort to establish a School of Theology. In the minutes of the Trustees, dated December 1779, is the record that:

"A written motion was made by Mr. Kunze concerning a Professorship of Divinity in the University, ordered to lie on the table for consideration."

Both the minutes of this German institution and a newspaper reference to Bodo Otto, under the date of 1773, credit him with membership in the American Philosophical Society, organized by Benjamin Franklin. The Society rosters, however, are confusing on this subject. It has been stated that their early papers were damaged by a burst water pipe, which destroyed some and made others difficult to read. In any event, the available lists contain a Dr. Otto, without a Christian name, who was made a member in 1769, but his residence is given as Bethlehem. A Moravian physician of the name of Otto then lived in that settlement, but in no other details do the Society records check with him.

Late in 1759, an advertisement appeared in a Philadelphia German newspaper that approximately dates the beginning of the Reading Apothecary shop that Bodo Otto purchased in 1773.

"Adam Simon Kuhn, of Lancaster, hereby makes known that he has reopened his Apothecary in Reading, since several years located near Adam Wittmann's, and which he was compelled to close owing to the fact that he had been unable to engage an efficient representative, and he further makes known that the Apothecary is stocked with the freshest materials from Holland and England; also that the best 'Simplicibus and Compositis have been multiplied; therefore, he is in a position to fill in the best and most efficient way, all and every receipt and other prescriptions of the most learned Doctors, through Daniel Adam Kurrer, the well known Druggist who has been in partnership with him in Reading.

"The Apothecaries in Lancaster and Reading will stay in constant correspondence with each other and will be managed with utmost care by persons who are well versed in the science of pharmacy.

"In these two Apothecaries shall be kept on hand at any time the famous medicines made in England, also the Universal Balsam De Maltha and Tinctura Solis as prepared by Mr. Stephani, Chemist in New York, also all kinds of paints and best varnishes for all kinds of work."

Dated: Dec. 7th, 1759.

Dr. Adam Simon Kuhn (Senior) was a man of many accomplishments, and he raised four sons to give him credit. One, his namesake, became a member of the first medical faculty of the College of Philadelphia, and two others served as Surgeons in the Continental Hospital during the Revolution, while the fourth was an ordained minister in the Evangelical Lutheran Church.

Again, no definite reason can be given for Bodo Otto's decision to abandon Philadelphia and move to Reading. His two older sons were married and well-established in New Jersey. John Augustus was then studying medicine in his father's Philadelphia office and attending lectures at the College, but he, too, decided to accompany his parents and complete his medical training in Reading.

The newspaper, as previously, was used to announce: "Penna. Staatbote, August 3rd, 1773.

"Bodo Otto, the Elder Medical and Surgical Practitioner living in Front Street, hereby makes it known that he shall shortly be removed from Philadelphia and therefore requests such people who have any claims against him to bring their accounts for settlement; also those who are indebted to him, are asked to make payment.

"He takes this opportunity to extend his warmest thanks to his patrons for their past kind favors."

Not long after the appearance of this notice, another appeared in several editions of the Philadelphia Penna. Staatsbote, "Doctor Bodo Otto hereby announces that he is now settled in Reading and has taken over the Apothecary Shop of Dr. Kuhn, where one and all may be supplied with good medicines.

"He will also continue his practice as heretofore and take mental cases for treatment, as well as others."

Reading can claim a unique distinction among Colonial towns in that it was conceived, located, plotted and exploited to serve a large number of already settled people who had no convenient place in which to sell their products or where they might obtain their necessities. Lebanon and Lancaster, situated twenty-eight and thirty miles from the center of the section that was to become Berks County, were too far away to satisfactorily service these 10,000 German farmers, so with the approval and help of the

Pennsylvania Proprietor, the streets of Reading were duly laid out, and the first public offering of land was made in 1749, with a second auction three years later. Many of the original purchasers became owners with the intent of becoming identified with the proposed town, while others bought lots with speculative intent. Among those registered in the 1752 sale was Adam Simon Kuhn of Lancaster, who took title to plot Number 105, located on the North East Corner of Penn Square and what is now Sixth Street. Conditions of sale of property located here required that the erection of a building be started within one year's time, so it is probable that Dr. Kuhn's Apothecary Shop came into being in 1753 or 54, to be continued by three generations of Dr. Otto's, as an adjunct to their medical practice, until finally sold in 1858, after the death of Dr. John Bodo Otto. An added impetus and importance were given to the Village of Reading in 1752 when it was made the County seat and became the residence of a number of Philadelphia attorneys. Berks County was distinctly German in character and speech, even more so than Germantown, and this circumstance and the fact that it contained approximately 20,000 inhabitants and very few qualified physicians, may have influenced Bodo Otto's decision in 1773 to pull up stakes again and change his residence. Dr. Jonathan Potts, who was destined to be closely associated with Dr. Otto in the cause of the Revolution, had obtained his M.D. degree abroad two years before and was now practicing medicine in Berks County. Others of prominence living in the district who influenced the opinions of the inhabitants were the Biddles, Collinson Read, Daniel Clymer, Alexander Grayson, Edward Scull, and young Neddie Burd, though the German population was more inclined to look to their own people for guidance. Among the latter were Mark Bird, Joseph Bower, Michael Bright, Daniel Brodhead, Henry Christ, Gabriel and Joseph Hiester, David Hunter, Nicholas Lotz,

Jacob Morgan, and Adam Witman, all of whom were to make names for themselves in the struggle for Independence and public affairs that were to follow. Many of these men lived on or in the neighborhood of Penn Square, which then had been built upon all sides and was bordered by a beautiful row of sycamore trees. A majority of the early Reading homes also served their owners as shops and offices, and many attained venerable age before being demolished to be replaced with buildings more suitable to the demands of business. A three-story brick house, erected on the north side of Penn Square, east of Fifth, not far from Bodo Otto's Apothecary Shop and home, became the residence of Dr. John Otto after his marriage in 1776, and this building remained standing until 1895.

Faithful to youthful training and life-long association, Bodo Otto and his family became members of the Reading Lutheran Trinity congregation. Old parish books contain many respectful references to the progenitor of the American Ottos and his descendants through more than one hundred years of its history. Even while engaged in the confining duties of a surgeon in the Continental hospitals, Bodo Otto found time to give some attention to the problems of his church, for the records of the Lutheran Synod and the diary of the Rev. Henry M. Mühlenberg contain many notations of visits and communications received from this honored member. Many of Bodo Otto's medical preparations had been well known throughout the Colony, and to encourage their continual use, an advertisement was inserted in the German paper published in Philadelphia.

"Aug. 2nd to 16th, 1774.

DOCTOR BODO OTTO, who now resides in the Apothecary Shop of Dr. Adam Simon Kuhn in Reading, where he continues his practice, makes known to the Public in general, and especially to the County Physicians, that besides a variety of chemical and medical supplies, the following, prepared according to his own prescriptions and under his personal supervision, may be obtained at reasonable prices.

"1. A Balsam Salve that has given as good results in fresh and old wounds as the famous Turlington Balsam or Balsam de Maltha.

"2. A wonderful oil that will soften and cure hard old tumors and swelling, even double chins (Goiters), if such are not too ancient.

"3. A Liquid, which has not its equal in the treatment of Gout and other similar ailments, such as rheumatism; to be taken internally, as well as applied externally.

"4. A Powder, which in case of Epilepsy (a disease that is not entirely curable) will certainly have extraordinary effects; also, in the treatment of Hysteria and Female Trouble, it has given immediate relief.

"5. A Plaster, which is highly recommended for bruises, fresh and old sores, Fistulas, Cancer, Sciatica, Back-ache, Bladder disorders, Toothache, and so forth.

"6. The famous Strassburger Horse Powder, which, because of its value in diseases of horses, is renowned in Germany and well known in America, will also be prepared in this Apothecary.

7. A health-giving Tea, which purifies the blood and is pleasant to drink. Also, a very strong Snuff for headaches and dizziness, Worm Pills for children and old people.

"The genuine Gold Tincture conceived by the chemist, Herr Stephani, and other medicines too numerous to mention are likewise available.

"With each article sold, full directions for use will be supplied."

News from the outside world came to Reading through travelers, privately delivered letters and an occasional newspaper, and it often became distorted. Vague rumors of serious conditions in Boston, resulting from reported encounters between the Colonists and British troops quartered in the town, reached this German settlement and occasioned a letter on the subject from Edward Burd to Edward Shippen in Lancaster.

"Reading, Sept. 10th, 1774.

"Dear and Honored Sir:

"We have been lately alarmed here with the most afflicting news that could happen to America; no less than that a civil war has actually commenced between us and the people of Great Britain.

"As the first accounts that we received did not contain absolute certainty of the fact, we sent an Express, in order that he be in Philadelphia when the Post arrived, that we might be the sooner put out of suspense and have good intelligence. He returned this morning with an account that the story had been false and that there was no disturbance at all in Boston."

The open break came at Lexington seven months later, and the Pennsylvania Germans' sympathy with the people of Boston was expressed in public meetings and demonstrated by collecting supplies and recruiting a company of soldiers to be sent to their assistance. Then followed a realization throughout the country of a need to guide and solidify the sentiment of all the people, that they might be prepared for any emergency, so the leading men of each community met and organized local Committees of Safety. They, in turn, appointed others to services in different activities, such as observation, correspondence, and supplies. Bodo Otto was selected as one of Berks County's Controlling Committee, and his signature as such was attached to the following:

"Committee of Berks County to Council of Safety, 1775 (Phila.)

Reading, Dec. 14th, 1775.

"Gentlemen:

"The Commissioners of Berks County have been informed by the Committee of Correspondence that the persons employed in the making of firearms for the use of the Province complain they cannot go on with the work, for want of ready money to purchase the necessary material. We take the liberty, at their request, to acquaint you that we conceive it will be very difficult (if not impossible) for the Commissioners to comply with the recommendation of the Honorable Assembly unless they are furnished with a sum of money to enable them to do so, and as Mr. Bright, one of the Commissioners will apply to you for that purpose, we beg leave to recommend him to you, as a gentleman on whose representation of the matter you may depend.

"We are, Gentlemen, your very humble servants,

Thomas Youngman, Christopher Witman, Jonathan Potts,
Henry Haller, Collinson Read, Bodo Otto."

Prompt action followed this communication and at a

"Meeting of Committee of Safety, Dec. 18, 1772, Phila.

"By direction of the Board, an order was drawn agreeable to a Resolution of Sept. 26th, in favor of the Commissioners and Assessors of

"Berks County, for 400 pounds, and this day it was delivered to Mr. Michael

Bright of that County."

One month later, some of the finished products, for which the money had been sent to buy raw materials, were received in Philadelphia, and again, the Philadelphia Committee recorded:

"Dr. Jonathan Potts, having sent 20 Provincial Muskets, accompanied with his account of sundry repairs made by different people from whom he collected them, has applied for payment. It is therefore resolved that an order be drawn on the Treasurer of the Board for same."

Then followed those turbulent days in July of '76, when Berks enrolled ten percent more than its quota of 600 men and the march of these German patriots toward New York to take part in the disastrous Battle of Long Island. Years afterward, Bodo Otto wrote:

"At the beginning of the War, I was chosen Surgeon of the Battalion of the Flying Camp Troops by the Committee of Berks County, and in the unexpected attack of the enemy at Long Island, our troops retired in great haste, and I lost all my medicines and instruments."

Bodo Otto was sixty-five years old when he assumed this service toward his friends and neighbors, an age when few men were willing or able to undertake the hardships of a campaign. The need for medical practitioners at home, his extensive practice, and the many patriotic services he could still render would have justified his remaining outside the active strife of war, but he felt that a further debt was payable to his adopted country for the opportunities, honors, and material things of life it had brought him.

CHAPTER SEVEN

THE PROVINCIAL CONFERENCE • Committees • Unions • Correspondence • Declaration of Independence

THE SEVEN YEARS' EUROPEAN WAR, in which the American Colonies participated in the New World against the French, left Great Britain heavily laden with debt. Under the theory that part of this had been incurred in protecting and retaining the land of English pioneers, Parliament enacted several laws devised to place part of the financial burden upon overseas citizens. This action was bitterly resented and actively resisted by the Colonies as "taxation without representation." Protests by resolution were adopted in many provincial meetings, and when these communications were continually ignored and troops were sent to enforce the Parliament's objectionable measures, the idea of a complete separation from Great Britain took form.

The sentiment that favored the severing of all ties with England developed more quickly in the North and South than it did in the Middle Colonies. Many who conceded that independence might eventually be declared thought the time had not yet arrived, and before taking any decisive step, believed that further efforts should be made to adjust existing differences. Several of the Colonies, among them Pennsylvania, were governed by laws defined in the original charters, with responsibilities directed to the King. Their Provincial officers and members were required to take oaths of allegiance to the English Government and fidelity to the Sovereign; so, not only their consciences but fear of the charge and penalty of treason restrained them from any step that would brand them as traitors.

When the agitation for separation began in Pennsylvania, the Quakers were in political control of the Colonial Government. They had established and maintained a system of representation in the Assembly based on a property qualification for suffrage, which gave a preponderance of members to Philadelphia against the outlying counties. The Quakers' scruples against fighting and the fear of the merchant class that war with England would destroy European trade greatly influenced the actions of many in the Assembly.

The resentment against Great Britain and approval of active resistance to the Parliament had been early evidenced in the Pennsylvania country districts by their sending material assistance and some well-equipped troops to the relief of Boston. These sturdy pioneers entertained no hope that England would abandon efforts to enforce her laws and adopt a more liberal policy toward America. The Pennsylvania Assembly was either indifferent or had no appreciation of the extent of the belief that the differences with the Crown were too fundamental to be surrendered or compromised. Otherwise, they would not have issued the following instructions to the Pennsylvania Delegates in the Continental Congress:

"November 9th, 1775. "Though the oppressive measures of the British Parliament and Administration have compelled us to resist their orders by force of Arms, yet we strictly enjoin you that you, on behalf of this Colony, dissent from and utterly reject any proposition, should any be made, that may cause or lead to a separation from the Mother Country, or a change of the form of the Government."

Several Congressional delegations from other Proprietary Colonies received similar orders from their assemblies, and this combined opposition to any action by the Continental Congress greatly hampered those in favor of the separation movement. However, by May 1776, there developed sufficient strength among the representatives from New England and the South to force the issue by means of a Congressional resolution addressed directly to the citizens of all the Colonies. Commenting on the action, John Adams wrote to a friend in Boston on May 15, 1776:

"This day the Congress has passed the most important Resolution that has ever been taken in America. It is, as nearly as I can repeat it from memory, in these words:

"RESOLVED-That it be recommended to the several Assemblies and Conventions to institute such Forms of Government as, to them, shall appear necessary to promote the happiness of the People. "This Preamble and Resolution are ordered to be printed, and you will see them immediately in all the newspapers upon the Continent. I shall make no comment upon this important and decisive Resolution."

The reaction was anxiously awaited. If the people of the Colonies, represented by stand-pat assemblies and delegates, indicated their approval of Congressional action by authorizing conventions to overthrow their existing form of government, the contemplated declaration of independence was assured; if not, the dissension in Congress was likely to increase, and a Union of the Colonies would be postponed and even jeopardized. The first Pennsylvania expression of approval of the resolution occurred at a public meeting held in the State House yard in Philadelphia on

May 20, 1776. Here, the Act of Congress was read in the following words:

"WHEREAS—His Britannic Majesty in conjunction with the Lords and Commons of Great Britain has, by a late Act of Parliament, excluded the inhabitants of the United Colonies from the protection of the Crown, and whereas no answer whatever to the humble petition of the Colonies for redress of grievances and reconciliation with Great Britain has been or is likely to be given, but the whole force of that Kingdom, aided by Foreign Mercenaries, is to be exerted for the destruction of this good people of these Colonies and whereas, it appears absolutely irreconcilable to reason and good conscience, for the People of these Colonies now to take the Oaths and Affirmations necessary for the support of any Government under the Crown of Great Britain, and it is necessary that the exercises of every kind of Authority under the said Crown should be totally suppressed, and all the Power of Government under the authority of the people of the Colonies for the preservation of internal peace, virtue and good order, as well as for the defense of their lives, liberties and properties, against a hostile invasion and cruel depredation of their enemies—

"THEREFORE Resolved:

"That it be Recommended to the Assemblies and Conventions of the United Colonies where no Government sufficient to the exigencies of their affairs has been hitherto established, to adopt such Government as shall be, in the opinion of the Representatives of the People, most conducive to the happiness and safety of their Constituents in particular, and America in general. "BY ORDER OF CONGRESS.

JOHN HANCOCK

President."

The assembled people then unanimously agreed:

"That a Provincial Convention ought to be chosen by the people, for the express purpose of carrying the said Resolution of Congress into execution."

The "Committee of Philadelphia" thereupon issued a broadcast to be circulated throughout the Province, reading:

"Friends and Fellow Countrymen: "The question which will come before you is short and easy: we know not how it may have been disguised or misrepresented to you by designing persons, but to prevent your being deceived, we tell you concisely, until we can prepare the matter fully for you, that you either are or will be called upon, to declare whether you will support the Union of the Colonies, in opposition to the Instructions of the House of the Assembly, or whether you will support the Assembly against the Union of the Colonies: We have declared for the former, and we will, at the hazard of our lives, support the Union; for, if the Union be broken, every Province on the Continent will be upon us. We have been open in our affairs; the sense of this City hath been publicly taken, and we will not be belied by Tories. We protest against private machinations, and we shall consider the authors of such as enemies and treat them accordingly. Let the men come forth who are endeavoring privately to undermine the Union; we will seek to find them out; we dare them to do it, at their peril.

"Seven thousand who appeared at the State House have sworn to support the Union."

At the same time, another letter was addressed to the different County Controlling Committees, saying:

"Gentlemen:

"We have, in a former letter to you, referred to the Instructions given by the Assembly of this Province to their Delegates, and they are published in the 'Votes of the House'; you will, therefore, not be surprised to hear that the Delegates of

Pennsylvania *did not* give their voice in Congress 'for establishing Governments throughout the Continent, on Authority of the People, but, by declining to vote on the momentous occasion, did, as far as was in their power, withdraw the Province from the Union of the Colonies, both in Council and in Action.

"By the enclosed papers, you will perceive the City and Liberties have been convened, and have expressed their sense on the whole resolve of Congress. We judge the number of People met on this occasion exceeded four thousand and consisted of that Class of men which are most to be depended on, in times of danger. A change of such importance as is now proposed is not brought about without some contest arising from the opposition of interest and the force of prejudice in favor of old and established form. . . . The Committee have thought the object before us of such consequence to the safety and happiness of the Province as to induce us to send some of our Committee and fellow citizens into each County to incite such of the good people as are friends of Liberty and determined to oppose the Cruelty and Injustice of Great Britain, to a spirited and manly exertion of their undoubted rights and privileges in the present favorable opportunity to establishing them forever. . . . . . We recommend to you, to nominate such a number of your Committee as you may think proper to meet Delegates from the other Counties in Philadelphia on Tuesday, the 18th Day of next month, in order to agree upon and direct the mode of electing members for a Provincial Convention to be held at such time and place as may be agreed upon... for the express purpose of forming and establishing a new Government on the Authority of the People only, and for the security of their Peace, Liberty and Safety, according to the enclosed recommendations of the Honorable Continental Congress!"

The Berks County reply was received under the date of Reading, June 1, 1776:

"Gentlemen:

"Agreeable to the assurance in our last, your letter of the 21st Ult., with several papers therewith sent, was laid before the General Committee of this County, and I am now directed to acquaint you that they have appointed a number of gentlemen of their body, to attend the Conference proposed to be held in your City on the 18th of this month, in order to agree upon and direct the mode of electing members for a Provincial Convention, a measure which they conceive to be extremely proper in itself, and mighty necessary in the present situation of our affairs. "

The gentlemen nominated by the Committee are:

Dr. Bodo Otto Henry Haller Jacob Morgan Charles Shoemaker
Benj. Spiker Joseph Hiester
Daniel Hunter and myself

"By order of the Committee Mark Bird, Chairman."

The Pennsylvania Assembly, realizing the indignation of the people regarding their previous position and convinced that drastic action was about to be taken, withdrew their standing instructions to the Continental Delegates on June 14th, just four days before the appointed conference, after which they immediately adjourned.

Ninety-seven of the one hundred and three appointed Pennsylvania delegates assembled in Carpenters Hall, Philadelphia, on June 18th and sat continuously, day and evening, until June 25th. The roll-call records show that Bodo Otto absented himself twice on Wednesday evening and Sunday morning, and it might be safely assumed that it was for the purpose of attending church services with his old St. Michael's friends.

By Sunday, the 23rd, the Conference was ready to act on the request of Congress, and on that day, they resolved that an election be held throughout the Colony on July 8th to select delegates to a Constitutional Convention.

The Pennsylvania Assembly having adjourned, with many important matters requiring immediate discussion, the assembled Provincial delegates presumed to consider and dispose of a number of matters, even though they lacked lawful authority. Seeking approval and endorsement of their action, they addressed a letter to the "Associators of Pennsylvania:"

"Gentlemen:

"The only design of our meeting was to put an end to our own power in the Province by fixing upon a plan for calling a Convention to form a Government under the authority of the People. But the sudden and unexpected separation [adjournment] of the late Assembly has compelled us to undertake the execution of a Resolve of Congress for calling forth 4500 of the militia of the Province to join the militia of the neighboring Colonies to form a camp for our immediate protection. We presume only to recommend the plan we have formed for you, trusting that in a case of so much consequence, your love of virtue and great zeal for liberty will supply the want of authority delegated to us expressly for that purpose.

"We need not remind you that you are now furnished with new motives to animate and support your courage. You are now about to contend against the Power of Great Britain in order to displace one set of villains to make room for another. Your arms will not be enervated on the day of battle with the reflection that you are about to risk your lives or shed your blood for a British tyrant or that your posterity will have your work to do over again.

You are about to contend for permanent freedom, to be supported by a Government which will be derived from yourselves, and which will have for its object, not the emolument of one man or class of men only, but the safety, liberty and happiness of every individual in the community. We call upon you, therefore, by the respect and obedience which are due to the authority of the United Colonies, to concur in this important measure."

The conference also appointed a committee to draft a resolution respecting the sentiments of the assembled delegates regarding independence, and the minutes record that:

"The conference met on June 24, 1776, P.M., and the committee ap pointed for that purpose, brought in a draft of a declaration on the subject of the independence of this Colony of the Crown of Great Britain, which was ordered to be read; by special order, the same was read a second time and being fully considered, then it was with the greatest unanimity of all the members agreed to, and is in the words following--viz:-- WHEREAS: George the III, King of Great Britain, in violation of the principles of the British Constitution and the Laws of Justice and Humanity, hath, by an accumulation of oppressions unparalleled in history, excluded the inhabitants of this and other American Colonies from his protection; and WHEREAS, he hath paid no regard to any of our numerous and dutiful petitions for a redress of our complicated grievances, but hath lately purchased foreign troops to assist in enslaving us, and hath excited the savages of this country to carry on a war against us, as also the negroes to embrue their hands in the blood of their masters, in a manner unpractised by civilized nations, and has lately insulted our calamities, by declaring that he will show no mercy until he has reduced us; and WHEREAS, the obligations of allegiance (being reciprocate between a King and his subjects are now dissolved, on the side of the Colonists, by the despotism of the said King, inasmuch that it now appears that loyalty to him is treason against the good people of this country; and WHEREAS, not only the Parliament, but there is reason to believe, too many of the people of Great Britain, have concurred in the aforesaid arbitrary and unjust proceedings against us; and WHEREAS, the public virtue of this Colony (so essential to the liberty and happiness) must be endangered by a future political union with, or dependence upon a Crown and Nation so lost to justice, patriotism and magnanimity, we, the deputies of the people of Pennsylvania, assembled in full Provincial Conference for forming a plan for executing the resolve of Congress of the 15th of May last, for suppressing all authority in this Province, derived from the Crown of Great Britain, and for establishing a Government upon the authority of the people only, now in this public manner, in behalf of ourselves and with the approbation, consent and authority of our constituents, unanimously declare our willingness to concur in a vote of the Congress declaring the United Colonies free and independent States; provided, the forming the Government, and the regulations of the Internal Police of this Colony, be always preserved to the people of said Colony; and we do further call upon the Nations of Europe, and appeal to the great arbiter and Governor of the Empires of the World, to witness for us, that this declaration did not originate in ambition, or in an impatience of lawful authority, but that we were driven to it in obedience to the first principles of nature, by the oppressions and cruelties of the aforesaid King and Parliament of Great Britain, as the only possible measure that was left us to preserve and establish our liberties, and to transmit them inviolate to posterity.

"'ORDERED:—that this Declaration be signed by all at the table, and that the President deliver it in Congress."

The business of the Pennsylvania Provincial Conference having been completed on June 25th, the delegates returned to their homes; some to raise and command troops, others to become delegates to the Constitutional Convention, and all to take some part in the struggle that confronted the Colonies.

The Provincial resolution for separation from England, adopted in the Pennsylvania Convention, anticipated the Declaration of Independence of the Continental Congress by nine days and showed a personal courage quite equal to that displayed by the "Signers."

That the actions and results of this assembly of Pennsylvania Colonial leaders are not better known or given commensurate credit for their accomplishments, is undoubtedly due to the greater importance of the immediately following Declaration of Independence by the Continental Congress.

Next to a pardonable pride in personal achievements or success of immediate family comes satisfaction in the attainments and prominence of ancestors. Yet few descendants of the delegates to the Pennsylvania Provincial Conference of June 1776 are aware of the noteworthy and determined part played by their forbears in making the thirteen American Colonies a free and independent nation.

CHAPTER EIGHT

THE MEDICAL DEPARTMENT • Continental Army • Hospital Reports • Wounds • Typhus Fever • Inoculation

PRIOR TO THE REVOLUTION, the medical men of New England and the Middle Colonies held many important positions and exercised great influence on public opinion in their respective communities. Of the Massachusetts Provincial Congress, no fewer than twenty-one members were of that profession, while six signed the Declaration of Independence. Ten physicians took part in the skirmishes of Lexington and Concord, and many eventually commanded regiments, brigades, and even divisions of Continental troops. Frequently, physicians who became officers in the Army served in both capacities when the need arose. Family traditions are that Dr. Bodo Otto's son, Bodo Junior, who commanded a New Jersey militia regiment, spent his furlough periods as assistant to his father in the Hospital of Valley Forge.

Notwithstanding the importance of the Medical Department of the Revolutionary Army, its history and the service of the personnel have never been fully recorded. It is also unfortunate that the different Directors-General, whose official contacts should have enabled them to tabulate all hospital institutions with a complete list of officers, have left but few writings of historical value. The destruction of United States Government buildings by the British in the War of 1812 increased the difficulties of compiling official records into a complete story, for many documents that might greatly enrich our Revolutionary medical history were burned.

It has been stated that there were thirty-five hundred practicing physicians in the Colonies at the outbreak of the war. It has also been estimated that of this number, probably fewer than 200 were graduates of European medical institutions and the recently established Colonial professional schools. These figures are interesting as indicating the large proportion of apprenticed trained medical men who responded to the call of Congress for the care of the American soldiers. An incomplete roster of physicians and surgeons of the Continental Army includes approximately fourteen hundred names. It is probable that a search of Colonial pension files of the thirteen original states, as well as those of the United States Government, would increase the number on this list, uncover interesting records of service, and locate many emergency hospitals. Unfortunately, research in this field has not appealed to historical writers. Incidents of strategy, of camp, and of fighting men have always held greater possibilities of interest than have the less conspicuous incidents connected with service to the sick and suffering soldiers, so no historiographer has come forward to do justice to the heroes of the hospitals.

The regular periodical reports from the senior physicians and surgeons on the number of hospital patients and the diseases involved are dry reading. They contain a duplication of afflictions that may explain a book issued for the use of the less experienced regimental mates and detached troops unaccompanied by medical officers. After enumerating various symptoms, this thesis prescribed several medicines that were supposed to be available in all regimental medical chests. Some of the precautions suggested and treatments recommended are unique. For rheumatism, it was directed that ten ounces of blood be taken from the arm on the affected side. In case the water was suspected of being contaminated, six ounces of vinegar was prescribed to be mixed with every three quarts, and under no circumstances should drinking water be drawn from near the bank of a stream.

The hospital reports recognized many different kinds of fever. Among those listed are typhus: putrid, jail, intermittent, inflammatory, nervous, slow, bilious, hectic, and remitting. Typhoid was not found among those reported, but it undoubtedly existed under some one of the other classifications. Most of the reports included cases of diarrhea, dysentery, rheumatism, venereal complaints, jaundice, rash, itch, measles, mumps, scurvy, piles, scrofula, lumbago, fits, angina, asthma, paralysis, erysipelas, consumption, ague, cholera, smallpox, cholera morbus, whooping cough, rupture, sore eyes, hip gout, abscess, and gravel. Many of the patients were admitted for a "good purging." Dr. Benjamin Rush's observations on the sick of the Army were so full of information and suggested precautions that they were ordered, published and distributed throughout the Army. Among his conclusions were that men were more sickly in tents than in the open air and more healthy when kept in motion than when in camp, that those under twenty years of age were subject to a greater number of camp diseases and that Southern troops were more sickly than Northern ones. He also contended that soldiers older than thirty years were the hardiest and that those who wore flannel shirts next to their skin generally escaped fevers and diseases of all kinds, while drunken men and convalescents were the most subject to fevers. He remarked that fever patients with large ulcers on their backs or limbs generally recovered and that the disease was frequently conveyed from hospitals to camp by means of lice carried in blankets or clothing.

The wounds of the Revolutionary War were principally caused by musket balls. The British rifle was a smooth, long-barreled gun which fired a round ball of about ¾" diameter. Its effective range was little more than one hundred yards, but it did considerable damage within that distance. Very few wounds resulted from artillery fire. Solid shot and grape were the ammunition used, but these guns were comparatively small bore and short range. The bayonet was seldom employed, though many wounds were recorded from clubs, knives, and hatchets, especially in campaigns where Indians supplemented British troops. There was no organized system of collecting or conveying the wounded to the hospital, so much suffering often resulted in the transfer.

To the dangers of contagion from disease and infection from wounds, the physicians and surgeons of the Continental hospitals were constantly exposed, and they encountered greater risks in the performance of their duties than officers of the line who faced the enemy. It is a matter of record that more hospital medical men died in proportion to their number than those in command of troops. A soldier had ninety-eight chances out of a hundred of escaping death in battle, but the odds of his leaving a hospital alive were but seventy-five percent. The pitiful part of this greater hazard was that serious afflictions which carried men off were often contracted in the hospital where the soldiers may have gone for treatment of some simple malady. Many fatal illnesses occurred as a consequence of ill-advised visits of convalescent soldiers to other patients who were seriously sick with contagious diseases. The precautions and sanitary protections of modern times were unknown in Revolutionary hospitals, so few physicians and surgeons served for any length of time without experiencing a serious spell of sickness. Dr. Bodo Otto's term of hospital duty from 1776 until 1782, between his sixty-fifth and seventy-second years, indicates both a robust constitution and immunity from disease, or perhaps a better knowledge of precautions, for no record exists of his having been ill or of his taking extended leaves of absence. Dr. James Tilton wrote:

"Six surgeons and Mates had been seized with Typhus in the Hospitals of Princeton and at Bethlehem; not an Orderly Man or Nurse escaped and but a few of the Surgeons."

Dr. John Augustus Otto stated, in his pension application made when eighty-two years of age, that after three years of service, he was unable to continue because of extreme disability caused by an attack of violent fever.

Dr. Thomas Bond, Jr., wrote his friend, Dr. Jonathan Potts:

"I have been on my back since Sunday with the Epidemical Broken Bone Fever three nights past. I have been delirious, and, indeed, my Friend, I never experienced such a disease in all my life. I would not wish the greatest enemy I ever had twelve hours of the pain. The discomfort of my pain and fever has abated a bit, but I expect severe returns."

Many such stories with more serious results could be told of the physicians and surgeons of the hospitals.

The greatest scourge of the army was typhus fever. The crowded conditions of the hospitals and inadequate ventilation and sanitary protection combined to make the disease fatal. The result of this combination of adverse features was that "their own stinking clothes and foul linen, etc." were enough to suffocate the patients, as well as others who were obliged to approach them. Smallpox was the one serious affliction that Colonial men understood, but until inoculation was ordered for all soldiers who had not experienced the disease, it caused great havoc in the Continental Army and influenced the result of several important campaigns. The casualty record for victims of natural Smallpox exceeded sixteen percent, while deaths from the disease taken through inoculation averaged but one in three hundred patients. Many regiments of five hundred men went through the treatment without the loss of a man. Subjects were usually prepared for the ordeal by systematic dosings of medicine, and Dr. John Augustus Otto's notebook contained the following:

"General direction for the regimen or diet necessary to be observed and used in the course of preparation for Smallpox by inoculation, etc., tea, coffee, chocolate in the customary manner; wheat bread of any kind, biscuit is generally used. Gruel, sago, ripe fruit and all kinds of vegetables, particularly potatoes, turnips, cabbage, carrots, radishes, pickles of any kind (peppers excepted), apple pies, dumplings, shortened with thin milk or molasses, etc. All the above to be taken at different times as agreeable to the constitution."

Should this liberal diet, as described, offend any of the "Faculty" who may read, it might be mentioned that there is a large "X" marked across the entire page, which may mean that it was discarded or that the doctor was testing a quill pen.

Official action on the matter of wholesale army inoculation had been delayed because Colonial differences of opinion had long existed on the subject. In some Provinces, inoculation was frequently practiced, while in others, it was prohibited by law and in a few, it was permitted under restrictions, and then only in specified towns. The presence of Smallpox in the Eastern and

Northern Armies had materially reduced the number of available troops, and the fear of it had discouraged recruiting, so, in February 1777, Congress and the Commander-in-Chief finally decided for a general inoculation.

Virginia was one of the Colonies opposed to inoculation, and in April 1777, General Washington wrote to Patrick Henry, then Governor of that State:

"I am induced to believe that the apprehension of the Smallpox and its calamitous consequences have greatly retarded enlistments. But may not those objections be easily done away with by introducing inoculation into the State? Or shall we adhere to a regulation preventing it and reprobated at this time? Not only by consent and usage of the greater part of the civilized world but also by our interest in and experience of its utility. You will pardon my observation on the Smallpox because I know it is *more destructive to an Army in the natural way than the swords* and because I shudder whenever I reflect upon the difficulties of keeping it out and that in the vicissitudes of war, the scene may be transferred to some Southern State."

There was no doubt in General Washington's mind of the value and comparative safety of the inoculation treatment, and seven months after addressing Patrick Henry, he wrote to John Augustus Washington:

"I congratulate you very sincerely on the happy passage of my Sister and the rest of your family through the Smallpox. Surely, the daily instances that present themselves with the amazing benefits of inoculation must convert the most rigid opposers and bring a repeal of the most impolitic law that restrains it."

In April of 1776, General Washington had written from New York:

"Mrs. Washington is still here and talks of taking the Smallpox, but I doubt her resolution."

Smallpox made its appearance in the New England Army early in 1775, and on June 27, the Massachusetts Provincial Congress directed that a hospital be established to care for such patients and that consideration be given to the problem involved. On July 21, 1775, shortly after taking command of the Army at Cambridge, General

Washington wrote to Congress:

"I have been particularly attentive to the least symptom of the Smallpox, and hitherto, we have been so fortunate as to have every person removed, so soon as noting, to prevent any communication, but I am apprehensive it may gain in the Camps. *We shall continue the utmost vigilance against this most dangerous enemy.*"

As early as February 21, 1775, the Massachusetts Provincial Congress took heed of the necessity of being provided with medical supplies should a skirmish occur with the British, and so appointed Doctors Church and Warren a committee to submit a list of necessities and on April 18, 1775, directed that medical chests be sent to Concord, Sudbury, Groton, Mendon, Stow, Worcester, and Lancaster. Later, they provided that each regiment of four or five hundred men should have a surgeon and surgeon's mate. On April 29, 1775, a permanent hospital was authorized and thus came into existence, the Medical Department of the Army.

In May 1775, the Massachusetts Provincial Congress appointed a committee to examine such persons as those who had applied for the positions of surgeon in the regiments and then formed. These examinations covered Anatomy, Physiology, Surgery, and Medicine and were very thorough; the thoroughness causing no little nervousness among the applicants. On June 2,

1775, Dr. Benjamin Church of Boston presented himself before the President of the Continental Congress with credentials from Massachusetts reading:

"Resolved, that Dr. Benjamin Church be ordered to go to Philadelphia and deliver to the President of the Honorable American Congress, there sitting, the following application to be by him communicated to the members thereof, and that the said Church is also directed to confer with the said Congress respecting such other matters as may be necessary to the defense of the Colony and particularly the State of the Army therein."

The result of Dr. Church's visit to Congress was the adoption of a Continental Hospital Plan for an Army of 20,000 men, the organization to consist of one Director General and Chief Physician, four surgeons and one apothecary, twenty surgeon's mates, one clerk, two storekeepers, and one nurse for every ten sick. Dr. Church was unanimously elected Director and Chief Physician on July 27, 1775, with authority to appoint his apothecary and four surgeons who, in turn, were to select their own mates.

Much of the medical service to troops in the early days of the war was rendered by physicians who lived in the neighborhood of the camps.

Connecticut regiments sent to join the Army in Canada were not accompanied by surgeons, and there are many resolutions on record, both in the Continental Congress and in the Provincial Assemblies journals, approving bills for such emergency requirements.

In the Spring of 1776, the Pennsylvania authorities sent a detachment of soldiers to reinforce the New Jersey Militia in protection of the Delaware Capes. These Pennsylvania troops were apparently unaccompanied by a surgeon, for on August 21, 1776, the Council of Safety at Philadelphia directed its

"Treasurer, John M. Nesbitt, Esq, to pay Dr. Frederick (C) Otto (of N.J.) 6 £ 11 s. 3 d. for attendance on a man wounded at Cape May, N.J., in the service of this (Pennsylvania) State."

The diary of Aaron Leaming also recorded an accident at a training camp in New Jersey when Dr. Bodo Otto, Jr., and others were summoned in the absence of a regimental surgeon. It reads:

"Thomas Godfrey, having his gun charged with stones, accidentally shot James Parker in the leg. The bone was much splintered and shattered, and it was judged necessary to amputate. For this purpose Dr. Otto was sent from Gloucester County. On the afternoon of May 12th, Dr. Otto performed the amputation, assisted by Dr. McGinnes of Philadelphia and Doctors Hunt and Benj. Stites. On the 17th of May, he died."

A book on military surgery published in Philadelphia in 1766 described the treatment of many different kinds of wounds. Amputation was usually necessary for compound fractures, especially those affecting the joints. Tradition tells us that soldiers about to undergo amputations were given bullets to chew, and many have been found with the marks of human teeth deep upon them.

The story of the Medical Department of the Revolutionary Army is one of intrigues from within and attacks from without. Reputations were assailed, and charges were made in speech and print that today could result in libel suits if not personal encounters. Some of the criticism made was justified, though much was unwarranted, but of this more will be told in its proper place. The beneficial results that can be recorded are the reorganization of the Department that followed when many legislative mistakes were corrected, and the expected needs of the hospitals were recognized.

Dr. John Cochran, the last of four Directors General of the Medical Department, who served the Revolutionary Army, was the only one who left the service with an unsullied record and was the exception who received the whole-hearted cooperation of the entire medical organization.

CHAPTER NINE

SMALLPOX • British Plan to Spread Infection • Precautionary Measures • Correspondence with Washington

THE MASSACHUSETTS PROVINCIAL ASSEMBLY quickly recognized the danger of Smallpox becoming prevalent among the New England troops, so provided for its treatment. Shortly after assuming command, General Washington reported to Congress the precautions taken to keep it under control.

The methods adopted were apparently quite satisfactory until early fall (1775) when a British deserter brought information to the Cambridge Headquarters that there were 2,000 sick among the English troops in Boston, many of them ill with Smallpox.

On November 27, 1775, General Washington reported to Congress: "General Howe has ordered 300 inhabitants of Boston to Point Shirley

in a destitute condition. I have ordered provisions to them until they can be moved, but am under dreadful apprehensions of their communicating the Smallpox as it is rife in Boston. I have forbidden any of them from coming to this place on that account."

On the following day, November 28, 1775, he again wrote:

"As the Smallpox is now in Boston, I have used the precaution of prohibiting such as lately came out from coming near our Camp."

Again on December 3, 1775, Robert H. Harrison addressed the Council of Massachusetts from Cambridge with:

"I am commanded by His Excellency to inform you that four deserters have just arrived at Headquarters, giving an account that several persons are to be sent out of Boston this evening or tomorrow that have lately been inoculated with the Smallpox with the design to spread the infection in order to distress us as much as possible."

General Washington confirmed this report to the President of the Continental Congress the following day, December 4, 1775:

"By recent information from Boston, General Howe is going to send out a number of the inhabitants in order, as it is thought, to make room for his expected reinforcements; there is one part of the information that I can hardly credit: a Sailor says that a number of them coming out have been inoculated with the design of spreading the Smallpox throughout the Country and Camp."

Six days later, on December 10, 1775, he notified the Massachusetts Legislature:

"This moment received from Mr. Thos. Croft the letter I have enclosed, from which it will appear that some of the people who came out of Boston are infected with the Smallpox. As the disorder, should it spread, may prove very disastrous and fatal to our Army and the country around it, I should hope that you will have such necessary steps taken as will prevent the infection being further communicated."

The following day, December 11, 1775, he notified Congress:

"The information I received that the Enemy intended spreading Smallpox among us, I could not suppose them capable of. I now must give

some credit to it as it made its appearance on several of those who last came out of Boston. Every necessary precaution has been taken to prevent its being communicated to the Army, and the General Court will take care that it does not spread throughout the Country."

Again on December 14, 1775, he wrote:

"About 150 more of the poor inhabitants are come out of Boston. The Smallpox rages all over the Town. Such of the Militia as had it not before *are now under* inoculation."

The next day, December 15, 1775, General Washington added a postscript to his letter to Congress saying:

"The Smallpox is in every part of Boston. The soldiers there who have never had it are, we are told, under inoculation and considered as a surety against any attempt of our (to attack). A third shipload of people is coming out to Shirley Point. If we escape the Smallpox in this Camp (Cambridge) and the country around about it, it will be miraculous. Every precaution that can be is taken to guard against the evil."

Just what precautions were taken and how effective they were are not recorded, nor is the success of the British in combating the disease among their own men. Later orders issued by General Washington from Cambridge indicated that General Howe had contended with the problem up to the time of his evacuation of Boston.

General Howe's decision to withdraw was known on March 7, 1776, and he notified General Washington that he would burn the town if he were attacked. The strength of the Continental

Army besieging Boston was then about 18,000 men, of whom 2,500 were sick in camp. General Washington published an Order from Cambridge Headquarters dated March 13, 1776, that read:

"As the Enemy with a malicious assiduity has spread the infection of Smallpox throughout all parts of the Town, nothing but the utmost

caution on our part can prevent that fatal disease from spreading through the Army and Camp to the infinite detriment of both. Therefore, no Officer or Soldier may go into Boston when the Enemy evacuates the Town."

On the following day, March 14, 1776, the Headquarters Orders announced:

"The General was informed yesterday evening by a person just out of Boston that our Enemies in that place have laid several schemes for communicating the infection of the Smallpox to the Continental Army when they get out of the Town. This shows the propriety of yesterday's Order."

The British evacuated Boston on March 17, 1776, and on the 19th, General Washington reported to Congress:

"As soon as the Ministerial Troops had quitted the Town, I ordered 1,000 men who had had the Smallpox, under the Command of General Putnam, to take possession."

The General Headquarters Orders of March 20, 1776, recited:

"Every possible precaution will be taken to destroy the infection of the Smallpox."

On the following day, March 21, 1776, General Washington notified the Massachusetts Legislature:

"Notwithstanding all precautions which I have endeavored to use to restrain and limit the intercourse between the town and the Army and Country for a few days, I greatly fear that the Smallpox will come to both."

Cambridge Headquarters Orders of March 25, 1776, directed that:

"Hospital and Regimental Surgeons are to examine carefully the state of the sick, and whenever they discover the smallest symptom of Smallpox, they are without delay to send the patient to the Smallpox Hospital in Cambridge."

In spite of all efforts, the infection found its way into the country, and many towns adjacent to Boston took precautions to restrict intercourse with the city. The town authorities of Salem, Mass., on July 18, 1776, registered a protest with a letter that read:

"Sir:

I am directed by the Selectmen and Committee of Safety of this Town to inform you that the inhabitants are very uneasy and urge the erection of a Gate at the entrance of the Town to secure them against the Smallpox of which they think themselves in danger by means of persons coming from Boston unexamined and uncleansed, which they do to this day, and it is feared will continue to do unless the Honorable Council take some effective order to prevent it."

The Council of Massachusetts sitting at Watertown was also disturbed, and on July 20, 1776, it addressed a communication to the Selectmen of Boston saying:

"Gentlemen:

It appears that there is a great uneasiness in the minds of the people in various parts of the State that no great care has been taken to prevent the spread of the Smallpox, and unless such care should now be taken as may be reasonable and satisfactory, great mischief must certainly ensue and still greater if the distemper should prevail over the country Towns."

Under date of July 9, 1776, the Council of Massachusetts wrote General Artemus Ward from Watertown:

"Sir

The Board was this day informed that you had given liberty to a number of Continental Troops now stationed at Winter Hill to receive the Smallpox by inoculation. The Board is unwilling to credit such a report as there is an act by *this* Colony prohibiting inoculation except in the Town of Boston. They, therefore, request, if you have given any such orders out, that you will immediately recall them that the good people of Medford, etc., may be relieved of their apprehensions and desire your Honor would not permit any of the Troops under your Command to receive the Smallpox inoculation in any other Town except the Town of Boston."

The Colony of New Hampshire also had restrictive legislation, for a petition was filed with the Honorable Committee of Safety of that Colony reading:

"That the Subscribers, the Selectmen of said Town of Portsmouth your Petitioners, have been requested by a number of the inhabitants of the Town forthwith to call a Town meeting to know whether the said in inhabitants will vote to have a Hospital opened for inoculation for the Smallpox under necessary regulations."

It might be assumed from the following exchange of letters between Dr. John Morgan, Director General, and General Washington that on the withdrawal of the British from Boston, certain personal property of avowed Tories was appropriated for official use. Dr. Morgan's letter reads:

"General Washington:

Having received a present of an exceedingly Handsome and good Horse, he thinks it too elegant and accomplished an animal not to wish General Washington Master of it. He, therefore, begs the General's acceptance. He shall think himself very happy to have had it in his power to furnish him so noble a steed when he may have more particular occasion for a good riding horse for his own use of that of Mrs. Washington.

"Dr. Morgan's servant now attends with the horse to deliver to whomsoever the General shall order to take charge of it.

"Tuesday, March 19th, 1776"

This letter still exists and bears the General's endorsement:

"From Dr. John Morgan, March 19, 1776. The offer is not accepted."

General Washington, however, graciously acknowledged the honor intended and, under the date of March 22, 1776, replied with:

"The General presents his best respects to Dr. Morgan: Upon inquiry of Col. Mifflin concerning the Horse (the Doctor very kindly made a tender after him), he is given to understand that the Horse did not belong to the King or any of his Officers but was the property of a Dr. Lloyd, an avowed enemy to the American Cause. As the General does not know under what predicament the property of these kinds of people may fall—in short, if there is no kind of doubt in the case—as the horse is too much of value for the General to think of robbing the Doctor off, he begs to leave to return him, accompanied with the sincere thanks for the politeness with which he was presented and this request—that the Doctor will not think the General meant to slight his favor."

The Continental troops started their movement toward New York the day after the British evacuated Boston, and on April 4, 1776, General Washington left, accompanied by the last brigade. Two regiments were left for the defense of Boston, and the remaining troops, as well as the inhabitants, were inoculated.

Three hundred sick were left behind, and in less than six weeks, all were discharged, but few had died.

In spite of the dangers of infection which it had experienced, the Army of Boston was comparatively healthy, for typhus was seldom encountered, and although dysentery was present, it was seldom fatal. Dr. Rush made the interesting observation that:

"It is very remarkable that while the American Army at Cambridge, in the year 1775, consisted only of New England Men (whose habits and manners were the same), there was scarcely any sickness among them. It was not until the Troops of the Eastern, Middle and Southern States met at New York and Ticonderoga in 1776 that the Typhus became universal and spread with such mortality in the Army of the United States."

On April 3, 1776, Director General Morgan received his orders for the hospital organization, reading:

"As the Grand Continental Army . . . will as soon as practicable be assembled at New York, you are, with all convenient speed, to remove the General Hospital to that city. The medicine, stores, bedding, etc., not immediately wanted in the General Hospital, should be loaded in carts and sent to Norwich, Connecticut, by a proper Officer or Officers of the Hospital. Upon their arrival there, they will find His Excellency's Orders and how and in what manner to proceed from thence, whether by land or water."

Then began the serious problems of the Continental Army hospitals, the solutions to which were a long way off. And then, too, began the troubles and griefs of Dr. John Morgan, which greatly embittered his later life.

CHAPTER TEN

THE NORTHERN CAMPAIGN • Benedict Arnold • Misery of Army • Retreat of Northern Army • Hospital Plan

WHILE THE CONTINENTAL ARMY lay at Cambridge, Mass., two American expeditions were sent against the British in Canada. One under Benedict Arnold was accompanied by a hospital organization composed of Dr. Isaac Senter and several assistants, but the other, consisting of four New York regiments and two from Connecticut, was without hospital attendants. On August 6, 1775, General Schuyler, the then Commanding Officer of the second Army, wrote to Congress:

"Out of 500 men that are here, near 100 are sick, and I have no kind of Hospital Stores, although I had not forgotten to order them immediately after my appointment.

"The little wine I had for my own table I have delivered to the Regimental Surgeons. That being expended, I shall no longer bear the distress of the sick... I shall take the liberty immediately to order a Physician from Albany to join me with such Stores as are indispensably necessary."

General Schuyler's communication also contained a statement that if Congress would not assume the expense involved in his request, he would personally accept responsibility for the payment of his obligation. General Schuyler's action for the care of his men was promptly approved by Congress, and on September 14, 1775, it endorsed his selection of a medical man with a resolution providing:

"That Samuel Stringer, Esq., he appointed. Director of the Hospital and chief Physician and Surgeon for the Army of the Northern Department."

Dr. Stringer was also authorized to enlist four surgeon mates to assist him, but this number was woefully inadequate, and by October 25, 1775, he requested permission from Congress to enroll additional surgeons and mates.

General Schuyler, because of illness, was obliged to relinquish active command of the Northern Department. In September 1775, the Army of 2,000 men under the leadership of General Montgomery began their march toward Montreal. Two British advance posts (Chambly and St. Johns on the Sorel River) and many prisoners were taken while en route, and finally, in November, the American troops successfully reached and captured their Montreal objective. By this time, however, the Continental force, through sickness, desertions, and expiring enlistments, was reduced to barely 500 men.

Meanwhile, Benedict Arnold, with a heroic band of 1,100 men, had cut his way through dense New England forests and, using available water routes under terrible handicaps and hardships, reached his goal—the St. Lawrence River. The exertions and exposures of the march caused some sickness among the soldiers, consisting principally of rheumatism and camp diarrhea, but fortunately, neither fever nor smallpox made an appearance. By the middle of November 1775, General Arnold had transported his Army across the St. Lawrence, but their number being too few to successfully attack Quebec, he withdrew further up the river and made camp. Here, on December 1, 1775, Arnold's men were joined by Montgomery's troops from Montreal. These soldiers brought with them the germs of the dreaded smallpox and thereby started an epidemic that greatly reduced the number of available fighting men, besides introducing into the Army the infection that was the greatest contributing factor in the failure of the Canadian campaign.

With the increased number of men and cooperation of troops under Montgomery's and Arnold's command, an attack was soon made on the British garrison at Quebec. The results were sad and disastrous to the American cause, for Montgomery was killed, Arnold wounded, and many important Continental officers captured. Sometime previous to this assault, Arnold had requested that additional troops be sent to him, and while awaiting their arrival the American Army maintained a siege of the walled city. Fresh New England Colonial militia reached the besieging army in March 1776, but many of these soldiers were sick and therefore incapacitated. On May 1, 1776, of 1,900 men confronting Quebec, 900 were unfit for duty, and of these, the great majority were victims of smallpox. When British reinforcements appeared in troop ships on May 6, 1776, panic seized the Americans, and the entire Army fled, abandoning camp, equipment and hospital, leaving some 200 of the most seriously ill unattended. About 150 smallpox patients left their beds and joined the fleeing soldiers. This panic-stricken, disorganized Army was finally halted and made camp at Sorel, where smallpox became a serious menace.

Congress quickly sent a commission to investigate and report on conditions in the North, and on May 15, 1776, General Arnold wrote to this delegation:

"I shall be glad to know your sentiment in regard to inoculation as early as possible. Will it not be best, considering the impossibility of preventing the spread of Smallpox, to inoculate 500 to 1,000 men immediately and send them to Montreal, and as many more every five days, until the whole Army receive it: which will prevent our Army being distressed thereafter; and I make no doubt we shall have more effective men in four weeks than by endeavoring to prevent the infection spreading."

The commission promptly approved General Arnold's suggestion of inoculation, and a large house having a capacity of six hundred patients was commandeered for hospital use.

The distressing condition of the American Army's retreat from Quebec is well described in a letter from Charles Cushing to his brother. It was written day by day over a period of time and under many dates. He wrote in part that: The line of retreat extended near thirty miles distance and a great part of them sick with the Smallpox. I am creditably informed no less than thirty Captains died of it, and not more than one in three that took it in the natural way lived.

Writing further of the retreat, he said speed was absolutely necessary, and great confusion existed, for everyone was trying to escape—

"As well as he could, leaving the sick to the mercy of the enemy though many of them who had the Smallpox out thick upon them, came off and went through the greatest fatigue, being exposed to the wet and cold without blankets or anything to cover them, and I afterwards saw them at Sorel.

"The New England men began to be very uneasy about the Smallpox spreading among them, as but few have had it. It was death for any Doctor to attempt inoculation. However, it was practiced secretly as many were willing to run that hazard rather than take it in the natural way.

"Some inoculated themselves, and several Officers and myself began it in our Regiment at Sorel... I was then under a Mercurial Preparation for the Smallpox.... General Sullivan's Brigade beginning to come in, and detachments sent up from Sorel; our Regiment was ordered over to St. John to have the Smallpox... General Thomas took the Smallpox in the natural way, came up to Chambly, and there died.

"We had been in St. Johns but ten days when we had orders for as many Regiments as were able to go to Sorel. Accordingly, a Petty Senior Mate was sent to examine the Men (not trusting our own Doctor who was a good Physician) who reported 200, who had been off duty but ten days for the Smallpox, fit for duty. Although they had the disorder lightly, no one could think of them as fit to go through so much fatigue... We have lost a vast number of men through Smallpox, it being very mortal to those who took it in the natural way."

Under the date of July 10, he added:

"We have now been at Crown Point eight days and since then have buried great numbers—some days not less than 15 or 20, but few have died except of the Smallpox. Some Regiments which did not inoculate have lost many, and Col. Read, in particular, says that by the time it has gone through the Regiment, he shall have lost one-third of them."

Dr. Stringer had been making continuous efforts from the time of his appointment to enlarge his hospital staff and finally appealed to General Washington for authority to engage "four Senior Surgeons, twelve Mates, one Matron and one or two Clerks, one or two Stewards, Surgeon Men and Apothecaries." General Washington replied he had directed Dr. Morgan to forward hospital supplies and would request the necessary authority for the increase. Congress approved Stringer's petition under date of

May 22, 1776, and five days later, the Commission in the North confirmed the serious situation as claimed, reporting:

"The Army is in a distressed condition and is in want of the most necessary articles... Three-fourths of the Army have not had the Smallpox... We cannot find words strong enough to describe our miserable situation."

Then began a series of American encounters with the British forces from Canada, and on June 11, 1776, in consequence, General Arnold ordered all the sick soldiers removed from Montreal. At the same time, he reported their number at St. John and Chambly as being 3,000. General Schuyler, writing to General Washington, said:

"If the Militia ordered into Canada should not have had the Smallpox, they will rather weaken than strengthen the Army."

One of the Congressional Committee wrote to a friend:

"Our misfortunes in Canada are enough to melt the heart of stone. The Smallpox is ten times more terrible than the British, Canadians and Indians together. This was the cause of our precipitate retreat from Quebec."

In three months, the American Army lost 5,000 men through disease and desertion, and of an equal number still remaining, 2,000 were sick. Dr. John Morgan's official return revealed an even worse condition, for on June 26, 1776, he reported 1,800 men incapacitated by smallpox and the total number of sick and unfit for duty in the Northern Army to be 3,300. It was shortly after this date that Dr. Jonathan Potts of Reading, Pennsylvania, was sent to assist Dr. Stringer, and there then began a systematic effort to eradicate the infection from the Northern Army. How desperate the situation was is indicated by the report from Fort George, where an official tabulation showed the Army to have had 5,247 men fit for duty; with 3,917 sick in camp, besides 915 lighter cases sent away to convalesce.

British men-of-war appeared in the St. Lawrence River on June 14, 1776, and the American Army withdrew to Crown Point, N.Y. Joseph Hewes wrote of this retreat under date of July 8, 1776, saying:

"Our Northern Army has left Canada and retreated to Ticonderoga and Crown Point. The Smallpox has made great havoc among them. Several Regiments had not enough well men to row all their sick over the Lake and men were drafted from other Regiments to do that service. In short, the Army has melted away in a little time as if the Destroying Angel had been sent on purpose to demolish them as he did the children of Israel."

Needless to say, the desperate condition in the North caused great anxiety throughout the entire country, and the fear existed that this prevalent disease might create a national crisis. John Adams wrote from Philadelphia on July 7, 1776, saying:

"I hope that measures will be taken to cleanse the Army at Crown Point from the Smallpox, and the measures will be taken in New England by *tolerating and encouraging inoculation*, to render that distemper less terrible."

Governor Jonathan Trumbull's apprehension over the situation was expressed in the following letter written to General Washington on July 4, 1776:

"The retreat of the Northern Army and the present situation has spread great alarm.... The prevalence of the Smallpox among them is in every way unhappy; our People, in general, have not had that distemper. Fear of the infection operates strongly to prevent soldiers from engaging in the service, and the Battalions ordered to be raised in this Colony fill up slowly. Are there no measures to be taken to remove the impediment? May not the Army soon be freed from that infection? Can the reinforcements be kept separate from the infected? Or may not a detachment be made from the Troops under your Command and the Militia raising in the several Colonies be ordered to New York, sending such men as have had the Smallpox to the Northern Department? Could any expedient be fallen upon that would afford probable hopes that this infection may be avoided? I believe our Battalion would (then) soon join the Northern Army."

Several days later (July 9, 1776), Governor Trumbull further unburdened himself in a letter to General Schuyler, saying:

"The Smallpox in our Northern Army carries with it greater dread than our Enemies. Our men dare to face them but are not willing to go into a Hospital. I wish to have every precaution taken to prevent the spread of that infection. Surely, by care and good discipline, the infection may be cleared and a stop put to its progress. To promote this design and afford every assistance in my power, I have sent up Major John Ely, a Gentleman skilled in that distemper, whose fidelity may be relied upon, to consult and assist in the matter.... Three Battalions from this Colony will soon come up; they may be preserved from the infection."

General Schuyler, writing from Albany on July 13, 1776, said that the main body of the Army was removing to Ticonderoga, where fortifications were being erected, and added:

"This disposition (of troops) will eventually prevent the Smallpox from being conveyed to the Militia by the now infected Army."

General Gates reported to General Washington from Ticonderoga on August 7, 1776, and declared:

"The very great desertion from this Army has, I believe, been principally occasioned by the dread of the Smallpox."

By August 1776, a plan for combating the disease involving group inoculation in segregated camps and hospitals was adopted. General orders were also issued forbidding soldiers and officers from secretly inoculating themselves as had become a custom, for it endangered the other men in the camp. Dr. Jonathan Potts received a report of an infraction of this order from Nicholas Scull, who, writing from Fort George, said:

"I received a letter yesterday from Dr. Johnston informing me that there were Three Villains detected in inoculating a Sutler (they belonged to Col. Warner's Reg.): a Surgeon, the Paymaster and a Lieutenant. They were secured, and I hope will be severely punished."

The result of this disobedience of orders was a military trial of the offenders, and a record of the punishment has been preserved in a letter written to General Horatio Gates:

"Sir:

"My son, who was Paymaster in Col. Warner's Regiment, writes to me that he has been cashiered by a Court Martial for inoculating a man, not belonging to the Army, who brought the infectious matter to him and promised immediately to go to a place about 30 miles distant from the Camp where inoculation was allowed under the inspection of a Committee;--that he did it inadvertently without any ill design.

"As he has always been a Friend to the American Cause, he seems much grieved to leave the Service under a censure, and though the emoluments of that Office are not worth the seeking, yet for the sake of his reputation, he wishes to be restored. I never heard, but he had been faithful in his public trust; he served some time as an Ass't. Paymaster in Canada, where he went as a Volunteer. . . If you, on consideration of the case, shall think fit to afford him relief, it will oblige him and be gratefully acknowledged by

Your Obdt. Humble Servant

Roger Sherman."

This appeal evidently had the desired result, for William Sherman, Jr., was reinstated in the Continental Army and remained in service until January 1, 1781.

Unauthorized inoculation must have been quite frequent, for William Williams wrote to Governor Trumbull of Connecticut as late as November 6, 1776, and after saying an officer had reported many soldiers dissatisfied because of not receiving their pay, added the explanation:

"It was suggested the probable reason was that the men had gone into inoculation contrary to Orders, etc., and that was alleged as a sufficient reason to cut them off and that the crime, if one in the circumstances, was treated with impolitic severity, I think, to say no more. I am greatly concerned that it will have a very ill effect on men in the Northern Service; the distressing feeling of the men under certain prospects of taking and dying with that disease, etc., in my opinion, pleads strongly in their excuse and in such cases allowance ought to be made, and faults winked at, especially when men are so wanted; things appear in a very different light to me than to some here."

The beneficial results of the hospital plan of treating the infection after preparation were soon apparent, for on September 2, 1776, General Gates wrote from Ticonderoga to the President of Congress:

"Thank Heaven the Smallpox is totally eradicated from amongst us; not I can assure you without much vigilance and authority being previously exerted."

Perhaps General Gates had in mind some prompt and decided action he had taken the previous month to prevent the disease from being again brought into the Northern encampments by arriving recruits. The story can be better told by quoting the correspondence. On August 10, 1776, General Gates had written from Ticonderoga to Max Hawley:

"Dear Sir:

"A Villain of a Surgeon (or what is commonly known as Doctor) is inoculating the Militia as fast as they arrive at Number

Four. Such a slave to private gain who would sacrifice this Army for the sake of obtaining a few dollars for himself deserves to be immediately brought to condign punishment; were he himself within my reach, it would not be many minutes before he would feel the weight of my resentment. That not being the case, I must apply to you to beg you would write to the Chairman of the Committee of Number Four directing him to exert his utmost power to stop this pernicious practice and, if possible, to send the Doctor instantly to jail.

"As fine an Army as ever marched into Canada has this year been entirely ruined by the Smallpox. If the Militia, which ought long ago to have been here are once infected, the Country will infallibly be exposed to the invasion of the Enemy. Such Officers as have stayed upon the way to be inoculated shall, they may depend upon it, be brought to a Court Martial as soon as they arrive at Skenesborough."

General Gates must have written other letters of the same character, for on August 12, 1776, Brigadier General David Waterbury, Jr., wrote from Skenesborough to "the Captain and Company of Carpenters at Williamstown" saying:

"I have received a line from Gen'l. Gates concerning you who have been inoculated which I will communicate with you. The Company of ship carpenters from Rhode Island who have been inoculated at Williamstown should be discharged and not suffered to come forward.

"The foregoing are the words of the General—I think as much as to say you are not to come into the Service. We don't intend to let anyone come into this place that has lately had the Smallpox (for you know that has been the bane of the Northern Army), and we have got it out of this place and out of Ticonderoga and we are determined to use every precaution to keep it clear; for your men to go and inoculate and presume to come here among fresh

Troops, we think is monstrous."

General Gates' letter regarding "the Villain of a Surgeon" evidently found its way to the culprit through the Town Committee of Safety, for the Doctor wrote in his own defense:

"Dr. Phineas Stephens to General Gates:

Charlestown-#4-Aug. 26, 1776

"Sir:

"May it please, your Honor, I was on the 23rd inst. summoned before the Committee of this Town in consequence of a letter addressed by your Honor to the Rev. M. Olcott, which letter, together with the copy of one to Major Hawley, enclosed in it, was read to me. The proceedings of the Committee and an account of my conduct, as far as it respects the crime whereof I have been accused, will be by them communicated. I should not, therefore, at this time trouble you in this manner were it, not the undoubted right, and I think I may add the duty of every individual, when injured in his character or property, to speak in his own defense that the defending party may be brought to justice. You are pleased to say in your letter to Maj. Hawley that 'a Villain of a Surgeon (or what is commonly called a Doctor) is inoculating the Militia as fast as they arrive at #4.' As I know of no person who answers your description I must think you have been grossly deceived and imposed upon by some ill-minded person from sinister views. You are pleased to add further that 'were he (viz., the Surgeon) within my reach, it would not be many minutes before he should feel the weight of my resentment.' I can, therefore, make no doubt but that some part, at least, of the resentment, will be felt by the Person who hath so greatly discomposed you by false information. I think I have a right to expect (I had almost said to command) that the informer be pointed out to me that I may know where to seek a reparation of the injury done me, which can't be considered as trifling since it has, for the time (at least) brought on me the displeasure of a Person of your Rank. I can say, with truth, that the bad effects of the Smallpox in the Army are lost, which I feel in common with my Countrymen, and no one has better wishes for the prosperity of your Honor and the Army under your Command than your Honor's most Obedient Humble Servant..."

This is not a very convincing answer and gives one the impression the Doctor is resenting an accusation of being a "Villain" rather than denying a charge of inoculating the men and endangering the health of the Army.

Dr. Jonathan Potts was given much of the credit, besides a vote of appreciation from Congress, for the successful fight against the disastrous scourge of the Northern Army, and by August 28, 1776, the situation was so well under control that General Gates was ready to take the offensive against the British. On that date, he wrote to General Washington from Ticonderoga:

"As the Smallpox is now perfectly removed from the Army, I shall, in consequence of the intelligence received of the motion of the Enemy, immediately assemble my principal strength to maintain this important pass and hope General Waterbury in a week at farthest will be able to come with Three Row Galleys to Ticonderoga and proceed the instant they arrive and are fitted out to join General Arnold upon the Lake."

CHAPTER ELEVEN

MORGAN AND STRINGER• Congressional Appointments • Army and Public Complaints • Dismissal

THE APPOINTMENT OF "Dr. Samuel Stringer as Director of the Hospital and Chief Physician and Surgeon for the Army in the Northern Department" on September 14, 1775, predated by 31 days the Congressional selection of-

"Dr. John Morgan as Director General and Chief Physician of the Hospitals in the room [place] of Dr. Benj. Church."

This priority of Stringer's commission and the entire absence of any resolution defining the relative position and authority of these two men furnished an excuse for a constant controversy that was a factor in the cause for the removal of both officers from the service. Stringer's efforts were not so much directed at supplanting Morgan as they were at creating a Northern Department to operate independently, while Dr. Morgan's endeavor was to confirm Dr. Stringer in a subordinate relationship to himself for the good of the service, either through additional legislation by Congress or by means of an order from the Commander-in-Chief. General Washington very definitely recognized Dr. Morgan's authority over all the hospital departments of the Army, as is shown by his referring Dr. Stringer's frequent appeals to the Director General for his attention. In the absence of clarity of wording in the official appointments and resolutions, General Washington quite properly did not feel justified in interpreting Congress' intent, so Dr. Stringer received no rebuke or intimation of his precarious position until he was surprised by an official notice of his dismissal. The Journal of Congress for April 29, 1776, registers the receipt of a petition from Dr. Jonathan Potts of Reading, Pa., asking for an appointment with the Northern Army, and this communication, now among the manuscripts of the Library of Congress, reads:

"To the Honorable, the Delegates of the United Colonies in Congress assembled:

"The Petition of Jonathan Potts, Doctor in Physick, sheweth that upon an application lately made on behalf of your Petitioner to be appointed Director of the Hospital intended to be erected for the Army in the Middle Department, your Petitioner was encouraged by many Members of Your Honorable House to hope for such an appointment as soon as it should be found necessary to form such an Establishment but that by the Movements of the Army since that time it appears the Hospital under the Direction of Doctor Morgan will be placed in the Middle Department and your Petitioner is informed it will be necessary to establish one in Canada.

"He therefore Prays he may be appointed Director of the Hospital there and hopes by a constant and faithful discharge of the Trust reposed in him, he will merit the approbation of this Honorable House and he will Pray.

Jonathan Potts.

Philadelphia, April 29, 1776."

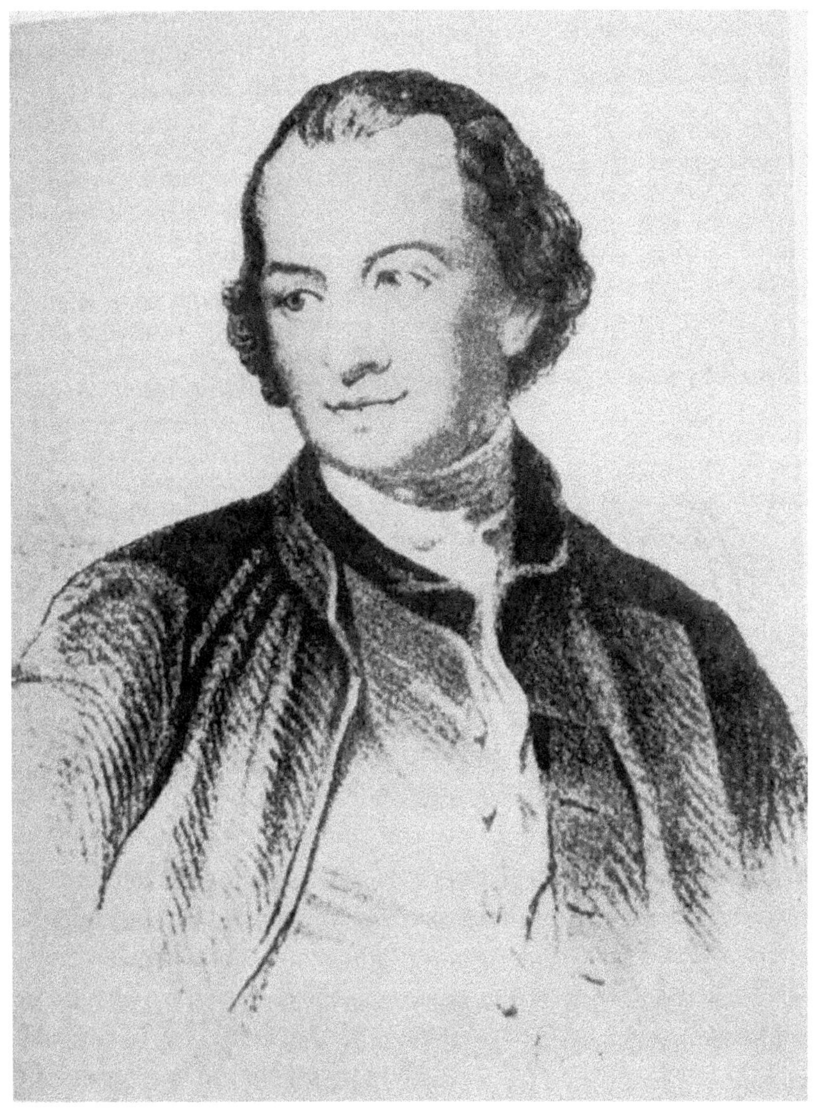

JOHN MORGAN

Director General of the military Hospitals and chief physician of the Continental Army, 1775-1777.

Pott's request for employment in the hospital service was promptly granted, for Congress resolved:

"That Dr. Potts be taken into the Pay of the Continent and be employed in the Canadian Department or at Lake George as General Schuyler shall think fit. But that this recommendation be not considered so as to supersede Dr. Stringer."

Dr. Potts did not set out for his appointed post until June 27, 1776, two months after his commission was received, and he then accompanied General Gates, who had been ordered to take command of the Northern Army. Dr. John Morgan's letter of July 28, 1776, addressed to Dr. Potts at Fort George, contains some instructions and advice that are worth recording:

"Sir:

"Herewith I send you the Resolution of Congress of July 17, of which you will please to take due notice, and in conformity thereto, you will be pleased to call upon the Regimental Surgeons within the immediate Department for an account of what Medicines & Instruments are in their possession and transmit to me, together with an exact return of the Number and Names of the Surgeons and Mates and other Officers in the Hospitals under you & their pay & an account of the Furniture & Expense of the Hospital; these Returns you are to repeat Monthly; the First Day of every Month that I may make reports thereof to Congress and the Commander in Chief when required. At your particular Desire and knowing how useful he may be to you. I hope you will find such an appointment particularly useful as it depends upon yourself to supply Medicines not only to your Hospital but to the Regi. Surgeons with you. It is experience in these matters that may stand you in great stead. Nay, without such a one I know not how you could either procure sufficient Medicine for your Department or dispense them when got.

"I have given a Warrant to Dr. McHenry, as a Surgeon under you, to take his orders from you. He has obtained Liberty to go to Phila. for a week & intends, by virtue of a letter he received from you, to bring you some Mates & to apply to Congress for some Medicines for you. I have also given a Warrant to Mr. Andrew Craigie to act as an Apothecary under you & to receive his Commands from you.

"Let me give you a piece of advice or hint that may be useful to you, which is to make it a part of the Duty of the Mates to assist the Apothecary in making up and dispensing Medicines. I call all mine 'Hospital Mates' & not merely 'Surgeon Mates' because I will not suffer names to mislead or allow any of them to refuse that Duty under a notion that they are 'Surgeon Mates' and that it is no part of their Duty to assist the Apothecary, who to all intents is to be looked on in Rank as well as pay in the light of a Surgeon and respected accordingly and he is capable he should in return do part of the Surgeon's Duty. If another piece of advice permit me to give you. Pay your officers regularly once a month & settle all your accounts monthly; let none remain beyond that period unpaid if you can help it. Any assistance or advice I can give, command freely.

"Before I conclude, I must tell you Mr. Craigie has leave of absence for about 11 days and will then join you. Pray make my best compliments to the Gen'l and all my Friends. I wish you all a happy and successful Campaign. I am,

Your affect.

Humble Servant

John Morgan"

A copy of the Act of Congress of July 17, 1776, regarding a Medical Departmental reorganization signed by Robert Harrison, Secretary, and attested by John Morgan, accompanied this letter.

Shortly after Dr. Morgan's communication was received, Dr. Potts was left in charge of the Northern Hospital Department while Dr. Stringer journeyed to confer with the Commander-in-Chief and his friends in Congress. Dr. Potts, in a letter to Dr. Morgan, tells of several hospital problems and, it might be inferred, of some dissatisfaction with the wording of his appointment by Congress.

"Fort George-Aug. 10, 1776.

"Dear Sir:

"I expected long ere this to have had Dr. McHenry at this Post with the Medicines I mentioned to you were to come from Phila., but have been greatly disappointed by his non-arrival; what has prevented him I know not; in a letter this day received from him he informs me he was then to set out from Phila, in order to procure those Medicines & some Mates and mentions your kind intention of assisting him both with advice and a supply of the Cartex,

"The distressed situation of the sick here is not to be described; without clothing, without bedding or a shelter sufficient to screen them from the weather.

"I am sure your known Humanity will be affected when I tell you we have at present upwards of one thousand sick crowded into Sheds & laboring under the various and cruel Disorders of Dysenteries, Bilious Putrid Fevers and the effects of a Confluent Smallpox, to attend this large number we have Four Seniors and Four Mates, exclusive of myself, and our little Shop does not afford a grain of Jalap, Ipecac, Bark, Salt, Opium and Sundry other Capital Articles and nothing of the kind to be had in this Quarter; in this Dilemma our inventions are exhausted for substitutes, but, we shall go on doing the best we can in hopes of speedy supply.

"Dr. Stringer left this place some few days since in order to lay this situation of the Hospital before his Excellency, General Washington & endeavor to procure relief.

"You may remember, Sir, when I left New York that I mentioned to you though the Resolution of Congress did not expressly say I was to be Director General of the Dept., yet I apprehended it was the intention of that Honorable Body, agreeable to my petition previous to my appointment, that I should act as such in Canada, but, on this side of that Province, I was not to supersede Dr. Stringer; as I have had since, the pleasure of Dr. Stringer's acquaintance and have been made acquainted by him of the nature of his appointment and have received those Resolutions of Congress made in his favor, I find he has full power to act as Director General of the Hospital for the Northern Department, which I knew not before; yet I shall still continue to act, as Director, under him until the matter is otherwise settled. I can assure you Dr. Stringer's conduct here and the great regard I have conceived for him from my short acquaintance influenced me in the wish we may be continued as at present, and more especially as I hope our army will be blessed with success and shall once more regain Canada when it will undoubtedly be necessary to have the two Hospitals in this wide extended Country. "I hope ere this reaches you, the line by which the different Departments are to act will be fixed. Dr. Stringer and myself have had some conversation respecting the expediency of acting under a Director Gen'l, of the whole; continuing thus, the Doctor was averse and mentioned some reasons which had weight with me: as you will see the Doctor need not take up your time by mentioning them for my part I am resolved to be governed by such regulations as our wise Congress shall think proper, wishing nothing more than to contribute my mite toward the relief of our Distressed County and assure the Glorious

Independent States of America, Pray present my most Respectful Compliments to His Excellency, General Washington, and General Mifflin and believe me to be,

"Dear Sir, your affect. & Most humble Servant

Jonathan Potts."

Congress was in session in Philadelphia when Stringer arrived with the double purpose of obtaining hospital supplies and of strength ening his official position and authority over his Department. The Journal of Congress of August 16, 1776, records the receipt of a petition regarding the matter from Dr. Stringer, which was referred to the Medical Committee of the House, and on the following day Dr. Stringer wrote Dr. Potts:

"Phila. 17 Aug., 1776.

"Dear Sir:

"Upon my arrival in New York, I found Morgan, after receipt of my letter, had procured a Resolve of Congress confirming his Superiority over the Department I am in & in consequence had sent me his instructions, and on my arrival here found he had procured the Resolve by virtue of a Petition: my objections were heard on the occasion & had my prior claim been attended to, he would not have succeeded; it was done inadvertently, as they told me. I have given in a Petition to support my claim and am told, by one of the Committee to whom it was referred, that Morgan is to have no power over me now to appoint my Surgeons or Mates & that I am, in no shape, to be controlled by him, only that for the sake of ease, in settling the Accounts & the convenience of the Commander in Chief knowing the State of the Army, I am to make a Monthly Return to Morgan, or rather through him, to the General in Chief & my Accounts are to be transmitted to him to be given in together, with his, to Congress. However disagreeable this still is, yet it is not so much as at first, & I am not determined whether I shall continue in the Service or not; my principal Friend here is Mr. Philip Livingston; when the Report is given in I shall consult his opinion respecting a Resig nation. "I delivered your letter to Mr. Hancock, which, if I recollect right, was also left to the same Committee that my affair is & by the same Member am told your appointment was nothing more than a First Surgeon & Physician your Friends, Mr. Miffin & Mr. Biddle, are both in the Service and at Camp. I have an order for Medicines which will begin to be packed the day after Tomorrow only, when you'll receive them. God knows I shall, however, wait for them. There went a box from Morgan for me, under the care of the Surgeon of Col. Wayne Regt. which he must have taken immediately. There will also arrive another box under the care of Doctor McHenry containing only articles, of which there is but 30 lbs. Bark and I think not a Purgative except some few pounds of Rhubarb and a little Fol Scord.

"I have just received yours of the 9th inst. & find the sick increase. You may be sure I am in great agitation. We expect, daily, to hear of the attack at York (N.Y.). Burgoyne, it seems, is run back again to Quebec-Men are crowding very fast to oppose Howe. God grant them the desired success.

"My sincere regard to all our Gentlemen.

I remain yours truly,

Samuel Stringer."

This letter has an unusual closing salutation for Colonial times, and in its form of "I remain yours truly," seems almost intentionally offensive in an age when "Your Obedient and Most Humble Servant" was the correct and courteous phrase. The Medical Committee to whom Dr. Stringer's communication was referred brought in their report on August 20, 1776, and Congress "Resolved, that Dr. Morgan was appointed Director General and Physician in Chief of the American Hospital; that Dr.

Stringer was appointed Director of the Hospital in the Northern Department only."

"That every Director of a Hospital possesses the exclusive right of appointing Surgeons and Hospital Officers of all kinds, agreeable to the Resolutions of Congress of the 17th of July in his own Department unless otherwise directed by Congress."

This Congressional ruling was not sufficiently clear or comprehensive to define the official relations between the two men and really only settled one question: that of authority over appointments. Stringer's immediate action following the congressional resolution was a refusal to recognize or confirm some of the Northern Army Hospital assignments made by Dr. Morgan in response to Stringer's own appeal to General Washington for much-needed medical men. Dr. McHenry, who we have seen, was appointed Dr. Potts' assistant by Dr. Morgan and directed to proceed to Philadelphia and purchase supplies for the Northern Hospital Department, was promptly dismissed by Stringer and on the day following Dr. McHenry wrote to Dr. Potts:

"Sir:

"A turn in affairs renders my coming any further altogether uncertain. My Commission for your Department, made out by Dr. Morgan, is considered as idle & nugatory by Dr. Stringer. He, as Director, will probably have the appointment of Surgeon for his quarters in his own hands. I feel the full force of my disappointment and lament that I cannot join you-except my Commission be recognized by Dr. Stringer; this I have no hope of.

"Who is to pay the expense I incurred in providing the Medicines which you requested me to procure. I know not. I do not blame you. A tissue of misunderstanding and mistake seems to be the fate of your District. May they soon end. And may you meet every form of success in your Department.

With Compliments to Dr. Brown, I am, Dear Sir,

Your Most Obt. Humble Servant

James McHenry. New York, 21 Aug. 1776"

Yet at the same time that Dr. Stringer was planning this vindictive and unjust action, he wrote Dr. Potts:

"Surgeons and Mates are hard to get: 1 doubt if any [can be had]."

Dr. McHenry immediately laid his situation before Congress, resulting in its declaration-

"That Congress have a proper sense of the Merit and Service of Dr. McHenry and Recommend it to the Directors of the Different Hospitals, belonging to the United States, to appoint Dr. McHenry to the First Vacancy that shall happen of a Surgeon's Berth in any of the said Hospitals."

Dr. Benjamin Rush sent a copy of this action to Dr. McHenry with the following letter:

"Dear Sir:

"The above Resolution of Congress does you as much Honor as if they had made you a Director of a Hospital.

"I need not hint to you after this, how unjust it will be in you to desert the Service, especially at this present juncture.

You will please furnish Dr. Morgan, Dr. Stringer, and the other Directors of the Hospitals of the States with a copy of the above Resolution. If there is at present a Vacancy in any of their Departments, you are authorized to demand a Warrant for it. "Wishing you much Health, Honor and Happiness, I am, with great.

Regards,

"Your most affectionate

"Humble Servant

"B. Rush."

Among the Potts papers in the Pennsylvania Historical Society is a letter from Dr. McHenry expressing chagrin over his dismissal and making a very reasonable request, though the epistle does not show to whom it was addressed:

"Sir: "The Congress, taking into consideration my peculiar disappointment from the new disposition of Directors, have obliged me with a Resolution in my favor, a copy of which I enclose. I would only beg leave to inform you that the Warrant for your District made out by Dr. Morgan bears date the 24th of July, 1776; that under that sanction, I took a journey to Phila. to procure some Medicine which Dr. Potts had written to me concerning but that I do not look for the expenses to be paid without you have it in your power to do it out of the Public Money. All in short, I expect is that my Commission from you will be of the same date as Dr. Morgan's. I shall wait your answer at Headquarters in Kingsbridge. I shall be glad to execute any of your Commands and am.

Sir, Respectfully your most obt. and humble Servant,

Camp near Kingsbridge

12th Sept. 1776."

Dr. McHenry immediately received an appointment as surgeon of the Fifth Pennsylvania Battalion commanded by Colonel Robert McGaw and was among the American prisoners captured by the British at Fort Washington on November 16, 1776. General Washington appointed McHenry his personal secretary while the Army was encamped at Valley Forge and later, Secretary of War, when he became President. McHenry also served in the same capacity in John Adams' cabinet, and Fort McHenry at Baltimore was so named in his honor.

Dr. Stringer's inexcusably long absence from his hospital post so aroused General Gates' displeasure and anxiety for the condition of his men that he wrote to Egbert Benson under date of August 22, 1776:

"Dear Sir:

"The 29th ult. I granted Dr. Stringer, at his earnest request a, permission to go to New York with all expedition to procure Medicine for the General Hospital and Army in the distance returning to his butylene promise he would not delay an instant in Predicinal Stores so much wanted, and which the Troops here are almost ready to mutiny to obtain. I am this day informed that Dr. Stringer, instead of fulfilling his promises and returning with all dispatch to his Duty, is gone Preferment Hunting to the Congress at Phila, while the Troops here are suffering inexpressible distress for want of Medicine "I entreat you, Sir, you will instantly lay this letter before General Washington and receive his Commands for sending a supply of Medcines to Dr. Potts at Lake George. Many of the Regiment Surgeons have not had any Medicines nor cannot be long answerable for the consequence of the shameful neglect of the Army in this

Department. "The U. S. expects the same good service from these Troops here as everywhere else. This they cannot have unless they command the same attention as is paid the health of their Soldiers elsewhere.

"I am Dear Sir, your aff. humble Servant,

"HORATIO GATES"

"P.S. Copy to Dr. John Morgan, D. G. of the Hospital!"

The sending of a copy of this letter to the Director Genenl, who had been deprived of authority over the Northern Medical Department, carried the inference that General Gates believed Dr. Morgan to be in some measure responsible for conditions. Its receipt must have aroused a feeling of indignation against Dr. Stringer, as well as of regret that the indefinite wording of the Congressional ruling deprived the recipient of a right to apply disciplinary measures.

"There was little Morgan could do to improve conditions in the North, but this was not understood in the Army or by the public. Indignant complaints and bitterness against Director General Morgan were expressed throughout the country, and finally, the demand was loud and angry that he be relieved of his commission. Yet as early as August 13, 1776, Morgan endeavored to clear up the hospital difficulties through an official action of Congress, for on that date, he wrote its President:

"Sir:

"Sensible of the value of your time, I should not now encroach upon it were it not that some further regulation of Congress is necessary, or at least some explication of those already formed respecting the appointments and subordination of Officers in the General Hospital... "If I have exceeded my Commission, it has been for want of knowing the design and resolve of Congress or their being misunderstood. Should the Congress on that footing annul my appointments and make others, I must at least stand acquitted of intentionally going beyond the line of duty, and it will behoove Congress to be more explicit in respect of its intentions, for if the Congress does not suppose the appointments of any new Surgeons rests with me, of what use is it to recommend one to me for my approbation?

"Be that as it may, wherever the path of duty is plain, I shall endeavor to walk steadily in it, having no design or inclination to exceed those bounds which the good of the service or the wisdom of Congress may present to me."

And so the difficulties and troubles of Morgan and Stringer accumulated. Congress was greatly overworked, much worried and irritated. Members of Congress were receiving frequent complaints and constant protests from the officers and soldiers of their Colonies. The problems of the hospitals might have been solved, and Morgan's recognized ability as an able executive retained in the service had Congress taken the time and trouble to investigate conditions and pass the required corrective legislation. Some purging and bleeding in the medical organization were inevitable and undoubtedly advisable, but the performance of a major operation insofar as Dr. Morgan was concerned was both cruel and unnecessary. Samuel Adams, writing on January 9, 1777, to John Adams from Baltimore, where Congress was sitting, said:

"Great and heavy complaints have been made of abuses in the Director General's Departments in both our Armies: some, I suppose, without grounds, others with too much reason. I have no doubt, but as soon as a Committee reports, which is expected this day, both Morgan and Stringer will be removed as I think they ought."

To this letter was added a postscript saying:

"Drs. Morgan and Stringer are dismissed without any reason assigned which Congress could of right do as they held their Places during pleasure. The true reason, as I take it, was the general disquiet and the danger of the loss of an Army arising therefrom."

Dr. Morgan did not accept his dismissal from the office of the Director General without a protest and presented a "Vindication" in his own defense accompanied with a demand for an investigation of his official acts and a verdict on the evidence to be submitted. Congress finally granted both requests and, after an inexcusably long delay, exonerated Morgan on all charges, but not before the injustice of their action and disgrace which he felt because of the discharge had embittered his life. It seems strange that Dr. Morgan's resentment should have been mainly directed against an old friend and associate whom he suspected of being the cause of his troubles rather than toward those members of Congress who had openly condemned and judged him without a hearing.

The revenge Morgan sought because of unproved suspicion against Dr. William Shippen, Jr., through a public charge of malpractice in office, was unfortunate in many respects, though it probably brought about many needed reforms in the Medical Department of the Army.

It is the hope that in another chapter, some new evidence may be offered concerning the Rush-Morgan-Shippen controversy that will present Dr. Shippen in a better light than history has conceded him, for while a court-martial officially acquitted him, a tradition has been maintained throughout the years that he was really guilty of the charges made by Doctors Morgan and Rush.

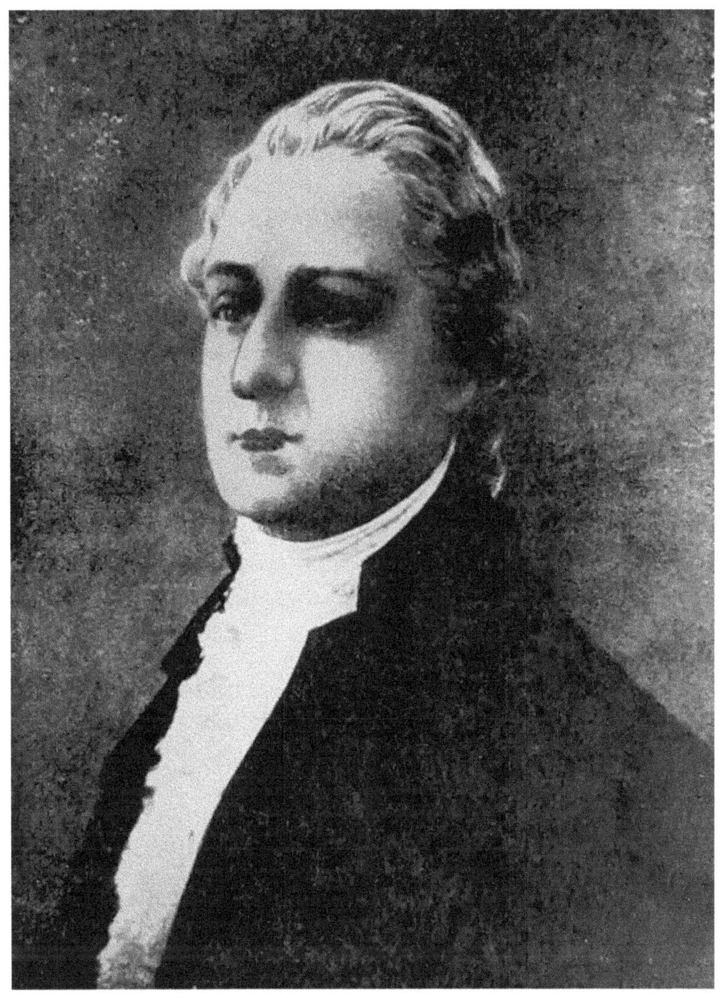

BENJAMIN CHURCH

Director General and Chief Physician of the American Hospital, 1775.

CHAPTER TWELVE

DEPARTMENT FRICTION • Courts of Inquiry Morgan's Reports and Problems • Appeals Dismissal

ON JULY 10, 1775, just seven days after General Washington assumed command of the Army at Cambridge, his Excellency wrote to Richard Henry Lee, a member of Congress:

"We want a hospital upon a proper establishment and a proper Director with good surgeons to take care of and be in charge of it; it therefore rests with Congress to consider the matter. I would not wish to see an expensive one set on foot, and I have no doubt of Dr. Shippen's recommending such gentlemen for surgeons as he can answer the ability of."

Friction among medical men of the New England Army had begun before the Commander-in-Chief's arrival, and on July 21, 1775, he wrote:

"Disputes and contentions have arisen and must continue until it [the Medical Department] is reduced to some system."

Dr. Church, the newly appointed Director General of the Medical Department, assumed command with a difficult task confronting him. Many regimental physicians had established hospitals for their own men and claimed they were not allowed proper or sufficient supplies for their sick. To these charges, Dr. Church replied that regimental hospitals were generally wasteful and, as a rule, unnecessary, for when a soldier was too ill to be properly cared for in the camp, he should be sent to a neighboring Continental hospital.

The Massachusetts Provincial Assembly was largely responsible for the discord that existed, for early in May 1775, it approved a report:

"That great uneasiness may arise in the Army by the appointment of Surgeons who may not be agreeable to the officers and soldiers in their respective Regiments; therefore, it was voted to allow the Colonel of each Regiment to nominate the Surgeons for his Regiment. and unless some material objections were made that they be accordingly appointed."

The result of this action was that selections were made among friends and neighbors of men in the ranks. Presuming upon the method of their appointment these physicians ignored or evaded all authority save that of their own regimental officers, who in turn shielded them in every controversy with the Director General. The situation finally became so annoying that General Washington was consulted, and on September 7, 1775, he issued an order reading:

"Repeated complaints being made by the Regimental Surgeons that they are not allowed proper necessities for the use of the sick before they become fit subjects for the General Hospital and the Director General of the Hospital complains that contrary to the rule of every established Army these Regimental Hospitals are more expensive than can be conceived, which plainly indicates that there is an unpardonable abuse on one side or an inexcusable neglect on the other. And whereas the General is exceeding desirous of having the utmost care taken of the sick wherever placed and in every stage of their disorders, he is at the same time determined not to suffer any imposition upon the public. He requires and orders that the Brigadier Generals, with the Commanding officers of each regiment in the Brigade do, sit as a Court of Inquiry into the causes of these complaints and that they summon the Director General of the Hospitals and the several Regimental Surgeons before them and have the whole matter thoroughly investigated and reported. When a soldier is so sick that it is no longer safe or proper for him to remain in Camp, he should be sent to the General Hospital. There is no need of a Regimental Hospital within the Camp when there is a General Hospital so near and so well equipped."

Brigade courts of inquiry were immediately organized under Generals Thomas, Spencer, Heath, Sullivan, and Greene, and apparently, Dr. Church was well satisfied with the outcome of the hearings, for under date of September 14, 1775, he wrote a letter in the third person, to one of the Brigadiers which reads:

"Dr. Church presents his most respectful compliments to General Sullivan and most heartily felicitates himself on receiving so honoring a testimonial of Gen'l. Sullivan's approbation as he met with last evening at Headquarters.

"The Doctor esteems himself peculiarly happy that the undeserved prejudice against him is so totally removed which from frequent intimations he was apprehensive had possessed the General's mind. He flatters himself that his whole conduct will bear the strictest scrutiny. A regard for place, popularity or the more detestable motive of avarice never influenced his conduct in Public Life. The sole object of his pursuit, the first wish of his heart, was ever the salvation of his country."

These were strong sentiments coming from a man who, even then, was in treasonable correspondence with his country's enemy. Dr. Church's removal by Congress from his post of Director General followed soon and occurred at a time of great confusion in the hospital organization and irritation among the medical men of the Army. Congress was urged to promptly fill the vacant office, and on October 17, 1775:

"Dr. John Morgan of Phila. was elected Director General and Chief Physician of the Hospitals of Massachusetts Bay."

Circumstantial evidence indicates that Dr. William Shippen not only refused this appointment but recommended Dr. Morgan for the position; this, however, will be presented later. That General Washington had a preference for Dr. Shippen for the post may be inferred from a postscript he added to a letter to Richard Henry Lee, saying:

"Tell Dr. Shippen that I was in hopes his business would have permitted him to come here as Director of the Hospital."

Dr. Morgan apparently did not report for duty as promptly as he might, for a full month after the election of the new director, General Washington wrote:

"Dr. Morgan is exceedingly wanted at this place and ought not to delay a moment as many regulations are being delayed and acts postponed till his arrival."

Immediately upon reaching camp, Dr. Morgan made an inspection of the hospital and medical organization and, in a report to General Washington, said:

"On my arrival at Cambridge, I set about to establish rules for the general Hospital Surgeons. I had heard of many abuses being practiced by enormous drafts of expensive stores from the General Hospital to which... I put a stop and Imited the demands of to such articles as Regimental Surgeons Indian meal, oatmeal, rice, barley, molasses and the like: I required that such sick as wanted other [supplies] should be sent to the General Hospital that these things might be delivered out under my own directions. The next information I attempted was to call upon all the mates in the Hospital to undergo an examination of their abilities in order to select from their number those that were best qualified for the service. This was followed by your Excellency's orders to see that all regimental surgeons and mates should have a like examination. I began the task, but the movements of the Army, the aversion of the surgeons to undergo their examinations, from which they were often screened by their Colonels, and the increasing business on hand prevented my proceeding far in it."

Morgan's problems and the resistance to his authority were even greater than those encountered by his predecessor. Departmental disputes had increased and resentment even arose over hospital surgeons outranking those of the line. The efforts to correct the troubles were further complicated through the complaints and appeals made directly to the Colonial delegates by regimental surgeons and staff. Many members of the Continental Congress became violent partisans in petty issues involved, losing sight of or ignoring the important problems to be solved. The entire medical policy of the Army became a subject of such controversy that some Colonies intimated they would not send any more troops into service until the care of the sick was better organized.

Morgan's problems were complicated. Their solution required the reconciliation of existing differences, establishing cooperation and discipline in and among different medical department branches, and obtaining authority to purchase much-needed hospital equipment and supplies. Congress was greatly to blame for the difficulties and confusion that existed, for it had not officially granted the Director General the necessary authority to cope with the issues and apparently had no real appreciation of the needs of a medical department.

The rate of pay for surgeons, etc., was so low as to make it difficult for members of the profession to engage in army service and maintain their families at home. In addition, hospital paydays were uncertain and often far apart. Besides, no adequate appropriation had ever been made by Congress for medicines and hospital stores. The Army's daily or monthly need for equipment and sustenance could be fairly well calculated and anticipated, but the requirements of the hospitals depended on and varied with the number of sick and wounded soldiers. So, without a proper margin of supplies in reserve, the Medical Department was often short of actual necessities and even entirely without essential articles.

Most of the charges of neglect and inhumanity lodged against Morgan in 1775-6 and later involving Shippen could rightfully have been filed against Congress. Official letters exist, written as late as 1779, when Congress had more experience, reciting that Dr. Potts, Purveyor General, had requested certain specified sums for the hospitals but that the amount requested was denied for the reason he had previously been allowed large sums for that department. Apparently, the question of whether the hospitals really required the supplies the money would purchase did not enter into the question or discussion.

The physicians and surgeons of the hospitals were well aware of the Congressional parsimony and neglect, for they had not only seen their sick and wounded patients suffer as a result, but they themselves had often gone without pay and subsistence allowance for many months. Perhaps the knowledge of Governmental responsibility for the lack of hospital necessities was one of the reasons why many medical men, quoted by Morgan and Rush as complaining against Shippen and expected to give evidence to prove charges made, appeared at the court-martial as witnesses for the defense instead of the prosecution.

Of course, the Continental Congress had no experience to guide it in providing for hospitals and, in its ignorance, had followed the British practice, which, while satisfactory abroad, did not apply to American conditions. Even General Washington, who was always anxious that the sick should have everything needful for their comfort and quick convalescence, showed little understanding of the real amount of money necessary for the hospitals. On December 31, 1775, his estimate to Congress for one whole year was only £6,000, which he wrote would provide hospital maintenance for an army of 15,000 men! True, the care of the sick of the forces in New England was not expensive compared to the requirements when the campaign was transferred to New York, New Jersey, and Pennsylvania, for the Eastern Army was comparatively healthy.

Dr. Benjamin Rush observed that the history of diseases furnished many proofs that a body of men from a given neighborhood might assemble and remain perfectly well, while the introduction of others with different habits into that group would result in much sickness. This was the situation in the New York campaign, which followed the evacuation of Boston when troops from different Colonies were consolidated into one army then made its appearance and became a serious epidemic. Besides caring for the sick, the hospitals were soon obliged to treat the wounded of many engagements which began with the Battle of Long Island. A report of the New York Army in September 1776 showed the number of sick to be 8,528, a full third of the muster roll.

Dr. Morgan was indefatigable in his efforts to properly organize the Medical Department to meet the situation, but resistance came not only from the regimental surgeons but from the commanding officers as well. One colonel stated that if it were in his power, no soldier of his command would be sent to a general hospital. Many of Dr. Morgan's staff were so discouraged that they attempted to resign.

General Washington wrote to Congress on September 24, 1776:

"No less attention should be paid to the choice of surgeons than to other officers of the Army... They should undergo a regular examination, and if not appointed by the director general and surgeons of the hospital, they ought to be subordinate to and governed by his directions.

"The regimental surgeons I am speaking of, many of whom are very great rascals countenancing the men in sham complaints to exempt them from duty and often receiving bribes to certify indispositions with a view to secure discharges or furloughs.

"But independent of these practices, while they (regimental surgeons) are considered as unconnected with the general hospital, there will be nothing but continual complaints of each other, the director of the hospital charging them with enormity in their drafts for the sick, and then for denying such things as are necessary. In short, there is a constant bickering among them, which tends greatly to the injury of the sick and will always subsist till the regimental surgeons are made to look up to the director general of the hospital as a superior. There is a necessity for it, or the sick will suffer.

"The regimental surgeons are aiming, I am persuaded, to break up the general hospital and have in numberless instances drawn for medicines, stores, etc., in the most profuse and extravagant manner for private purposes."

The regimental surgeons also appealed their case to Congress, often aided by their commanding officers, and Dr. Morgan's efforts to obtain a conference with Continental leaders for the purpose of reconciling differences met with no encouragement. General Nathaniel Greene attempted to bring the seriousness of the situation to Congressional notice in a letter reading as follows:

"The sick of the Army, who are under the care of Regimental Surgeons, are in a most wretched condition; the Surgeons being without the least articles of medicine to assist nature in her efforts for the recovery of health. There is no circumstance that strikes a greater damper upon the spirits of the men who are well than the miserable condition the sick are in. They exhibit a spectacle that is shocking to human feelings, and as the knowledge of their distress spreads through the country, it will prove to be an unsurmountable obstacle to recruiting the new army.

"Good policy as well as humanity, in my humble opinion, demands the immediate attention of Congress upon the subject that the evil may be sought out and the grievance redressed.

"The sick of the Army are too numerous to be all accommodated on the contracted plan of the General Hospital. The Director General says he has no authority by his commission to supply the demands of the Regimental sick, and the General Hospital, being too small to accommodate much more than half the remainder, lies without any means of relief than the value of the rations allowed to every soldier. Many hundreds are now in this condition and die daily for want of proper assistance, which means the Army is robbed of many valuable men at a time when reinforcements are so exceedingly necessary.

"Both officers and men join in one general complaint at this evil which has prevailed so long.

"Some measure should be taken to justify the director general or to empower the Commander in Chief to qualify him to furnish the Regimental surgeons, under the direction of the Colonel of the regiment, with such supplies as the state of the sick may demand.

"The Director General complains of the want of medicines and says his stocks are but barely sufficient for the General Hospital. I can see no reason, either from policy or humanity, that the stores for the General Hospital should be preserved for contingencies which may never happen and the present regimental sick left to perish for want of proper necessities. It is wholly immaterial, in my opinion, either to the state or to the Army, whether a man dies in the General or Regimental Hospital."

Shortly after this letter was received, Oliver Wolcott, a member of Congress, wrote:

"The Medical Department will undergo a reform of men, at least if not of measures, that not so much complaint, which I fear has been too well grounded, may be heard respecting the conduct of that department, but after all that can be done, I still fear that the interesting business will go slowly and sorry I am that the late encouragement for that purpose was not earlier made."

The Hospital Department of the Revolutionary Forces had definitely broken down, and Congress was irritated by the many complaints that were received. A reorganization was absolutely necessary, but this also applied to every other division of the Army, so Dr. Morgan was sacrificed to satisfy a popular protest.

Morgan's tireless energy, his solicitude for the sick and wounded soldiers, his efforts to organize the medical departments into a cooperating entity and his attempts to obtain authority and help were all forgotten.

By comparison, the Medical Department was as well managed as other divisions of the Army, but public clamor had to be appeased, and Dr. Morgan was dismissed without a hearing and even without a considerate notice or expression of regret

CHAPTER THIRTEEN

HOSPITAL REORGANIZATION • Army's Despondency Shippen-Washington • Correspondence Hospital Districts

THE EXPANSION OF THE Medical Department of the Continental Army started with American campaign activities in and around New York before General Washington began his precipitous New Jersey retreat. Emergency hospitals had already been established on the west side of the Hudson River, and when the American troops retired and occasionally halted to fight or rest, the sick and wounded soldiers were hurriedly sent on ahead. Thus, temporary hospitals became necessary at Hackensack, Amboy, Fort Lee, Newark, Elizabethtown, Morristown, Brunswick, and Trenton. When General Washington eventually crossed the Delaware River on December 8, 1776, with a depleted force, his command's sick and wounded men were distributed among more permanent hospitals, then established in Easton, Allentown, Bethlehem, and Philadelphia. The additional discomforts that these poor creatures endured by reason of frequent transfer from one place to another, defy description.

Dr. Shippen accompanied the larger number of his patients from the Morristown hospital to Bethlehem and neighboring Pennsylvania towns, while Dr. Morgan assumed the direction of those diverted to Philadelphia. An old hospital account book, with a record of pay for nurses who served in the Philadelphia Bettering House, furnished the proof that Bodo Otto had been given charge of this commandeered hospital, located in the square bounded by 11th,12th, Spruce and Pine Streets. A number of Philadelphia gentlemen were appointed to cooperate with Army officers in the distribution and care of distressed soldiers who were arriving daily. Authorized to take possession of empty houses, stores or any other buildings suitable for hospital purposes, this committee secured the Sneider, Shields and Carpenter residences, the Elroy, Semples, and Sproat stores and some accommodations in the Pennsylvania Hospital and the smallpox pesthouse.

The authorities had not anticipated the many necessary supplies required for these hospital patients, so patriotic people of the city were importuned to furnish the much-needed articles. Many of these unfortunate soldiers died during the winter of 1776-77, and it has been written that two thousand of them were buried in the Philadelphia potter's field.

When General Washington crossed the Delaware at Trenton, the British Army was close behind but was prevented from following by a lack of necessary ferryboats and the fear of having a river at their rear.

The American situation was then desperate, for the Continental Army had melted away during the New Jersey retreat, and it was debatable whether sufficient numbers remained to defend Philadelphia should the British succeed in passing over the Delaware. Congress hastily removed its headquarters from Philadelphia to Baltimore, and all Government papers and supplies were transferred to places of greater safety. Dr. Benjamin Rush afterwards wrote in his journal:

"Nothing but the signing of the Declaration of Independence preserved the Congress from a dissolution in December 1776, when Howe marched to the Delaware."

The British commanding officers were well aware of the existing fears and despondency that prevailed through Tory sympathizers. This opportune time was then chosen by the English authorities to publish an offer of a full pardon to all former American subjects of the King who would admit their mistake, agree to lay down their arms and cease resistance. Many took advantage of this proffer, and among them was Col. Charles Read of Burlington, New Jersey, commander of a regiment in the Flying Camp, of which Bodo Otto's son, Bodo Junior, had been appointed Surgeon by the New Jersey

Assembly. Colonel Read's yielding to the British appeal has never been understood, for all his previous activities had manifested a conspicuous sympathy with the American cause. His acceptance of an English pardon can only be considered indicative of the general discouragement that then prevailed. Some American troops soon apprehended Colonel Read, and Christopher Marshall wrote in his diary:

"Phila., Jan. 21st, 1777. "It is said that several more Tories were brought in this day from the Jersey; among them is Col. Charles Read."

During this time of uncertainty in Philadelphia, Dr. Jonathan Potts arrived in Pennsylvania from his Northern post to visit his family, and to him, the Philadelphia Committee of Safety wrote on December 5, 1776:

"Sir:

"The Council requests your aid and assistance with other physicians, in taking care of and administering to the relief of the sick, returning from the Army; to see they have proper quarters, medicines and provisions, and that they be furnished with every necessity for their relief."

This communication to Dr. Potts was immediately followed by another, saying:

"You are requested to remove all the sick soldiers to Potts Grove or some other place of security, for which purpose you are to procure wagons and every other necessity."

Before the order could be put into execution, another was issued, changing the destination of the patients. This may have been because of a realization that a very large number of the sick and wounded soldiers were already quartered on the inhabitants of Pennsylvania and that the Philadelphia patients had better be sent southward. The information regarding this change was found in a letter to Dr. Potts from Dr. Morgan.

"Order Dr. Tillotson and the Mates you have employed in this service to take a list of all the sick of the Army now in Philadelphia, distinguishing those of the Flying Camp belonging to Maryland from those of the standing Army-the former to be removed to that part of Maryland you think most proper, and where they can be best accommodated in every respect. Let no necessary expense for nurse attendants and refreshments be spared or for procuring sufficient covering or warm lodgings.

"If the sick can be well accommodated at Wilmington, Newport or Christeen, free from danger from the enemy, ny, seek quarters for them in those and other neighboring villages. Committees of Safety ought always to be applied for their safety and assistance. If a place thought to be safe becomes afterwards exposed to the enemy, let the sick be expeditiously removed to places of greater security. Apply to the Asst. Quarter Master and Commissaries of Supplies for whatever is needful.

"For the sick now in Philadelphia that cannot be removed without endangering their lives, in case the enemy should take possession of the City, I have appealed to the humanity of the gentlemen of the faculty, who do not propose to leave and who may be solicited by the inhabitants, to extend their charitable care till the charge is superseded by order of the gentlemen of the British Hospital. Wherefore, let a list of them be made out and delivered to Dr. Clarkson.

"With a view to preserving the drugs, medicines and other hospital stores and furniture belonging to the American Army, I have had all I could not transfer to Bethlehem and Newton by land carriage, shipped to Christeen. Remove from thence, if needful, to the head of Elk or to Elk Ridge landing in Baltimore County or to the Town of Baltimore, as emergency requires."

Meanwhile, Dr. Shippen had settled his patients and established headquarters in Bethlehem, Pennsylvania, a place destined to be associated with many of the shortcomings in the Continental Medical Department. Here the Doctor was joined by his family on December 12, 1776, and there they remained until the following March, when the Bethlehem hospital was closed.

When the medical authorities took possession of the Brethren House of the Moravian Order on December 3, 1776, it was obvious that the entire 2,000 patients expected from Morristown could not all be sheltered in Bethlehem without completely disrupting the peaceful communal life of the village and turning the citizens out of their homes, so, many of the soldiers were diverted to neighboring towns.

While all loyal Americans were willing to make sacrifices and help any unfortunate victims of the war, the prospect of having a hospital established in any quarter where suitable buildings existed was the constant dread of every community, not so much on account of the inconveniences that resulted, as because contagious hospital diseases invariably spread and took their toll from among the peaceful citizens. It was in December of 1776 that a committeeman of the town of Reading vaguely wrote and expressed a hope they might be spared that catastrophe.

"We have heard that a hospital is to be made at this place. Strange this, when we have no unoccupied houses in town, for many families have come hither from Philadelphia."

On December 17, 1776, Dr. Shippen wrote of his hospital conditions and enumerated the troops assembled thereabouts to reinforce General Washington's Army, then encamped on the west side of the Delaware River:

"After much difficulty and expense, I have removed all the sick to Easton, Bethlehem and Allentown.

"There is no paymaster or General near us, and I am almost out of cash. I must, therefore, beg the favor of you to procure me 5,000 dollars and send them by the bearer, Dr. Halling, for the use of the hospitals...

"I saw about 4,000 of General Lee's troops this morning, marching from Easton, about two days [distance] from General Washington; all were in good spirits and much pleased with their General Sullivan. General Gates, with 900 men, marches from this place this afternoon and tomorrow. We hear that General Heath is within four days' march, with 3,000 men.

"God send that all who joined may save Philadelphia and disappoint the cursed Tories this winter."

The Christmas night surprise attack on the Hessian garrison at Trenton and the following successful engagement with the British at Princeton compelled the enemy to make a hurried retreat toward the Hudson for the protection of their base camp and supplies.

General Washington's Army closely followed the British troops, and on January 6, 1777, established a permanent encampment at Morristown. Then, some of the old New Jersey emergency hospitals were reopened, and new ones were organized for the better convenience of the Army.

There were very few Americans wounded at Trenton but many at Princeton, so a hospital was organized there in Nassau Hall of the College. The Hessians at Trenton were not so fortunate as the Continentals, for they lost 17 killed, 78 wounded and surrendered, 84 officers, 25 musicians, and 759 enlisted men. The wounded foes were immediately paroled and hospital facilities under their own surgeons were furnished them. Proof of this is contained in a letter from one of the Continental Hospital officers to Dr. Potts:

"The amputating instruments which you sent for the use of the Hessian Surgeon were taken away yesterday by Mr. Wood, and I am told by the former that they were so bad that he could not make use of them had they been left. There are four or five men here who must soon submit to an operation or lose their lives. I therefore beg you to send a complete set."

Among the Hessian wounded soldiers was a young officer who finally became a patient of Dr. Otto in the Old Barracks. Included with the family's cherished relics is a "German Improved Song Book for use in public worship as well as private edification," with this inscription on the flyleaf:

"Lieutenant George Saltzmann gave this book to John A. Otto as a present on the 18th of July 1777, at Trenton."

A German sword also figures among the treasures of the war, and the tradition is that this, too, was presented to Dr. Bodo Otto by this same unfortunate victim of the conflict, in which his services had been bartered by his sovereign for gold. Possibly Lieutenant Saltzmann belonged to some Brunswick troops and came from the section of Germany where the Otto family had lived, so sympathy and friendship had resulted.

News came to America in June 1776 of George III's contracting for an army of mercenaries to fight against the Colonists. This naturally aroused a feeling of anger and resentment, and when it was followed later in the year by a British effort to induce Continental soldiers to renounce the American cause, lay down their arms and accept an English pardon with a reward for so doing, the United States Congress decided to retaliate.

The Journal of Congress records the first action taken on August 9, 1776:

"Resolved that a Committee of three be appointed to devise a plan for encouraging the Hessians and the other foreigners employed by the King of Great Britain and sent to America for the purpose of subjugating these States, to quit that iniquitous service.

"The members chosen were Mr. James Wilson, Mr. Thomas Jefferson, and Mr. Richard Stockton."

On August 14, 1776, the minutes read:

"The Committee appointed to devise a plan for encouraging the Hessians and other foreigners to quit the British Service brought in a report which was taken into consideration; whereupon, the Congress came to the following resolution:

"Whereas, it has been the wise policy of the States, to extend the protection of the laws to all those who should settle among them, of whatever nation or religion they might be, and to admit them to participation in the benefits of civil and religious freedom;

and, the benevolence of this practice as well as its salutary effects, have rendered it worthy of being continued in future times.

"And whereas, his Britannic Majesty, in order to destroy our freedom and happiness, has commenced against us, a cruel and unprovoked war; and, unable to engage Britons sufficient to execute his sanguinary measure, has applied to certain foreign Princes who are in the habit of selling the blood of their people for money, and from them has procured and transported hither, considerable numbers of foreigners.

"And it is conceived that such foreigners, if apprised of the practice of these States, would choose to accept of land, liberty, safety and communion of good laws and mild government, in a country where many of their friends and relations are already happily settled, rather than continue to be exposed to the toil and dangers of a long and bloody war, waged against a people guilty of no other crime than that of refusing to exchange freedom for slavery; and that they will do this the more especially when they reflect, that after they shall have violated every Christian and moral precept, by invading and attempting to destroy those who have never injured them or their country, their only reward, if they escape death and captivity, will be a return to the despotism of their Prince, to be by him again sold to do the drudgery of some other enemy to the rights of mankind.

"And whereas, the Parliament of Great Britain has thought fit by a late act, not merely to invite our troops to desert our service, but to direct a compulsion of our people taken at sea, to serve against their country.

"Resolved, Therefore, that these States will receive all such foreigners who shall leave the Armies of his Britannic Majesty, in America, and shall choose to become members of any of these States; that they shall be protected in the free exercise of their respective religion, and be invested with the rights, privileges and immunities of natives as established by the lawright privileges and, moreover, that the Congress will provide for every such person, 50 acres of unappropriated land in some of these States, to be held by him and his heirs in absolute property.

"Resolved: That the foregoing resolution be committed to the Committee who brought in the report and that they be directed to have it translated into German and to take proper measures to have it communicated to the foreign troops.

"In the meanwhile, that this be kept secret."

Various methods were adopted to circulate American propaganda among the foreign mercenaries. Patriotic citizens of German birth visited different Hessian camps for one excuse or another and told stories of opportunities in the new republic. German translations of the Congressional resolutions were packed with tobacco and put in canoes that were set adrift in tides calculated to carry them to the enemy's camp. Haym Salomon, who later became Robert Morris' trusty assistant in financing the Revolution, was one of those who were helpful in persuading Hessians to quit the British service. Salomen's opportunity came through being engaged by the British in New York to act as a German interpreter. Dr. Benjamin Rush informed Congress of a request from a German-born American citizen for authority to attempt a visit to the Hessian camp, in a belief that he could return with 200 deserters. The real chance to convince the Hessians of opportunities that were present in America came when a large number were captured at Trenton.

Christopher Ludwig, 'the Director of Baking for the Army of the United States,' then said to the Commander-in-Chief:

"Parole and turn them over to me! I'll march them to Philadelphia and show them the fine churches and people, farms and barns, where they eat beef every day, and I'll say to them:

"Now you know the difference between a German slave and an American freeman."

The Philadelphia Committee of Safety also realized the potential advantages that might result and wrote to General Washington:

"December 28th, 1776.

"We cannot avoid mentioning that we don't think it advisable to exchange your Hessian prisoners at this time. We think their capture affords a favorable opportunity of making them acquainted with the selection and circumstances of many of their countrymen, who came here without a far farthing of property and have by care and industry acquired plentiful fortunes, which they have enjoyed in perfect peace and tranquillity until these invaders have thought proper to disturb and destroy those possessions."

So well planned and executed was this effort to win the sympathy of the foreign troops for the American cause that when the war was over, 10,000 mercenaries who came to fight England's battles remained to become United States citizens.

The year 1776 was a disastrous one for the American cause. It has been written that, while 47,000 Continental troops were in the field, they had only enlisted for one-year periods. In addition to these, 27,000 militiamen served short terms of duty, resulting in many soldiers of both classifications leaving the Army at some critical time in a campaign. Of this grand total of 74,000, it was estimated that 1,000 were killed in action, 1,200 were wounded, 6,000 were taken prisoners, and 10,000 died from disease. Truly, many of the latter expired in British prisons, the result of English indifference and neglect, but our own Continental hospital methods were responsible for a great majority of these casualties. It was universally admitted that a change in methods and organization was necessary, and it was hoped that a more generous Congressional policy toward the Medical Department might correct major difficulties. But of this, more later.

Immediately on General Washington's establishing his headquarters at Morristown on January 6, 1777, he wrote Dr. Shippen of a decision to attack the greatest enemy of the Continental Army.

"Finding the smallpox to be spreading much and fearing that no precaution can prevent it from running through the whole of our Army, I have determined that the troops shall be inoculated.

"The expedient may be attended with some inconvenience and some disadvantages, but yet I trust in its consequences, will have the most happy effects. Necessity not only authorizes but seems to require this measure, for should the disorder infect the Army in this natural way and rage with its usual virulence, we should have more to dread from it than from the sword of the enemy.

"Under these circumstances, I have directed Dr. Nathaniel Bond to prepare immediately for inoculations in this quarter, keeping the matter as secret as possible, and request that you will, without delay, inoculate all the Continental troops that are in Philadelphia and those that come in as fast as they arrive. You will spare no pains to carry them through the disorder with the utmost expedition and to have them cleansed from the infection so that they may proceed to camp with as little injury as possible to the country through which they pass. If the business is immediately begun and favored with the common success, I will fain hope they will soon be fit for duty and that in a short space of time, we shall have an Army not subject to this, the greatest of all calamities that can befall it, when taken in a natural way."

On January 28, 1777, the Commander in Chief again wrote Dr. Shippen:

"In your last, you mentioned your intention of inoculating all the recruits that had not had the smallpox. This would be a very salutary measure if we could prevent them from bringing the infection into the Army, but as they cannot have a change of clothes, I fear it is impossible. We shall soon have the troops from the Eastward, and as few of them have had that disorder, we should have a great part of our Army laid down. I have, therefore, ordered General Gates to suffer no more of the Southern troops to come into Philadelphia but to march them into Germantown and let them remain there until they are equipped and ready to march; all that now have the disorder to be perfectly cured, and before they are suffered to join the Army, to have new clothes if possible, and if not, the old ones well washed, aired and smoked.

"As I would have the smallpox entirely out of Philadelphia, suppose all the patients that could be removed, were carried down to the hospital upon Providence Island and make that in the future the smallpox hospital, except their numbers should be too great.

"P.S. The Barracks upon Fort Island might be likewise made use of."

General Washington probably meant 'Province Island' instead of 'Providence,' which was located at the mouth of the Schuylkill River in the Delaware. Fort Island, situated nearby, is now known as 'Mifflin.'

In General Washington's first letter to Dr. Shippen, he gave positive orders for treating the Continental troops, but in the second, he indicated a doubt that recruits about to join the Army could be similarly protected. Evidently, a solution to seeming difficulties was soon found, for on February 10, 1777, the Commander-in-Chief informed the New York Legislature:

"The Physicians are now making preparations to inoculate all, at the several posts in this quarter, and Dr. Dr. Shippen will inoculate all the recruits that have not had the disorder, as fas as they come into Philadelphia. They will lose no time by this operation, as they will go through while their clothing, arms and accoutrements are preparing."

On February 12, 1777, the Continental Congress, sitting in Baltimore, took action on the same subject, and the following day Dr. Benjamin Rush, Chairman, wrote to General Washington:

"The Congress, apprehending that smallpox may greatly endanger the lives of our fellow citizens who compose the Army under your Excellency's command and also very much embarrass the Military operations, have directed their Medical Committee to request your Excellency to give orders that all, who have not had that disease, may be inoculated if your Excellency shall be of the opinion that it may be done without prejudice to your operation.

"Some battalions from Virginia are now on their march to join you and are ordered to take the upper route to avoid Philadelphia, where the infection now prevails."

Several days after the Commander of the American Armies had received Dr. Rush's communication, General Caesar Rodney, at his headquarters in Trenton, was handed the following letter:

"General Hospital, Phila., Feb. 17th, 1777.

"Dear General: "General Washington has directed that all the Continental troops shall be inoculated. I have [therefore] sent Dr. [Bodo] Otto to Trenton upon this business, as well as to take charge of ye Military hospital at that place; whether the General means the Militia of the different States [also] or not, I can't tell, but all the regular troops should, I imagine, be immediately inoculated, in such a place as you and the Surgeon think proper. This, I submit to your judgment and discretion, and am, Dear General,

"Your very humble servant, "Wm. Shippen, Jr."

The intention of a general smallpox inoculation created considerable anxiety among the people living in town adjacent to the various camps, and General Washington showed his consideration for their fears in a letter to Dr. Shippen:

"Dear Sir:

"H. Q. Morristown, March 6, 1777.

"It ever was my desire to secure cities from any contagious disorders that may attend the troops that must pass through them, and I shall always be happy to execute such plans as their caution may suggest...

"Dr. Shippen had evidently been anticipating a medical departmental reorganization, for in December 1776, he wrote Richard Henry Lee from Bethlehem and inquired as to the advisability of then offering his plan to Congress. Lee replied with the suggestion that an outline be submitted directly to General Washington, who, he said, had just been given complete authority over all matters pertaining to the Continental Army."

The removal of Dr. John Morgan from the service on January 9, 1777, made the position of Director General vacant and gave Dr. Shippen his great opportunity. Under date of January 27, 1777, General Washington wrote from his headquarters at Morristown:

"For Dr. Shippen, Jr.

"I have yours without date, favoring me with a plan for the formation of General hospitals, for which I am obliged.

"Although the Congress has vested me with full power to make all military arrangements, and I dare say would approve whatever appointments and salaries I should fix, yet I do not think myself at liberty to establish hospitals upon such extensive plans and at so great an expense, without their concurrence.

"I have no doubt but the number of officers that you propose are necessary and will be allowed, but I am afraid you have rather over-rated their pay. By your regulation, the pay of a Director [considerably] exceeds that of a Major General, and the rest in proportion. I shall, however, lay the plan before Congress without mentioning any names, and as the nominations will lay principally with me, you may be assured of having the Director's [pay] considerably exceed that of a Major General and the Assts. attached to it, as are most agreeable to yourself...

"I have some particular gentlemen provide for in the new arrange to ment, but you may depend that those who have already distinguished themselves by their assiduity shall not be unnoticed. "As I am very anxious to have the great work set in motion, I shall desire Congress to give me their opinions as speedily as possible.

"By not dating your letter, I am not able to determine whether Dr. Cochran had reached Philadelphia when you wrote, but as I conclude he had not, I shall defer sending your plan to Congress till you have seen him, as I sent him down purposely to consult with you upon the subject...."

It was a week earlier, on January 20, 1777, that General Washington had given instructions to Dr. John Cochran, a member of his staff:

"To proceed from hence to New Town (Pa.), tomorrow, and there inquire into the state of smallpox, and use every possible means in your power to prevent that disease from spreading into the Army and among the inhabitants, which may otherwise prove fatal to the service. To that end, you are to take such houses as will be convenient in the most retired parts of the country and best calculated to answer that purpose.

"You will then proceed to Philadelphia and consult Dr. Shippen, the Director, about forming a hospital for the ensuing campaign, in such manner that the sick and wounded may be taken the best care of, and the inconveniences in that department so much complained of in the last campaign, may be remedied in the future.

"You will also, in conjunction with Dr. Shippen, point out to me in writing such officers and stores as you may think necessary for the arrangement of a hospital in every branch of the Department, as well as to constitute one for the Army in the field which may be styled a Flying Hospital; also fixed hospitals in such parts of the County as the nature of the service from time to time may require.

"Let your standard be for 10,000 men for one campaign, and so in proportion for a greater or lesser number as may hereafter be ordered."

General Washington presented the reorganization proposal to Congress in a letter dated February 14, 1777:

"I do myself the honor to enclose you a plan, drawn up by Dr. Shippen, in concert with Dr. Cochran, for the arrangement and future regulation of the General Hospital. As the plan is very extensive, the appointments numerous, and the salaries, at present affixed to them, large, did not think myself at liberty to adopt any part of it before I laid it Sore Congress for their approbation. I will just remark that though the expense of attending our hospital on the enclosed plan will be very great, it will in the end, not only be a saving to the public but the only possible method of keeping an army afoot.

"We are now at an enormous bounty, with no small difficulty recruiting an army upwards of 100 battalions. The ensuing campaign may, from the same causes, prove as sickly as the last. If the hospitals are in no better condition for the reception of the sick, our Regiments will be reduced to companies by the end of the campaign, and those poor wretches who escape with life will be either scattered up and down the country and not to be found, or if found, totally enervated and unfit for further duty. By these means, the bounty is not only lost, but the man is also lost, and I leave you to judge whether we have men enough to allow such consumption of lives and constitutions as have been lost in the last campaign. For my part, I am certain that if the army, which I hope we should have in the field this year, is suffered to smoulder away by sickness, as it did in the past, we must look for reinforcements from some other places than our own States.

"The number of Officers mentioned in the enclosed plan, I presume are necessary for us because they are found so in the British hospitals, and as they are established upon the surest base, that of long experience under the ablest Physicians and Surgeons, we should not hesitate a moment in adopting their regulations, when they so plainly tend to correct and improve our former want of method and knowledge in this important department.

"The pay affixed to the different appointments is, as I said before, great and perhaps more than you may think adequate to the service. In determining upon the sum that is to be allowed to each, you ought to consider that it should be such as will induce gentlemen of character and skill in the profession to step forth and in some manner be adequate to the practice which they leave at home. For unless such gentlemen are induced to undertake the care and management of our hospital, we had better trust the forces of nature and constitutions, rather than suffer persons entirely ignorant of medicine to destroy us by ill-directed applications.

"I hear from every quarter that the dread of undergoing these same miseries, for want of proper care and attention when sick, has much retarded the new enlistment, particularly to the Southward.

"There is another reason for establishing our hospitals upon a large and generous plan; we ought to make the service as agreeable and enticing as possible to the soldiers, many of whom (especially when we call forth the Militia) not only quit the comforts, but the luxuries of life.

"As no time is to be lost in appointing the necessary officers, fixing upon the proper places for hospitals and many other preparations, I would wish that Congress would take this matter under their immediate consideration and favor me with their sentiments as soon as possible."

This letter of General Washington is of unusual interest for two reasons: first, because he suggested the thought that, unless hospital conditions were improved, it might be necessary to look for mercenaries or foreign alliances before an army could be in the field, and secondly, because of the strong arguments he advanced in favor of a proposal, he apparently feared would be kept with Congressional opposition. Washington's correspondence with Congress throughout the war indicated a reluctance to try to influence legislative action. He was more inclined to simply make reports of conditions and needs and leave solutions to the wisdom of the Continental delegates. But in support of the proposed hospital plan, he appears as an advocate, and presented arguments that were hard to refute.

Shippen's and Cochran's collaborated plan was referred to the Medical Committee of the Congress, and they made their report on February 27, 1777, but no action was taken, and it was not until March 22, 1777, that the House considered and debated the proposal. Two days later, the submitted legislation was taken under consideration by Congress as a Committee of the whole and returned to the Medical Committee for further change. Final action occurred on April 7, 1777, when Shippen's plan, with certain minor changes, was enacted into law. On April 11, 1777,

Dr. William Shippen, Jr., was chosen "Director General of all the Military Hospitals for the Army" by the unanimous vote of the thirteen States. By the new arrangement the country was divided into four hospital districts: Eastern, Northern, Southern, and Middle, the most important, which included all territory lying between the Hudson and Potomac Rivers.

The compensation provided for Continental hospital officers under the new act, was most generous when compared with the pay authorized in the Army reorganization law for officers in command of troops. It might be here mentioned, however, that hospital paychecks were always in arrears, frequently to the extent of two years, and when Dr. Bodo Otto resigned his commission on February 1, 1782, he received a Government certificate of indebtedness for over two thousand dollars, representing pay, ration and clothing allowance that was overdue.

The Director General's pay was $6.00 a day and 9 rations; the various District Deputy Directors, $5.00 and 6 rations; Senior Surgeon, $4.00 and 6 rations; Junior Surgeon, $2.00 and 4 rations; and Surgeon Mates, $1.50 and 2 rations, while a Colonel of Continental troops received the equivalent of $2.50 a day; a Lieutenant Colonel, $2.00; a Major, $12/5; Captain, $11/3; a Lieutenant, less than $1.00; and an Ensign, 662/3 cents. On April 22, 1777, Congress resolved:

"That the Director and Deputy Directors General shall constantly publish in the newspapers, the names and places in which the Military Hospitals are respectfully kept."

A diligent search of the available files of 1777 failed to find any such public notice. This is greatly to be regretted, for official records of the location, time and extent of the hospitals of the Continental Army are woefully scarce.

Dr. Shippen did, however, announce the reorganization of the Medical Department in no uncertain language:

"The liberal provisions made by Congress in the new medical arrangements and joined with a humane desire to prevent the repetition of the distresses which afflicted the brave American soldiers the last campaign, have drawn men of the first abilities into the field, to watch over the health and preserve the lives of the soldiers, many of them from very extensive and profitable practice and every species of domestic happiness. Dr. William Brown of Virginia, Dr. James Craik of Maryland, and Dr. Thomas Bond, Jr. of Philadelphia, are appointed Assistant Director Generals. Dr. Walter Jones and Dr. Benjamin Rush of Philadelphia, Physician and Surgeon Generals of the Hospitals of the Middle Department. Under these, none but gentlemen of the best education and well-qualified are employed as senior Physicians, Surgeons, &. The Eastern and Northern departments are filled with gentlemen of the first characters in these countries, and the public may depend on it that the greatest exertions of skill and industry shall be constantly made and no cost spared to make the sick and wounded soldierly comfortable and happy. As a consequence of the above liberal arrangement of the Honorable Congress, we do with great pleasure and equal truth, assure the public (notwithstanding the many false and wicked reports propagated by the enemies of American liberty, and only calculated to retard the recruiting service) that all the military hospitals of the United States are in excellent order, and that the Army enjoy a degree of health, seldom to be seen or read of.

"W. SHIPPEN, Jun., Director General of the American Hospitals. "JOHN COCHRAN, Physician and Surgeon General of the Army in the Middle Dept." –Headquarters, Middlebrook, June 4, 1777.

"It is requested that the above may be published in all newspapers on the Continent."

(From the Pennsylvania Evening Post, June 5, 177).

It was the result of these better inducements that two of Bodo Otto's sons, Dr. Frederick and Dr. John, offered their services as HOSPITAL REORGANIZATION (139) Junior Surgeon and Surgeon Mate. Both were immediately commissioned and assigned for duty in their father's hospital at Trenton.

Applicants for hospital positions or preferment did not hesitate to make their appeal direct to General Washington himself. Early in March 1777, his Excellency replied to one candidate:

"The Doctor will undoubtedly find a place in the new hospital suitable to his merits and abilities, as it is proposed to have the new arrangement upon an extensive plan. As Dr. Shippen will probably be at the head of the Medical Department, he had better apply to him in time."

Even earlier than the above date, the Commander-in-Chief had answered a letter of similar character from Dr. John Warren:

"Morristown, February 23, '77.

"I have yours of the 18th inst. Your continuing to act in the hospital, upon the uncertainty of being provided for under the new arrangements, is very commendable, but I can assure you it was my intention to take particular care that those who had filled their old stations with reputation should not be degraded in the new appointments. The plan for the establishment of the general hospital is now before Congress, and whenever I receive their approbation, the officers will be appointed.

"I can not promise that you can be fixed at Rhode Island, but I dare say, in the settlement of the Surgeons and Physicians who are to superintend the different departments, the private convenience of the gentlemen will be attended to if thereby the public will not be injured."

To Dr. James Craik, an old friend whom he first knew as a Surgeon in the French and Indian Wars, General Washington wrote, on his own initiative:

"Morristown, April 26, '77.

"Dear Doctor:

"I am going to address you on a subject which may lay some claim to your attention, as I do to your candor, in the determination of the proposition.

"In the Hospital department for the Middle District, there are at present two places vacant, either of which I can obtain for you; one is Senior Physician and Surgeon of the Hospital, with the pay of 4 dollars and 6 rations per day and forage for one horse; the other is Assistant Director General, with the pay of 3 dollars and 6 rations per day, and two horses and traveling expenses found, according to Dr. Shippen, Director General's account. He also adds that he thinks the latter is the most honorable and desirable of the two.

"Had I expected that Congress would have proceeded to the appointments in the department at the time they did, I have no doubt but that it might have been in my power to have got you any other place (except that of Director General) but that is now over, and the matter in which I claim your candor is, that you will not let my introducing the present proposition to you have any undue influence.

"I have only to add, therefore, a request that you let me know the result of your determination by the return of the post or as soon as possible, as the places will be kept vacant till I hear from you."

Dr. Craik accepted the position recommended and became an important officer in the Middle Division. He served in the Medical Department until the end of the war when he returned to private practice in Virginia, and there attended General Washington in that great American's final illness.

Prior to General Washington's opening of the 1777 Spring Campaign at Morristown, the Continental hospitals located in the country districts of Pennsylvania were relieved of congestion by deaths and discharged convalescent soldiers. The remaining patients were transferred to Philadelphia, and the hospitals of Allentown, Easton, and Bethlehem were closed. Many of the soldiers, who had been serving as nurses and orderlies in the New Jersey hospitals, then received orders to return to their regiments for military duty. General Washington attempted to replace them with females in certain hospitals, and, by general orders dated June 17, 1777, issued at Middle Brook; he directed: "that a proportionate number of women, to the sick of each regiment, shall be sent to the Hospitals at Mendham and Black River, to attend the sick as nurses."

The sudden embarkment on July 23, 1777, of General Howe's Army from New York to an unknown destination threw the American command into confusion. The Morristown Hospital patients were immediately removed to Philadelphia, and General Washington put his troops in motion to the southward in anticipation of a British landing in the Delaware River or Chesapeake Bay.

On April 8, 1777, Congress had directed:

"That in times of action and any other emergency, when the surgeons are not sufficient in number to properly attend to the sick and wounded that can not be removed to the hospitals, the director or Deputy Director General of the District be empowered and required, upon request of the Physician and Surgeon General of the Army, to send from the hospitals under his care to the assistance of such sick and wounded, as many

Physicians and Surgeons as can possibly be spared from the necessary business of the hospitals."

Under this authority, many medical men were withdrawn from their regular hospital assignment and directed to attend General Washington in anticipation of an expected battle. Dr. John A. Otto was among those Surgeons ordered into the field, and in his writings, he told of necessary emergency operations performed on soldiers wounded at Brandywine.

A report of the condition of the Army, filed with Congress shortly before General Washington began his movements to protect Philadelphia, gave the number of the rank and file as 17,949, of whom 14,204 were fit for duty. With 4,745, or 26 percent, sick in the hospitals and a campaign starting, the problem of caring for additional casualties greatly disturbed the Medical Department. The important question was, what would be the outcome of a battle? If an American victory resulted, the location, safety and convenience of neighboring hospitals and towns might more easily furnish a solution, but what if success crowned the British? Such a misfortune to the American Army would not only involve the necessity of immediately removing patients from existing hospitals to distant points but would require the hasty creation of new ones to care for casualties.

The Continental losses at Brandywine, besides 300 killed, were 600 wounded, and all of the latter who could walk or be helped in the effort were immediately started toward Philadelphia, while those who were incapacitated but not seriously hurt were transported in open wagons. These, General Washington directed, should be sent through to Trenton, where Dr. Bodo Otto's Barracks Hospital was to be supplemented by such other buildings as might be required.

The soldiers, who were more seriously wounded, were given necessary treatment in nearby buildings. Some were unknowingly left on the field when they fell, and these were collected by the British and taken to Wilmington, where American medical men attended them under a flag of truce.

The remaining casualties of Brandywine were sent to Ephrata, Pennsylvania, where houses of the Monastic Community of Dunkards were taken, and here, 500 sick and wounded were located during the following winter of 1777-78.

The unfortunate defeat at Brandywine and the maneuvering of the British Army up and down the Schuylkill kept General Washington uncertain of General Howe's intent and made the retention of Philadelphia very doubtful. Congress, therefore, abandoned the city on September 18, 1777, transferring the capital to Lancaster, but not before the stores, supplies, ordnance, and hospital patients were sent to Trenton and other New Jersey localities. Even then, General Washington foresaw the risk in allowing these hastily removed necessities to remain so near to Philadelphia, and amid his worries and the uncertainty of his own position, he wrote to the President of Congress, the Commanding officer of the New Jersey District, the Quarter Master General and Committee of Safety, urging them to see that all Government property, as well as the hospital patients, be immediately moved to places of greater safety.

Thus, the sick and wounded, located in the hospitals of Bordentown, Burlington and Trenton, were soon again loaded into open springless wagons and taken to Bethlehem, Allentown, and Easton.

The Battle of Germantown, on October 4, 1777, which followed shortly after the Brandywine fight, settled the fate of Philadelphia. Four hundred and twenty-one American soldiers were then added to the number of Continental wounded, and emergency hospitals were set up at Evansburg, Trappe, Pennypacker Mills, Falkner Swamp, and in the houses of John

Jantz and Adam Golwals at Skippack. Eventually, these patients were transported to more distant and safer places, where permanent hospitals had been established.

It was on September 19, 1777, that a messenger from Dr. Shippen arrived at Bethlehem, informing the Reverend Ettwein, head of the Moravian community, of regret that the fortunes of what necessitated a return to their peaceful village and re-establishment of a hospital in their midst. The medical officers visited another Moravian community settlement at Lititz, and here, a hospital was organized in a three-story stone building belonging to that religious order. By December 19, 1777, it was recorded that all its rooms, and even the halls, were filled with sick and wounded soldiers transferred from New Jersey.

Hospitals were also established at Reading, in the Court House, Potters Shop, First Reformed Friends Meeting House, Bunkhouse, and the Trinity Church. Lutheran traditions are that Trinity was offered to General Washington for hospital use at the instigation of Bodo Otto, under his promise to personally take charge and protect the property. As Bodo Otto was then either in Trenton or had already been transferred to Bethlehem, it must have been his son, John, to whom credit is due, for the records are that he (Dr. John) served at this post until the Reading hospitals were closed.

These unfortunate victims of the war endured much unnecessary suffering because of the many changes in their hospital location. Perhaps they submitted to frequent transfers in the hope of reaching a permanent, safe place where rest and recovery could be realized. If the hospital staff had any such expectancy of a fixed post, where they might settle down with some domestic comfort, they were doomed to disappointment, for a constant shifting of hospitals or assignments seemed to have been the rule rather than the exception. In this respect, however,

Dr. Bodo Otto and his eldest son, Dr. Frederick, seemed to have been exceptionally fortunate, for they remained at one hospital for nearly four years.

Shortly after the British Army withdrew from Germantown and established their base in Philadelphia proper, the Continental Army approached nearer the city and made camp at Whitemarsh. Here, a council of war was held, and the alternative plans discussed attacking the enemy in Philadelphia or withdrawing a greater distance from the city and making a winter camp. The American troops remained at Whitemarsh from November 2 to December 11, 1777, when a decision had been made, and the Army marched toward Valley Forge. It was at Whitemarsh that General Washington offered a reward of $10 to any person who would produce the best substitute for shoes made out of rawhide.

On October 27, 1777, Dr. Shippen appealed to Congress, saying:

"The pressing necessity of the hospitals, which begin effects of cold and dirt, calls upon me to address you in a serious manner and urge you to furnish us with an immediate supply of clothing requisite for the very existence of the sick now in the greatest distress in the hospitals, and indispensably necessary to enable many who are now well and detained solely for want of clothing, to return to the Army."

The Congress's action on Dr. Shippen's communication was not very prompt, for it was not until November 19 that they ordered:

"That the Clothier General be directed to deliver to the Director General of the Military hospitals, etc., for the use of the sick and wounded of the several departments, a proportionate share of the blankets, shirts, shoes and stockings he shall from time to time procure, for the supply of the Army.

"(Also) That the Director General of the Hospitals be authorized to cause stoves to be erected in the different hospitals, in case he shall think such a measure will conduce to make up for the present scarcity of blankets and clothing, or to the greater comfort of the sick, and that wagons annexed to the Hospital Department be employed as much as possible, in the transportation of fuel for the respective hospitals."

The day prior to the above resolution, the orderly book of the Army at Whitemarsh contained the record that:

"The Government of the State of Pennsylvania, having appointed a Commission in each County thereof, to collect blankets and clothing for the Army, all officers sent out for this purpose are to be recalled with such clothing and the 200 blankets they have collected. The several brigades are to send for their quotas.

"The sick are to be sent to Hospitals, but before they are removed, the application is to be made of Dr. Cochran or other Directors of the Hospital for directions unless the place to which they are to be sent has been positively pointed out in General Orders.

"No more sick are to be sent to Buckingham Meeting House. A surgeon and twelve orderly men are to be sent to Buckingham in order to take care of the sick."

Again, on December 1, 1777, several days before the Army broke camp at Whitemarsh, it was ordered that:

"Returns are to be made early tomorrow morning of all men in the several Brigades and Corps who have not had the smallpox."

In General Washington's consideration of several possible sites for winter quarters, he requested an opinion from each of his Generals on three alternative proposals. First, a camp to be established at some point on a line between the Schuylkill and the Delaware; second, a base to be located at Wilmington; and, third, quarters in selected villages, between Reading and Lancaster. It was General Knox's suggestion that the Army encamp in huts to be erected at some spot about thirty miles from Philadelphia, but it was on General Mühlenberg's recommendation that Valley Forge, a neighborhood with which he was familiar, was definitely selected.

And so the men of General Washington's Army arrived at the site of the proposed encampment on December 11, 1777; their feet exposed through worn-out shoes; their bodies poorly clad in tattered remains of stockings, breeches and shirts; food was scarce, many of the soldiers were sick, and most of them disheartened. The weather was cold and rainy, and huts had yet to be built. Truly, these were discouraging circumstances of tribulation upon which to build a well-trained and determined Army with which to continue the war for liberty and independence. It was under such appalling handicaps of suffering and privation that our Continental soldiers at Valley Forge received the military training that enabled them to defeat the British and win the sincere admiration of those same French officers who, six months before, had called them an "undisciplined mob."

CHAPTER FOURTEEN

VALLEY FORGE • Care of Sick. Roster of Medical Men • Hospital Stores and Equipment Lists • Letters

THE DIRECTOR GENERAL'S REPORT of November 24, 1777, gave the number of sick, wounded, and convalescent soldiers being cared for in the hospitals of the Army as 4,167 and their locations as Princeton, Burlington, Trenton, in New Jersey; Buckingham Meeting House, North Wales, Skippack, Easton, Allentown, Reading, Bethlehem, Manheim, Lancaster, in Pennsylvania; and in addition, one at Baltimore, Maryland, and others not enumerated, in the Northern and Eastern Departments.

Dr. Jonathan Potts was on leave at Reading from his Northern post when the hospital patients were being transferred from New Jersey and the Philadelphia neighborhood to places of greater safety, and here he received a letter from Dr. Shippen, saying:

"Bethlehem, December 14, 1777.

"Dear Sir:

"You were so kind as to offer your assistance on your arrival from ye North. Now I have great need of your best exertions because the late movements of ye army make it necessary to move all our sick to the west side of the Schuylkill. All must pass through Reading, and you can do much toward making their stay there comfortable and their transportation to the places assigned for them easy and safe.

"I am sure that if your inclination is equal to your abilities, the business will be well done, and there is no doubt with me that you are an honest fellow, and I, in return, will be, as I ever have been, your affectionate friend."

"William Shippen, Jr."

The Director General's communication to Congress in December 1777 revealed that the Burlington, Trenton, Buckingham, and Skippack hospitals had been discontinued, and new ones opened in Ephrata, Rheimstown, Lititz, Warrick, and Shaefertown.

The following roster of medical men, though not submitted as a complete list, contains the names of surgeons and physicians who are known to have served in the Continental hospitals adjacent to Valley Forge.

Jonathan Potts (Pa.), P. G.

Wm. Shippen, Jr. (Pa.), D. G.

John Cochran (Pa.), P. & S. G. of the Flying Camp of the Army.

Thomas Bond (Pa.), ass't. D. G.

James Craik (Va.), ass't. D. G.

Wm. Brown (Va.), P. G.

Andrew Craigie (Mass.), A. G.

John B. Cutting (N. Y.), A. G.

The hospital surgeons and physicians, junior surgeons and mates were:

Bodo Otto (Pa.)	Bodo Otto, Jr. (N. J.)
Frederick Otto (N. J. & Pa.)	John A. Otto (Pa.)
Samuel Kennedy (Pa.)	Wm. Smith (Pa.)
W. P. Smith (N. Y.)	E. C. Smith
Hall Jackson (N. H.)	Jenison
Samuel Finley (Mass.)	Charles McKnight (N.Y.)
Acquila Wilmott (Pa.)	Joseph Harrison (Pa.)
John Hindman (Mass.)	John Cowell (Pa.)
Gilbert Fennent	James Finley (Mass.)
Robert B. Henry (N. J.)	George Draper (Va.)
Goodwin Wilson (Pa.)	Frederick Maus
Ennals Martin (Md.)	Gustavus Henderson
Garrison	Mathew Irvine (Pa.)
Frederick Ridgely (Md.)	J. Hutchinson (Pa.)
Thomas	James Tilton (Del.)
George Glentworth (Pa.)	James Fallon (Pa.)
Francis Alison (Pa.)	Barnabas Binney (Mass.)
John H. Latimer (Del.)	Moses Scott (N. J.)
Solomon Halling (Pa.)	Samuel Duffield (Pa.)
David Jackson (Pa.)	Rober Johnson
Cornelius Baldwin (N. J.)	James Houston (S. C.)
John Duffield (Pa.)	John Scott (Md.)
Ezekiel Bull (Pa.)	—White
Thomas Marshall (Md.)	Samuel Edminston (Pa.)
Moses Bloomfield (N. J.)	Nicholas Scull
Benjamin Snowden	John Reed
Henry Crow	John Witherspoon (N. J.)
—Wodgson	—Lugman
McCuryher	Ebenezer Crosby (Conn.)

George Ickman and Fraley served as assistant apothecaries, Samuel Morris as Commissary General of the hospital, with Hugh James acting as his assistant, and Joseph W. Shippen served as paymaster. The Reverends James Sproat and Spencer were the hospital chaplains.

The often-quoted diary of Surgeon Albigence Waldo of the Continental Line gives a good account of the condition of the soldiers when they arrived at the site of the Valley Forge encampment.

"December 14, 1777. The army, which has been surprisingly healthy heretofore, now begins to grow sickly from the continual fatigue they have suffered. Yet they still show a spirit of alacrity and contentment not to be expected from so young troops. I am sick, discontented, and out of humor. Poor food, hard lodgings, cold weather, fatigue, nasty clothes, nasty cooking, vomit half my time, smoked out of my senses the Devil's in it-I can't endure it. Why are we sent here to starve and freeze? What sweet felicities have I left at home: a charming wife, pretty children, good beds, good food, good cooking–agreeable, all harmonious; here, all confusion, smoke and cold, hunger and filthiness a pox on my bad luck. There comes a bowl of beef soup, full of leaves and dirt, sickish enough to make a Hector spue. Away with it, Boy! Here comes a soldier, his bare feet seen through worn-out shoes; his legs nearly naked from the tattered remains of only a pair of stockings; his breeches not sufficient to cover his nakedness; his shirt hanging in strings; his hair disheveled; his face meagre and discouraged.

"December 21, 1777 (Valley Force). Preparation made for the huts. Provisions scarce-heartily wish myself at home. My skin and eyes are almost spoiled with continual smoke. A general cry goes through the Camp this evening among the soldiers, 'No meat, no meat.'

"What have we for dinner, Boy?

"Nothing but cake and water, Sir.

"December 22, 1777. My eyes are started out from their orbits like rabbits' eyes, occasioned by great cold and smoke.

"I am ashamed to say it, but I am tempted to steal fowls if I could find them or even a whole hog, for I feel as if I could eat one.

"December 24, 1777. Huts go up slowly. Cold and smoke make us fret.

"December 25, 1777. Christmas day. We are still in tents. The poor sick suffer much in tents in this cold weather.

"December 28, 1777. Yesterday, upward of fifty officers in General Greene's division resigned their commissions. Six or seven of our regiment are doing the like today. All this is occasioned by officers' families being so neglected at home on account of provisions.

"December 29, 1777. So much talk about discharge among the officers his Excellency lately expressed his fear of being left alone with soldiers only."

Dr. Waldo's complaint about excessive smoke gives credence to another tradition that there once existed a Revolutionary wartime letter from one of Dr. Bodo Otto's sons, reading:

"My darling wife,

"I miss you and the children, and I miss your cooking. Here, we have to change the order of our courses to get a variety. For breakfast, we have bacon and smoke; for dinner, smoke and bacon; and for supper, smoke."

While it was a fact that many sicknesses prevailed among the soldiers throughout the entire encampment, their ailments, in the beginning, were closely related to exposure and malnutrition, while the serious illnesses, of which so much has been written, did not become a hospital problem until April 1778.

Dr. Waldo wrote in his journal in the early winter:

"Very few die, for they are used to exposure and hardship."

On December 23, 1777, 2,898 men at Valley Forge were reported sick or unfit for duty on account of lack of clothing. A later return dated February 1, 1778, increased the number of incapacitated to 3,989, and again, the scarcity of clothes was cited as the principal cause.

Congress recognized the great fortitude of General Washington's men on December 30, 1777.

"Resolved that in recognition of the soldierly patience, fidelity, and zeal in the cause of their country, one month's extraordinary pay should be given to each soldier."

General Washington issued an appeal to the farmers of the counties adjacent to Valley Forge to immediately thresh their grain so that the army and hospitals might obtain the resulting foodstuff and straw. Orders were also published apportioning the straw to the soldiers so that none might be wasted.

"Twenty pounds of straw shall be issued to every six men, including officers, but none will be allowed in the summer except in rainy weather, and for the sick, but not oftener than once in three days, in any season."

This same order likewise provided:

"One-quarter cord of wood per day shall be apportioned to every sixty men, including officers."

General orders of January 2, 1778, directed that:

"Every morning, the regimental surgeons shall make returns to the Surgeon General in camp, of all under their care, specifying names, company, regiment, and disease."

Under date of January 6, 1778, it was further ordered that:

"The regimental surgeons shall immediately make returns to Dr. Cochran, the Surgeon General of the Flying Camp, of all who have not had the smallpox. They are also directed to call upon Dr. Cochran for what sulphur they may need for their regiments."

Two days later, the reason for sulphur requisition was cited in the day's orders:

"Being informed that many men are rendered unfit for duty by the Itch, the Commander in Chief directs the regimental surgeons to look attentively into the matter, and as soon as the men (who are infected with the disorder) are properly disposed in huts, to have them anointed for it."

Almost a month before this was issued, Baron De Kalb wrote to his friend, Count De Broglio, in France:

"In Camp, 17 miles from Philadelphia, December 12, 1777.

"Our soldiers are infected with the Itch without the hospitals or anyone else troubling themselves. I have just been shown one of them, all covered with scabs. I have ordered that huts be hastily constructed to house these unfortunate ones in order to separate them from the rest of the troops."

December 12, 1777, was the date the army arrived at the Gulph, where it was first thought that winter quarters might be established. The army did not remain long enough, however, to permit General De Kalb's plan of treating his own men to be put into effect.

The Medical Department organization plan of April 1777 provided that a Flying Camp hospital should be attached to each army, and it decreed:

"There shall be a Director and a Surgeon General whose duties, in subordination to ye Director General, shall be to superintend and receive from him a suitable number of large, strong tents, beds, bedding, medicines, and hospital stores for such sick and wounded persons as cannot be transported to ye General Hospital with safety, or who may be rendered fit for duty in a few days.

"He shall also see that the sick and wounded, while in his hospital, are properly attended and dressed, and when able, to be conveyed to ye General Hospital, for which last purpose he shall be supplied by ye Director General with a proper number of convenient wagons and drivers."

To carry out these provisions, an order was issued on January 9, 1778:

"The Major and Brigadier Generals of each division are to fix on some suitable ground near the respective brigades, where hospitals may be erected; one for the sick of each brigade, and as soon as the men can be spared from working on the huts, they are to erect the hospitals."

Two days later, specifications were published that:

"The Flying Camp Hospital huts are to be fifteen feet wide, twenty-five feet long, and at least nine feet high; to be covered with boards or shingles, without any dirt. A window shall be made on each side and a chimney at one end. Two such hospitals are to be erected for each brigade, located in their rear as near the center as may be, and, if the grounds admit of it, not more than 300 nor less than 100 yards from it."

These small brigade hospital huts were used throughout the period of the encampment for treatment of simple ailments and as clearing houses for the seriously ill who were to be sent to the outlying hospitals, as directed by the proper officials at Yellow Springs or by Dr. James Craik, Assistant Director, stationed at Valley Forge.

A notice was published in the orders of January 21, 1778, to the effect that:

"It being impossible for the Surgeon General of the Flying Camp to make provisions for the sick, unless they are sent to places properly furnished for the purpose, all officers and regimental surgeons are therefore to apply to the chief surgeon (Assistant Director) present in the camp and take his directions where to send the sick. A contrary practice has been attended with great inconvenience to the sick and probably has occasioned the death of several men. Many have been sent to hospitals already crowded with patients or to places where no provision had been made."

On January 15, 1778, it was ordered that:

"Colonels Humpton and Gibson, Lt. Colonel Vose, Major Furnald, Vice Bassell, and Major Ball are appointed to repair the several hospitals in the Middle department. They will receive their orders at the Adjutant General's office tomorrow morning."

These assignments were evidently made for the purpose of directing necessary changes and additions where barns and churches had been taken over for hospital use.

Yellow Springs (now Chester Springs), situated some ten or twelve miles west of Valley Forge, was a health resort of reputation, with medicinal springs and baths. It had many advantages to recommend it for the army hospital headquarters, and possession was immediately taken. The springs and baths, with some usable houses, were located on a farm belonging to Dr. Samuel Kennedy, who was among the first physicians ordered to Yellow Springs, where he established hospitals in three barns. Dr. Kennedy be came an early victim of the malignant putrid fever. A year after his death, Congress directed that his widow be paid $5,000 for the use of the property.

By order of General Washington, the construction of a commodious building was immediately started to serve both as the Yellow Springs Medical Department headquarters and the principal hospital unit for the camp. "Washington Hall," as it was later called, was the only specially designed hospital erected for the soldiers of the Continental Army, with the exception of those small log huts constructed in various camps for temporary use. Washington Hall was 106 feet long, 36 feet wide, and three full stories and attic high. The third floor was divided into many little rooms, while the second contained two large wards. The kitchen, dining room, and all the utilitarian quarters were located on the first or ground floor. Nine-foot porches surrounded the Emergency quantities of constantly needed hospital stores. Remedies were carried in a commissary depot at Yellow Springs. Still, the main warehouse of supplies was located at Reading, where Dr. Jonathan Potts, the Purveyor General, maintained his headquarters. However, hospital drugs were prepared and compounded mostly in Apothecary General Craigie's shop in Carlisle, Pennsylvania. Three miles beyond Yellow Springs, at Red Lyon or Lionville, was located the Uwchlan Quacker Meeting House. This building was undoubtedly the first church in that neighborhood, commandeered for hospital use. The minutes of the meeting of the first month, eighth day, 1778, record that:

"A few days ago, the key of the Meeting House was demanded by some of the physicians of the Continental Army in order to convert the same into a hospital for their sick soldiers. The Friend who had the care of the house refusing to deliver it; forcible entry was made into the house and stable."

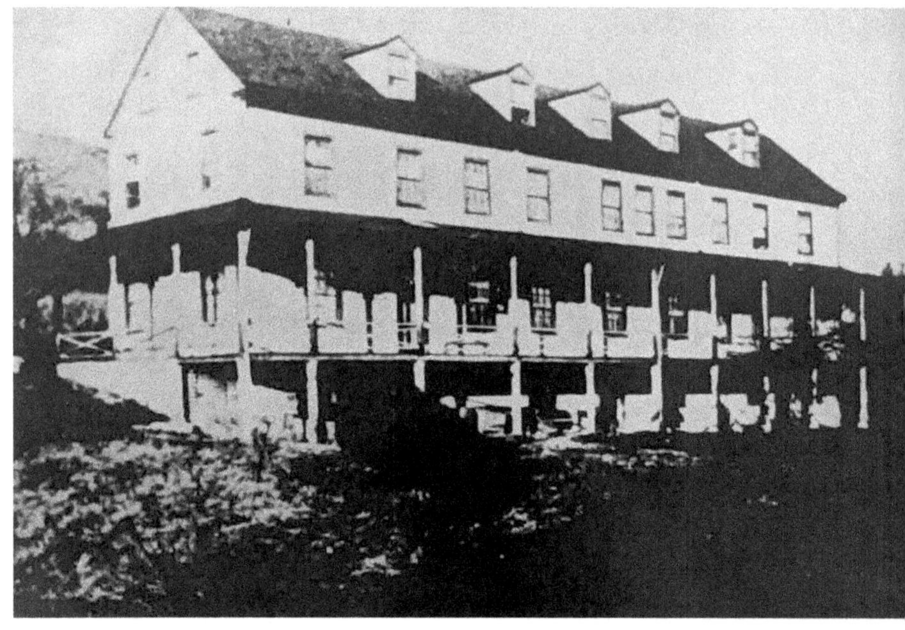

WASHINGTON HALL Medical Headquarters of the Valley Forge Encampment, located at Yellow Springs, Chester County, Pennsylvania. Erected 1778. Destroyed by fire in 1902.

Several months later, the Lutheran Zion Church and the German Reformed, with their common parsonage at French Creek, a few miles north of Yellow Springs, were also ruthlessly possessed. The Rev. Henry Melchior Mühlenberg, the patriarch of the Lutherans in America, thus related the circumstances in one of his periodical reports to the Halle Fathers in Germany:

"During the past winter, spring, and summer, he (the Rev. Ludwig Voight) has had a great deal of sorrow and trouble because a spiteful commissary and a surgeon of the American Army... both of his had taken over churches for hospital use and had put sick soldiers in them. Yea, they had even filled the parsonage also and had afflicted him with all kinds of persecution because he refused to publicly pray for the Congress and because he was thought to be a Tory. However, after a German chief surgeon (Bodo Otto), well known to us and belonging to our Church, was appointed to command this district, and before whom our complaint was laid, he immediately ordered that the house should be cleared of soldiers."

The newly established hospitals in the neighborhood of Yellow Springs must have been well organized before February 1778, for in that month, an order was issued at Valley Forge that:

"The commanding officer of each brigade shall appoint a Captain of the Day to visit the sick near camp and ascertain whether they are properly attended and furnished with everything their situation requires, as far as circumstances will permit."

It was in February 1778 that Dr. Jonathan Potts assumed his office as Purveyor General of the Hospital Department of the Continental Army, with the duty of paying salaries and dispersing money to cover incidental hospital expenses, besides purchasing and distributing all supplies and medicines. Dr. Potts' correspondence then became voluminous, and it is from his collection of letters that much of the data contained in this chapter was obtained.

Anticipating a great need for spirituous liquors for the hospital, a proposition was submitted to Congress in January 1778 for the erection and operation of two distilleries to be located in the Middle division. It was represented that a private citizen had offered to purchase and improve the necessary land if supplied with copper for making the stills and the working capital to carry on the business and that he would engage to repay the whole amount within three years in whiskey at one dollar a gallon and pork at seven dollars per hundred pounds. He also agreed to supply large quantities of vinegar at ten and two-thirds dollars per barrel. It was represented that private distillers were taking advantage of unusual demands and the fact that no whiskey could be imported; that this activity was also affecting the market price of grain. The statement was made that under existing conditions, whiskey was costing the hospital two and one-half dollars a gallon; vinegar twenty dollars a barrel; and pork thirteen to fourteen dollars per hundred pounds. Claims were made that the expense of fattening hogs would be negligible, as they could consume the refuse of the distilleries, and that the entire plan would effect a saving to the government of $60,000 a year.

Army departmental lack of cooperation evidently delayed the completion of the Apothecary General's shop at Carlisle, Pa., for on February 24, 1778, a letter was written to the President of the Board of War:

"There is a large quantity of oil and sulphur in the hands of the Commissary of Military Stores which they can spare and of which we stand in need. Our laboratory and stores for ye reception of medicines, etc., belonging to the Military Hospitals, cannot possibly be finished without we obtain assistance from the different magazines and artificers in this place. We, therefore, pray the honorable Board of War to give an order to Major Lukins to deliver those articles and such assistance as from time to time shall be required by the Apothecary General of the Middle department at Carlisle.

"We have the honor to be,

"Dear Sir,

"Your most obedient humble servants,

Wm. Shippen, Jr ., D. G. Jonathan Potts, P. G."

Carlisle, Pa.

The Apothecary Department, like all others, had difficulty in meeting the demands made upon it, and on May 1, 1778, Dr A. Craigie, the Apothecary General, wrote Dr. Potts:

"I did not find the medical stores in that order which I expected, and much exertion is necessary to so render it. We have many important medicines but by no means an assortment sufficient for the army. There are medicines in different places, of which I have no list, and I conceive it necessary for the person who has the immediate management under your direction to know what medicines, etc., are engaged in the department in order to ascertain the deficiencies.. for the department is at present in chaos no regularity-no system, but with your assistance, I will put it on a respectable footing.

"I beg leave to query whether this will not be the [adopted] plan.

To have the principal store at Carlisle, where all the medicines shall be prepared and the chests completed. Under the supposition that the general hospitals will be more collected and the number lessened, I would propose that an apothecary attend each with a complete chest of medicines, that the surgeon and physician general of the army be attended by an apothecary with a good chest, and that the regiments be supplied upon the Northern plan. I would have an issuing store at a convenient distance from the army, from which the hospital and regimental chests might occasionally be replenished.

"I enclose a list of our wants; they are great and many. We are destitute of almost everything necessary for regimental chests, among the rest, of bottles. Pray give me leave to urge the propriety of setting the glass works going at Manheim."

In March 1778, Dr. Potts began receiving reports and inventories from the different hospitals. One from Dr. Solomon Hallings, written on the sixth, from Rheimstown, recited:

"By bearer of this, you will receive, according to your order, a report of the sick with returns of the stores and medicines for the use of the hospital in this place.

"I have also sent a return of the clothing, as I did not know but that it might be necessary."

The Rheimstown hospital was among those that were hurriedly opened in December of 1777, and it is evident that it was continued for any great length of time, for the visiting chaplain recorded in his diary on April 16, 1778:

"This day rode to Rheimstown, where I supposed there was a hospital; continued the five miles to Dunker's Town (Ephrata)."

The Manheim hospital inventory, as taken on March 7th and reported by Hugh James, Hospital Commissary General, consisted of:

"11½ Pipes of Madeira Wine
2 Barrels of Port Wine
220 Gallons of Molasses
31/½ Hogsheads of Spirits
250 Pounds of Coffee
3 Barrels of Salt
7 Barrels of Herring
15 Barrels of Sweet Oil
3 Tierces of Rice
8 Tierces of Brown Sugar
250 Shirts
170 Pairs of Stockings
36 Pairs of Overalls
10 Blankets

"It should also be noted that to the above may be added 27 Tierces of sugar, 12 quarter casks of Port Wine, besides 77 Tierces of the same in the hands of Banet & Co. at that town."

The large and important hospital (established in Moravian Community Buildings) at Lititz was opened by Dr. Kennedy in December 1777. Here, he remained until transferred to Yellow Springs, probably in January of 1778; Dr. Latimer then became senior surgeon at Lititz. When Dr. Wm. Brown was elected Physician General in February 1778, he made this place his headquarters. The Lititz hospital was abandoned in August 1778, and its patients were transferred to Bodo Otto's hospital at Yellow Springs.

In the last part of February or the first part of March 1778, Dr. Shippen conferred with Dr. Brown regarding the needs of the entire medical department. The result was that the following tabulation, compiled by Dr. Brown, was sent to Dr. Potts bearing Dr. Shippen's endorsement:

20 Pipes-Madeira Wine	£ 18,000
20 do port	12,000
100 Tierces Rice	4.000
500 Barrels Indian Meal	3,000
100 Barrels Herring and Shad	1,000
300 Bushels Salt	1,800
50 hhd Muscovado Sugar	40,000
50 do Molasses	25,000
1000 pounds Loaf Sugar	1,500
1000 Coffee	750
1000 Bohea Tea	4,000

1000 Chocolate	1,250
300 hhd Vinegar	9,000
100 Barrels Barley	1,000
20 hhd Spirits	10,000
Lard; Soap, hard and soft; Candles	
Herbs, Cups, Bowls, etc.}	5,000
3000 Blankets	24,000
6000 Shirts and Sheets	24,000
Spoons, Dishes, Chamber Pots, Buckets,	
Pails, Tubs, Brooms, Scrubbing Brushes	
Iron Pots, Kettles, Ladles, Knives & Forks }	2,000
100 Reams of Wrapping Paper	500
1000 Fine and Coarse Teeth Combs	500
50 Reams Writing Paper	500
Pins for Bandages and Twine	500

	£192,300
Medicines, Vials, Corks, etc	20,000

	£212,300

Dr. Brown supplemented this list, as the result of further thought, in a letter under date of March 11, 1778.

"To Dr. Jonathan Potts, P. G.

at Reading, Pa.

"Dear Sir:

"Before you receive this, Dr. Shippen will have delivered to you a list of stores and medicines which we were of the opinion would be wanted for the hospitals during the present year.

"The list was made out by me at a time when my head was very unsteady and confused from the weak state in which the fever had left me. I have, therefore, no doubt omitted some very necessary articles. I have since recollected a few of them and dare say there are more which I hope you (knowing them to be necessary) will add as they occur to you or present themselves during your search for the rest. At present, you will oblige me by adding to the list:

"3 dozen sets small apothecary weights and scales

3 dozen Bolus (pills) knives

2 dozen sets large weights and scales (the latter may be made of wood) for use by the commissaries to issue sugar, rice, barley, etc., by weight

2 dozen measures from ???

6 dozen earthen vessels (deep) different sizes, with handles, of from two-quart to two-gallon capacities for boiling decoctions or two

dozen copper dittos of one gallon for the same purpose

1 dozen bedpans for the use of very weak patients who cannot get up

2 dozen spades or shovels

2 dozen common axes

6 dozen delftware tiles for mixing Bolus (pills), etc., on

"Our hospitals are very defective in these articles at present, and we are often at a loss what shift to make for want of them. Let me urge you to immediately add the above articles to your list when you receive this letter and before it falls aside and you forget it.

"P. S. I beg to leave to say one thing more; that I do not think we are upon a right plan for procuring lint from the Moravian Sisters, and as far as I see, those two houses at Bethlehem and this place are the largest and principal sources from whence we may expect supplies of that necessary article, which is used in our hospitals in such large quantities. I think that if particular persons at each place were employed and money put in their hands (perhaps three or four hundred dollars at a time) to receive and pay for the lint as fast as it is made and at the same time to urge that business, the effects would be great. At the present, they are careless about it. At this place, I believe they have entirely left off making it because there is no one to receive and pay for the lint. I don't know how it is at Bethlehem. If you think it proper to adopt this mode, I would recommend that Dr. Alison be employed for that purpose at this place... and Mr. Horsefield, the apothecary, at Bethleherpose at this, formerly employed for like service by Dr. Shippen and collected a large quantity of lint from the Sisters.

Yours, W. B."

Dr. William Brown, P. G., was born in Scotland and receivedhis medical degree at Edinburgh in 1770, after which he emigrated to Alexandria, Virginia. He was a friend of Washington and Jefferson and entered the Continental Army service in September 1776. In January of 1778 Dr. Brown was elected Physician General of the Middle division to replace Dr. Benjamin Rush. It was while living at his Lititz headquarters that he wrote a pharmacopœia for use in the Continental hospitals. The Physician General resigned his commission in the summer of 1780, and before leaving the army he wrote a letter to Dr. Bodo Otto, commending him for faithful and noteworthy service rendered. Dr. Shippen's call upon Dr. Brown at Lititz was made at the beginning of an inspection trip of the outlying hospitals in order that he might obtain a personal impression of conditions as well as to determine which, if any, might be abandoned. March 20, 1778, found the Director General in Allentown, where Dr. John A. Otto was then stationed, and from here he wrote Dr. Potts:

"All the commissaries hereabouts are out of cash. I shall advance them what I can spare, on your account.

"Beef is very scarce, and no assistance can be obtained from the Army Commissary. The thing to do will be to break up these (Allentown, Easton, and Bethlehem) hospitals as soon as possible.

"Do write to Mr. James to send immediately a wagon with stores, wine, rice, barley, and whiskey, etc., for these three hospitals."

On March 24th, Dr. Shippen again addressed the Purveyor General from Kingswood:

"Yours by Express found me at this place. The stores which you said were in Okely's hands, he told us were sent on to you, but Colonel Abell has found some wine which Bond will make use of.

"I found the hospitals at Easton and Allentown in such good order that not above sixty or seventy remain in them. All sick not fit to go to camp, I have ordered sent to Bethlehem.

"If you have an opportunity, do send to ye Yellow Springs for a return of everything there and keep it until I arrive in Reading, which will be in about ten days. Princeton Hospital returns will soon be sent in."

The hospital at Easton was immediately closed, but the one at Allentown remained open until after April 6, 1778, for on that day, the Rev. James Sproat recorded that he had then prayed with the sick.

Apparently, most of the patients cared for in this neighborhood were about ready to be discharged, for on April 3,

1778, the hospital chaplain reported he had that date addressed one hundred convalescents in the Bethlehem hospital.

This favorable condition and the fact that the army at Valley Forge required more hospital capacity resulted in the abandonment of the Brethren House and the transfer of the entire Bethlehem hospital staff to the neighborhood of Yellow Springs.

The history of the Brethren House Hospital with its overflow of patients into tents and an emergency constructed building, has been often recorded, but it is not generally known that a separate hospital unit was established in the Fulling Mill. Here, woolen cloth has been processed as a department of the Moravian activities. The building stood not far from the main hospital on a mill-race leading off Monocacy Creek. It was 108 feet in length and also contained a grist mill.

It is a matter of published records that part of the fuller's living quarters, located in the mill, was used as a surgeon's mess hall and that a Mr. and Mrs. Carr of Philadelphia had been quartered there when ill, but proof that the building was also utilized as a hospital for the continental sick was found in a very remarkable letter written by a soldier to his commanding officer.

"Major Johnson,

Sir:

"I do hereby accuse my wife of robbery committed on the body of Captain James Grier of the first Pennsylvania regiment, commanded by Colonel Chambers; said robbery consisting of one silver watch, two thirty dollar bills, one five dollar bill, and some small bills at present not remembered.

"The above thief, Mary Myler, lives at the Fulling Mill Hospital under Dr. (Bodo) Otto.

(Signed) Mat. Myler."

The morale of the Valley Forge Army was at a low ebb in March 1778. Food was scarce, soldiers were becoming more sickly, and many officers were demanding discharges or leaves of absence. On the 24th, General Washington wrote:

"As it is not improper for Congress to have some idea of the present temper of the army, it may not be amiss to remark in this place that since the month of August last, two or three hundred officers have resigned, and many others, with difficulty, dissuaded from it."

Among Dr. Rush's papers is a notation that the Valley Forge encampment in March 1778, was "dirty and stinking; the men filthy and ragged" and that they had been allotted only "three ounces of meat and three pounds of flour in seven days." He also wrote that "fifteen hundred horses had died for want of forage."

The official forage allowance at Valley Forge was fourteen pounds of hay and six quarts of oats for a saddle horse, but a draft animal was given twelve quarts of oats and sixteen pounds of hay. Regulations also provided that double rations of grain might be issued in lieu of any hay or a double weight of hay if grain were not available.

With lessened demands upon the hospital stores in the Northern department, an order directed that certain supplies be sent to Valley Forge for the use of the Flying Camp. Writing of them, as well as of other needs, Dr. Cochran, the Surgeon General of the army, said:

"To Dr. Jonathan Potts, P. G.

Reading, Pa.

"Dear Sir:

"Camp Valley Forge March 22, 1778

"I received yours of the 17th inst. with the articles agreeable to the invoice, for which we thank you. I sent all the articles to the Flying Hospital stores except the loaf sugar and spirits to be divided by our commissary among the sick in camp and the inoculated patients. I have also sent the commissary two barrels of brown sugar, chocolate, and wine which I brought in my return sleighs from Albany.

"A quarter cask of wine was stolen out of the sleigh on the way down. It was taken at a Committee man's house, where it was thought to be very safe.

"I thank you for your promise of the instruments; they are very much wanted, and the sooner you forward them, the better.

"Medicines are much needed here, particularly camphor, of which we have not a particle.

"A number of troops from the southward are expected in camp in the course of two or three weeks. They are ordered on without taking takin the smallpox and, consequently, will be inoculated somewhere near camp. Molasses in abundance will be expected for the purpose of supplying these people, and the sooner a small quantity for present use is forwarded, the better."

Dr. James Craik, A.D.G., from his stations in camp, sounded the first alarm that sickness among the soldiers was increasing and that resulting demands on the hospitals should be anticipated. In a letter to Dr. Potts dated April 7, 1778, he wrote:

"On my way to Manheim I visited Yellow Springs and Red Lyon hospitals, which I found in excellent order, and they have but few sick at present. However, as the army is becoming more sickly, we may expect they will soon be full.

"Dr. Fallon gave me the enclosed list of wanted stores. What you see checked on the paper arrived in a wagon while I was at Yellow Springs. Whether the quantity of wine ordered is not rather too much at a time, you will be the better judge. You will please have the needed stores sent as soon as possible.

"You will also find they are in want of a steward. If you have any in your eye, you may send him; if not, let me know, and I shall look out for one.

"Dr. Shippen requests that you immediately have wine laid in at Manheim for the hospitals at Lancaster and Lititz as they are in great want of it.

"When the army moves from Valley Forge, it is more than possible there will be at least one thousand soldiers to immediately go to hospitals. It will be necessary, therefore, that I know the ones you would choose to receive them, as well as the number each can take, that I may be ready.

"Tomorrow morning, I shall set out for Headquarters, where I shall be ready to receive your commands."

The list to which Dr. Craik referred read:

"Stores wanting at the Yellow Springs, Red Lyon, and Franch Creek Meeting House for the sick and wounded there:

"Common salt-one barrel arrived
1 Pipe, Madeira
2 Pipes, Port
1 Hogshead, Rum-arrived
1 Whiskey-arrived
1 Vinegar
1 Sugar-arrived
1 Barrel, Barley
Coffee
Chocolate
Soap and Candles
400 Shirts
100 Pairs Sheets

"N. B. Dr. Shippen is requested to supply this hospital with a steward of character; we have none now.

(Signed) James Fallon."

Another consignment of supplies from Reading reached Yellow Springs on April 24, 1778, and this was acknowledged by Alexander McCarake, the headquarters commissary, to Samuel Morris, Commissary General of the hospitals.

"Sir:

"I have received from John Hevener and Peter Hoover wagoners 428 gallons of vinegar, 47-bed cases, 58 sheets, one box of lint, and one box of bandages.

"There are two sheets and one-bed case wanting of the number you mentioned in the service.

"I have sent you two empty hogsheads and one pipe.

"I am just out of cash and want an immediate supply.

"N. B. The sick are suffering for want of wine."

Within three weeks from the date of Dr. Craik's warning to Dr. Potts of an expected increase in sickness, the hospital needs so expanded that the Purveyor General was hard-pressed to meet all the demands made upon him. The result was that while some requisitions were promptly filled, others were delayed. Dr. Craik's requests were evidently among those receiving deferred attention, for on April 26, 1778, he wrote impatiently:

"I have repeatedly written for stores to be sent down here immediately, particularly molasses and wine. I sent an Express to have those things hurried, and he returned without bringing me an answer whether I might expect them or not. I am now under the necessity of sending another Express to you upon the same account, for the army and hospitals are suffering for want of those things.

"The molasses here will not last longer than tomorrow, and there are at least one thousand under inoculation. Of wine, there has not been a drop in the hospitals for three weeks past. Unless these things are supplied directly, the greatest clamor will be raised that has ever yet been. I must, therefore beg and pray that you will instantly furnish us with them and that an Express may be sent to hurry them with all expedition.

"Ten or twelve hogsheads of molasses, at least, are needed. Wine, both in the Flying Camp hospitals and others, is exceedingly wanted.

"I wrote Dr. Bond, too, for a supply of necessities for opening new hospitals and have not received an answer whether or when I am to receive them. If I am not supplied with what I write for, it will be impossible for me to give satisfaction here, and the hospital service will suffer.

"In two days I expect complaints will be lodged, and I shall be at a loss what excuse to make.

"Dr. Tilton has written me for a junior surgeon and mate to assist

him at Wilmington. Please send two proper ones to be sent on to him. "The hospitals are now full of sick, and I have neither utensils nor the necessities required to open new ones. You may easily guess what distress I am in. The General will not have the sick sent to hospitals at any great distance from the army so that I shall have a number of barns and other houses to open, but this cannot be done without proper conveniences. You will please prevent the distress that must ensue from want of these things, by giving us a speedy supply.

"Please inform me by return of the Express when I may expect the molasses and wine and likewise the other things."

The requisitions from the surgeons at Lititz on April 27, 1778, were less important than many others but, nevertheless, were essential for the comfort of the sick.

"A few articles much wanted at this hospital, which Mr. Malsby informs me he brought from Bethlehem and left in Reading:

"6 Large Washing Tubs

2 Large Iron Pots

4 Dozen Wooden Bowls

1 Dozen Brushes (sweeping) Chamber Pots

Combs, etc.

"We have never been supplied with these things, consequently stand in great need.

"You will please send by the same wagon, the sugar and tea you were so kind as to promise me.

"Your very humble servant, Francis Alison

Senior Surgeon

"P. S. Dr. Brown presents his compliments to you and will also thank you for some tea and sugar."

The two following letters from Dr. Kennedy and Dr. Fallon, both written at Yellow Springs and on the same date (April 27, 1778), seem to be contradictory but may have reflected a shortage of certain supplies and a sufficiency of others. Then again, Dr. Kennedy may have thought he stood a better chance of having his needs promptly filled by expressing appreciation of past consideration rather than by registering complaints or demands.

"The bountiful supply lately given these hospitals (three barns) most certainly entitles you to ye hearty thanks of every person who wishes health to these brave defenders of the

American cause. Permit me then, Dear Sir, to tender you my grateful acknowledgment on behalf of the sick and, in the interim, to acquaint you that in consequence of Dr. Craik's order, we have opened a Convalescent hospital about two miles distant from here, for which we are in great want of furniture of almost every kind.

"Putrid fevers abound greatly, and the sick crowd in fast; hence, we are in great need of wine. Cider would also be very acceptable.

"To you, dear Sir, we look for the supply of all our wants, not doubting but that the same patriotic benevolence which has ever distinguished your character will still continue to render the brave sons of liberty as happy as possible.

"(Signed) Samuel Kennedy."

Dr. Fallon's plea was for present and future consideration, with no reference to what was past.

"I lately wrote a few hurried lines to Dr. Bond on the subject of our wants.

"To you, I make bold to repeat the same supplicating suit. We want, my dear Sir, wine above all things, for our sick are numerous, and our cases generally putrid. Officers, wounded in the conflict with worms as well as of Mars, crowd in upon us, and from the reputation of our hospitals, they call for wine and threaten excision if they do not get it.

"We also want sheets, shirts, iron spoons, candles, soap, writing as well as wrapping paper, pots, and every other kind of hospital utensils.

"Our number here at present is about 250; our hospital is neatly arranged, clean, and healthy. Dr. Cutting will tell you the reputation it is now in, with the whole army. I wish that you would soon come to visit us.

"Dr. Craik informs me that His Excellency will not allow any more sick to be sent from the camp to the back hospitals; therefore, a proportionate number of barns and meeting houses in this vicinity are to be taken over for that purpose.

"The commissaries of this place and the Red Lyon are in want of money.

"P. S. We are likely to lose Dr. Wodgson, a mate, of putrid fever."

General Washington had issued orders on January 21, 1778, that the Director of the Hospitals should furnish the regimental surgeons with medicine chests for camp use. The available supply of necessary drugs was then so limited that it was not until April that a start was made. On the 16th of that month, Dr. J. B. Cutting, Apothecary General, wrote Dr. Potts on the subject:

"Dear Sir:

"Yellow Springs.

"Our dispensing store is opened here, and we have begun to supply the regiments in camp, but I am very apprehensive that the several hospitals in this vicinity will render a further reinforcement necessary before we shall be able to complete the whole. Many regiments have no chests, and many who have them are deficient in surgeons.

"I have not yet been able to get a return of the number of regiments in the army but suppose at present there are at least eighty, including artillery. Dr. Cochran has given orders to the division on the left to bring their chests first, and we propose going through the entire army in the order in which they now lay. To give only a few of the capital medicines to each will be the work of time and a much more intensive piece of business than I first imagined. The best method that I can think of is to act immediately about preparing new chests at some convenient place for all such battalions that did not get chests from Dr. Craigie in the last campaign. When these new parcels are ready, let us call all the large chests into stores; these are too capacious for field service, so in lieu of them, we will issue smaller ones. By this exchange, the General Hospital will be well supplied with standing chests and acquire a great variety of useful articles which are not essential in camp."

Between the dates of April 19 and May 3, 1778, the commands of Generals Patterson, Leonard, the first and second Pennsylvania brigades, and those under Generals Poor, Glover, Scott, and Woodward, including the entire division of Lord Stirling, turned in their medicine chests to Apothecary General Cutting at Yellow Springs, and every regiment received a standardized field box containing a definite list and quantity of necessary drugs and supplies.

Following is the invoice of those things thought essential for the protection and health of soldiers in the field or camp:

Two fluid drams Tincture Cinnamon

Two fluid drams Elixir Paregoric

One and a-half fluid drams Spirits Lavender Compound

Two fluid drams Ol. Ricini (Castor Oil)

One and a half ounces Balsam Traumatic (Wound Balsam)

Twelve ounces Spt. Sal. Vol. Amon. (Aromatic Spirits of Ammonia)

Two fluid drams Elixir Vitriol

One and a half drams Ol. Tereb. (Oil of Turpentine)

Two fluid drams Bals. Capsici. (Balsam of Capsicum)

Twelve fluid ounces Tincture Myrth and Aloes

Two fluid drams Laudanum Liquid Two fluid drams Sal. Tart. (Salts of Tartar)

Three and a half drams Linimentum Saponis (Soap Liniment)

Two fluid drams Pulverized Cream of Tartar

Two fluid drams Elixir Bol. c. Op. (Elixir Bolus cum Opium)

Two drams Jalap

Three-quarters dram Cantharid. (Cantharides)

Twelve ounces Pulverized Ipecac One dram Fluid Oc. Cani Four drams Rhie (Rhubarb)

Four drams Sal. Nitri (Salt of Nitre)

One dram Comp. Cardiac 700 bandages

Ounce and a half Gum Myrrh Drams, three-quarters Gum Guaiac

Twelve ounces Gum Ammon.

Two drams Arabic

One dram Gum Opium

One dram Aloes Sac.

Two and a half drams Rad. Gentian

Two drams Rhei. (Rhubarb)

Four ounces Cont. Peruv. cort. (Peruvian Bark)

Two drams Fol Sena

One and a half drams Fl. Sulphur

One dram Nutmegs

One dram Cinnamon

Two drams Sago

Three drams Cort. Aurant (OrangePeel)

Six drams Sal. Ammon. So.

One dram Emp. Epispaticum

One dram Emp. Diach, C. G.

Two and a half drams G. Camphor

Two pewter Syringes
One-half dram Tart. Emet.
Two ounces Vit. Alb. (Vitrolum Album)
Two ounces Mercury (Corrosive sublimate)
Two ounces Merc. Precip. rub. (Precipitated Rhubarb)
One pewter, ounce and a half measure
Four ounces thread
Seven common needles
Six quires writing paper
One set scales and weights
One spatula
One pocket dido
One plaster knife
One scalpel
One steel director
One silver probe
Two pieces tape
One-half-thousand pins
Eight common Tourniquets with Ligatures
Thirty-four dozen splints
Six dozen compresses
One dram Stomach Magest
Two paper ink powder
One-half dram twine
One-quarter-hundred quills
One set amputating instruments
One dozen trepanning do.
One-quarter dram Cara Flav. (Yellow Caraway)

Six yards flannel

Four drams Ung. E. Lapis. Cal.

Three fluid drams Ung. E. Gum Elemi

Three fluid drams Alba Camp. (White Camphor)

Three drams lint

Two pairs shears

Four dozen worsted caps

One bundle rags

Three fluid ounces Flo. Chamomile

Chests, Bottles, Pots, etc.

Three drams Sperm Aceti

Six drams Sapo. Vir.

One loaf sugar

Two drams Emp. Diach. Sim. (Simple diachylon)

A Revolutionary period journal kept by one of the Hartman family who lived in the vicinity of Yellow Springs records how the German farmers of the neighborhood collected meat, flour, potatoes, cabbages, and other foodstuffs, together with straw and clothing, and presented them to General Washington for his men. It also tells how the farmers' wagons regularly returned from camp loaded with sick soldiers for distribution among the surrounding hospitals and how smallpox and putrid fever became epidemics.

Again, it related to the kindness of the neighborhood people and that the wife of Zachariah Rice died from a malignant fever contracted in the hospital where she had gone to distribute food.

In the spring of 1778, there was a strong suspicion of Tory sympathy among some of the personnel of General Washington's bodyguard. Stories have been handed down of plots to seize His Excellency and even of attempts by poison upon his life.

Acting on the recommendation of the Commander-in-Chief's own staff, a new guard was organized, composed almost entirely of Germans recruited from Berks and Lancaster counties. This body of men, known as the Independent Troop of Horse, was commanded by Major Bartholomew von Heer, a veteran officer of the Seven Years' War in the service of Frederick the Great. Faithful to their trust until the end of the war, General Washington chose twelve of the company to attend him on his homeward journey to Mount Vernon. In appreciation of their devotion to his person, his Excellency presented the twelve with their horses, arms, and accouterments, besides giving them many remembrances.

Scurvy must have prevailed in the army to some extent during April 1778, for in that month, a William Bell of Lancaster wrote Dr. Potts he was delivering two barrels of lime juice and holding five additional ones, subject to further orders.

Dr. James Tilton of Delaware entered the service as a regimental surgeon in 1776 and was later transferred to the General Hospital. He accompanied the Brandywine wounded sent to Princeton, and easy stages made the journey with rest stops in Philadelphia, Bristol, and Trenton. In February 1778, Dr. Tilton obtained leave of absence following an attack of putrid fever at Princeton, with permission to remain home until restored to health. He was then assigned to a hospital in Newport, Delaware, which was removed to the Nottingham Meeting House near Wilmington. From both places Dr. Tilton wrote to Dr. Potts of his hospital requirements and of some business he had undertaken for the Medical Department.

"Dear Sir:

"Newport, April 22, 1778.

"Since the first of March I have had charge of this hospital for the reception of sick from General Smallwood's division.

"I have just received a letter from Dr. Shippen directing me to expect my future supplies of medicines and stores from you. We have the occasion of an immediate supply of both. The stores we want are wine, coffee, and tea. The enclosed list will show you the medicines we need.

"The hospital is to be removed from this place to Nottingham brick meeting, where I shall be glad to receive a supply as soon as possible. Besides the ordinary sick of the garrison, we have about fifty recruits under inoculation and expect a great many more.

"Dr. Latimer requested me, in your name, to purchase a number of lancets of Major Aiken at some distance from this place. As soon as I could take the time, I waited upon the Major and purchased fifty (all he had) for twenty-nine dollars. I shall send all of them to you, except three or four, which will be necessary for the use of this hospital.

"I expect in a few days to have the Turner's business set up in a manner that will probably, in a short time, furnish as much of that kind of ware as you have occasion of. I don't know what the expense of the work will be and shall be glad of your direction whether it may go on to greater expense than the $300 sent me by Dr. Latimer. I am, dear Sir,

"Your most obt. Serv. James Tilton."

No attention was paid to Dr. Tilton's communication of April 22, 1778; another was forwarded:

"Dear Sir:

"Nottingham, May 8, 1778.

"Having received no return of my letter written to you about a fortnight ago from Newport, I expect it has miscarried.

"Several medicines absolutely necessary to our hospitals being entirely exhausted, I am under the necessity of sending an

Express Messenger and if you will be pleased to furnish them to the Bearer, he will bring them in his saddle bags.

"We have had no wine since the hospital was removed to this place. I have been obliged to substitute strong beer in many cases of great weakness.

"The Turning business is going forward at Couches' Mill near Christiana Bridge, but I don't know what progress they have made. Two Turners with two hands to help them are at work. I find there is a very good Turner in this neighborhood, and if you have the occasion of great dispatch in this business, he might probably be engaged.

"Our number of sick and wounded is commonly about eighty, besides which we have at this time 150 being inoculated, and the new recruits coming in daily will probably increase our number.

"I will thank you for some printed diet boards.

"P. S. Be kind enough to send everything prepared, for we have neither mortars, pestles, nor sieve to powder anything."

The "Turning business," which Dr. Tilton mentions in both letters, had been authorized by Dr. Brown, the Physician General, through his assistant, in an effort to establish a plant to manufacture wooden bowls, an article of many uses in the hospitals. It may be remembered that in a letter already quoted, Dr. Latimer once requisitioned four dozen for Lititz from a reserve supply in Reading.

Among Dr. Potts' papers were found many scribbled calculations and memoranda, which probably formed the basis of his numerous appeals to Congress for funds. One contained information that the pay of the surgeon officers and attendants at the hospital, including forage, vegetables, milk, etc., was running $20,000 a month.

Another, dated April 10, 1778, gave the

"Estimated expense of vegetables, milk, mutton, veal, and bread for 3000 sick under inoculation for three months £27,000

"Estimated expense for the pay of officers, surgeons, mates, matrons, nurses, orderly men, apothecaries, clerks, and forage for three months..27,000

£54,000"

A frequently depleted reserve of food available for hospital use greatly disturbed the Purveyor General, and when hurried attempts were made to purchase supplies in the common markets, hospital agents found themselves in competition with those of the army. In the hope that he might obtain his needs from the Continental storehouse or that some plan of cooperation might be adopted, Dr. Potts addressed a communication to the Commissary General of the army and directed Dr. Craik to seek a personal interview and discuss the subject. The result of the effort will be found in the letters which follow.

"Camp Valley Forge
May 2, 1778

"Sir:

"Your favor of the 27th of April received, and I am exceedingly sorry I cannot comply with your order respecting meat. Beef cattle are so scarce that it is almost out of my power to support the army from day to day, nor is it part of my duty to furnish the hospitals, though I have done so and have never refused when provisions were plenty of to spare in the neighborhood of camp. You have many persons engaged to furnish the necessary provisions wanting for your department they paid if proper might accomplish it, who, your people to be attention when they cannot procure provisions from but the application those you have appointed for that purpose. Lancaster County can produce good veal and mouton with some young cattle sufficient to supply a hospital of 2500 men this two months. If you expect any assistance from (which in meat cannot be before the month of June), you will dismiss all those persons whom you have appointed to purchase (and on which account the price of provisions has been raised ten per cent) and call upon me for what provisions you want for the hospital (or any article I can purchase in the Middle department), which shall be supplied regularly according to your demand or so far as I can procure it. Enclosed, you have an order on Major Edwards at Grubs' Works, who will furnish you with flour for the Lititz, Ephrata, and Schaefertown hospitals. Matthias Slough of Lancaster will afford you flour for that place and what small beer he can procure.

"When the Commissary General returns to camp and I have the opportunity of seeing you, we will adopt some mode of your being regularly supplied.

"Your most Obed't Servant, Eph. Blaine, D. C. G."

"To Dr. Potts Lancaster"

"Commissary Office May 1, 1778

"Sir:

"You will please furnish Dr. Jonathan Potts or his order with such quantities of flour as he may order from time to time for the use of the hospital at Lititz, Ephrata, and Schaeferstown, taking duplicate receipts for the same, and oblige,

"Your most humble Servant, Eph. Blaine, D. C. G."

"Major Thomas Edwards at Grubs Iron Works."

Dr. Craik's letter to Dr. Potts on May 2, 1778, six days after he had written a protest on having his requisitions ignored, reflected a more serene frame of mind due to the arrival of some greatly needed supplies.

"I have the pleasure to inform you that we have been supplied with some molasses by the Commissary General, which kept things easy until your supply arrived.

"Wine is what we are in great need of at present, and I wish you would immediately order two or three pipes sent down from Carlisle, one to camp and two to Yellow Springs.

"I have sent for rice today, Colonel Cox having promised to forward it immediately. It was ordered to be sent some time ago, but wagons could not be had. At present, we are entirely without in camp. However, I hope we shall be supplied in a few days.

"The oil came some ten days ago but went to the Commissary General, and he had disposed of a quantity of it before I knew. I never received your former letter about it as it fell into Dr. Cochran's hands.

"In opening the new hospitals, we shall be much at a loss for pots, caps, bed ticks, sheets, and shirts unless you can supply us. Perhaps you can do this from those hospitals you have broken up.

"No sick will be sent to any of the hospitals above unless we should move toward the enemy. Indeed, I do not know that any will be sent then as it is probable the huts will be employed for that purpose, as they will be much more convenient to the army.

"The hospitals here are in fine order and much approved of. If they are well-supplied, I hope they will keep up their character. We have not any barley, so sending some of that article will be proper.

"Agreeable to your request, I waited on the Commissary urging the necessity of supplying your hospitals above with flour and beef. He seemed very willing to do everything in his power to assist us but, at present cannot spare any meat to you. This, I believe to be true, for it is with much difficulty he is able to supply the army from day to day. If he undertakes to assist us with meat, he expects to have the doing of it exclusively as your purchasers and his interfere with each other. However, this you will see in the enclosed letter. The order he issued is also enclosed.

"We shall, I suppose, be soon preparing for tents. It will be necessary that the hospital tents be made ready and sent down. Lancets, pocket knives, and all other kinds of instruments are much wanted at present.

"I have been confined to the house [Moorhall] with a severe pain in my ear which has prevented my visiting the Yellow Springs, so I do not know what stores have arrived there within these few days. "The medicine chests are much wanted by the regiments. Dr. Cutting had best have them filled as soon as possible to prevent complaints. "I suppose you have had all the good news from France, so I need not repeat them. We are in great spirits and expect to have a Feu de Joie soon.

"James Craik."

News of the defeat and surrender of General Burgoyne's Army by the Americans reached France in December 1777 and was received with great rejoicing. Treaty negotiations with the French Government immediately quickened, and on the 16th, members of his Majesty's Council of State informed the Continental commissioners:

"That after long and full consideration of your affairs and propositions in after long and full consider, this Majesty was determined to acknowledge the independence of the United States and make a treaty with you." This information reached General Washington at Valley Forge on the 1st of May, 1778, and on the 5th, he announced in Orders:

"It has pleased the Almighty Rulers of the Universe propitiously to defend the cause of the United American States and finally by raising us up a powerful friend among the Princes of the Earth to establish our Liberty and Independence upon lasting foundations. It becomes us to set apart a day for gratefully acknowledging the Divine goodness and celebrating the important event that we owe to His benign interposition.

"The several brigades are to be assembled for the purpose at nine o'clock tomorrow morning when their chaplains will communicate the intelligence... offer up a Thanksgiving and deliver a discourse suitable to the occasion."

The following day was therefore spent in parades, the firing of salutes and general rejoicing, while his Excellency provided a collation for all the officers of the army and his guests. Another celebration was witnessed on May 11, 1778, when some of the officers at Valley Forge presented Addison's play, "Cato."

Dr. Craik's expectation that the Valley Forge huts would be used as hospitals after the army broke camp was not realized, for the records prove that all reports regarding the patients left behind came from Yellow Springs. It is possible that some soldiers were too ill to be moved, and a temporary hospital was maintained for their care. In fact, Dr. John A. Otto's pension application sustains such an idea, for he wrote that he had attended hospitals at both Yellow Springs and Valley Forge.

On February 3, 1778, Congress resolved:

"That every officer who holds, or shall hereafter hold, a commission from Congress shall take and subscribe the following oath or affirmation: I,______do acknowledge the UNITED STATES OF AMERICA to be a free, independent, and sovereign State and declare that the people thereof owe no allegiance for obedience to George the Third, King of Great Britain; and I renounce, refuse, and abjure any allegiance or obedience to him; and I do__________ that I will to the utmost of my power, support, maintain, and defend the said United States against the said King George the Third, his heirs and successors and his or their abettors, assistants, and adherents, and will serve the said

United States in the office of___, which I now hold, with fidelity according to the best of my skill and understanding.

"Dated ________

Signature.

"Witnessed__________"

For some unknown reason, no action was taken to comply with the requirements of Congress until May 7, 1778, when General Orders at Valley Forge provided:

"In order to accomplish the essential work of administering the Oaths of Allegiance as early as possible, the following officers are to administer the oaths and grant certificates to the officers of the Divisions, Brigades, or Corps set against their names, including the Staff.

"Major General Lord Stirling, to the officers of the late Conway Brigade.

"Major General de la Fayette, to that of Scott's and Woodford's Brigades.

"General Knox, to those of the Artillery in camp and officers of Military Stores.

"General Poor, to those of his own Brigade.

"Brigadier General Varnon, to those of his own Brigade.

"Brigadier General Wayne, to those of the First and Second Pennsylvania Brigades.

"Brigadier General Mühlenberg, to those of his own and. Weeden's Brigade

"Brigadier General McIntosh, to the North Carolina Brigade.

"Major General Greene, to administer the same oath and grant like certificates to the officers of his department.

"Printed copies of the oath will be lodged in the hands of the Major and Brigadier Generals to facilitate the business. The generals administering the oath are to keep a duplicate of the same and grant certificates when made.

"In the beginning of the oath the name, rank, and the corps of the party making said oath are to be inserted. The duplicate certificates are to be returned to headquarters by the generals."

On May 11, 1778, a supplemental order was issued to the effect that:

"The general officers are requested to meet at headquarters at 11 o'clock tomorrow A.M. that they may take the oath appointed by Congress published in the orders of the seventh."

Many of these original documents can be found in the archives of several different departments of the Government in Washington. Among them are the oaths of allegiance administered by Major General Greene on May 25 and 26, 1778, to Doctors Bodo Otto, Frederick Otto, Samuel Kennedy, and Ebenezer Crosby, all of Yellow Springs.

Dr. Craik again wrote to Dr. Potts on May 10, 1778:

"I had the pleasure of writing you two days ago when I mentioned the probability of our moving soon. I, this day, directed to have things in readiness to have all the sick of the army taken care of in case the army should make a sudden move, and to enable the Flying Camp hospital to go along with the army.

"Tomorrow morning, I shall send an Express to Dr. Shippen to send immediately all the surgeons, Juniors, and Mates that can be spared from above to attend the sick that will be left on the grounds, as there will not be less than fifteen or seventeen hundred. I scarcely believe the army will remain here three days longer.

"You will please order down everything you think will be wanted. If Dr. Bond could come down, I think it would be proper, for it is probable I shall go with the army or soon afterwards. I think from present appearance, we shall shortly be in Philadelphia, but how long we shall stay there is uncertain. Perhaps we may have a trip to New York.

"Send down bandages, lint, such instruments that you have, sugar, vinegar, and all necessities of which I wrote that can be got.

"As I expect, we shall be in a great bustle in a very little time. You may depend upon it I shall do everything in my power for the best.

"P. S. Send Dr. Latimer down immediately."

Dr. Craik's enthusiastic belief that the army would break camp within three days was not to be realized and by May 15, 1778, he was writing of the problems that then faced the hospitals at Valley Forge.

"As I am willing that there should be no cause for complaint against our department, I embrace every opportunity to inform you of our wants. I have just returned from Yellow Springs and that neighborhood where I have given directions that additional hospitals be opened. More stores, of course, will be needed and as the following articles are scarce, a fresh supply is immediately wanted of coffee, tea, chocolate, vinegar, writing paper, pots, kettles, and salt. All of these will be required in large quantities as a number of hospitals must be supplied. The Flying Hospital is in need of vinegar, so I wish you to send a couple of hogs heads directly.

"I am sorry Dr. Cutting went away before the regimental chests were finished, for there is great clamor about them, though a Dr. Lugman is as busy as possible. I am afraid there are not enough medicines here to keep the regiments supplied. I hope Dr. Craigie will soon have his chest ready.

"I should be glad to know how wagons are to be furnished to the different hospitals. They will require some one constantly with them to supply wood.

"Assistant commissaries will be wanted for the new hospitals. Let us be furnished with a quantity of beds, tubs, sheets, and blankets as soon as possible; otherwise, the sick can never be kept clean and comfortable. It will be necessary to send down a quantity of money, as the commissaries are in much distress from lack of cash. The surgeons are likewise anxious to have their pay. The money I brought down will go only a very little way. I think Mr. Morris had best come down as soon as he can and settle with the commissaries, for paying the people punctually will make them more ready to oblige besides keeping our credits good.

"I think if you would procure a person of character who can properly keep books, it would not be amiss to do so, for such a person could take charge of the stores at Yellow Springs, enabling Mr. McCarake to better attend to the outside business. When you send down a proper supply of stores, the care of them will be of considerable importance. It will be proper to keep us well supplied with vinegar, for there is much demand for it.

"His Excellency went out to the Yellow Springs two days ago to visit the hospitals and found them in fine order. He spoke to every person in their bunks, which exceedingly pleased the sick. He was highly pleased to find the hospitals in such order. If we can keep up this character, we shall do very well.

"I am sorry that the general store of necessities is at such a distance from the hospitals as it is a long time before they can be received after written for. A little time now will determine whether we shall get into Philadelphia. Various are the opinions at present. By all accounts, it would appear that the enemy is soon going somewhere. Forage and heavy cannons are being put aboard the transports, as well as wood and water.

"Many of our soldiers are ordered into tents. They begin to be more sickly than they have been, but wagons cannot be conveniently had to carry the sick to the hospitals.

"I wish that Dr. Cochran's dispensary chests could be sent soon, for he could then stop the mouths of the noisy."

Dr. Craik's request that money be sent for use by the commissaries in settling outstanding bills resulted in Dr. Potts sending Dr. Bond to obtain cash from Congress. On May 17, 1778, Bond reported:

"I have been to York Town and, by a steady attention to the Lords of the Treasury, received a warrant for $100,000. The cash, however, cannot be obtained until next Saturday. With great difficulty, I procured leave from Blodget, General Greene's aide, to let Helleges give me $12,000 for present necessities if only to keep the devil out of our pockets.

"Out of that sum I send you and Sheets $245 cash. I gave Craigie, the Apothecary, $4,000 more."

Anticipating a movement of the army, many soldiers who were serving in various hospital capacities were needed for military duty.

So on May 1, 1778, Dr. Craik informed Dr. Potts:

"The General desires all the orderlies to join their regiments by the first of June, and we have already had some scuffling with several colonels about them. I wish some method could be fallen upon to employ women that can be depended on. The General says we may enlist them for at least the same money as are paid soldiers, for he can no longer bear having an army on paper and not have them in the field.

"We still receive fresh accounts of the enemy's preparations to move somewhere, as they are putting their horses, cannons, and heavy baggage on board and seem to be in great confusion."

Considerable excitement prevailed throughout the Valley Forge camp on June 16, 1778, by reason of the information that the British were evacuating Philadelphia, and this was reflected in Dr. Shippen's hastily written note to the Purveyor General.

"Yours by Mullady just received. Dr. Craik is not here now. Mullady, wife, nurses, and furniture are wanted in the barns under Dr. Jackson between here and Reading. Let them come immediately.

"I wrote you this morning by Express that we expect to go to Philadelphia tomorrow morning.

"Two deserters, who have just come in, say that only the grenadiers were left in ye city to guard it and that they had orders to roll up their blankets and be ready to match this morning."

From several of these quoted letters, it is evident that the officers expected General Washington to occupy Philadelphia before making a move to contact the enemy. However, on June 18, 1778, the Commander-in-Chief led his men in their march through Bucks County across the Delaware at Coryell's Ferry to meet the English in the Battle of Monmouth on June 28, 1778.

Meanwhile, back in Valley Forge, the sick of the army had been left behind to be gathered together and quartered in the Yellow Springs hospitals or among the new ones established for the purpose. The executive officers of the Medical Department either accompanied General Washington into New Jersey or transferred their quarters to Philadelphia, so Dr. Bodo Otto was left in charge as director of all the hospitals in the Yellow Springs neighborhood.

The Library of Congress Collection of Revolution War papers includes a report from Dr. Shippen that:

"The total number of ye sick in ye different hospitals within the vicinity of the Yellow Springs together with the discharged and dead solders since the last return taken on August 10, 1778:

Brigades	Sick	Discharged	Dead
Woodford's	60	22	17
Glover's	23	30	4
Knox's	30	11	2
Scott"s	69	33	8
Leanerd's	48	16	5
Mühlenberg's	81	35	11
McIntosh's	57	14	12
Smallwood's	68	21	4
Weeden's	43	10	2
Varnum's	12	28	7
Wayzes'	5	18	7
Conway'z	74	22	7
Poor's	75	116	24
Patterson's	40	60	17
Manfield's	8	2	2
Total	725	445	124

In September 1778, Bodo Otto made a report of the Pennsylvania patients in his hospital at Yellow Springs, listing their names and regiments. They belonged to the second, third, fifth, sixth, seventh, ninth, and tenth regiments and totaled thirty-eight men. The hospital record of one individual was also included.

Private George Tilson, 1st Pennsylvania Line, was shot through the left leg at Trenton, New Jersey, on January 2, 1777;

transferred from General Hospital at Bethlehem to Lititz on December 20, 1777, and thence to Yellow Springs.

Seven years later, this soldier applied for a Pennsylvania state pension and requested an attestation of his wounds by the surgeon who had him in charge. The reply was:

"I do certify that George Tilson, a private soldier in Captain Willson's Company, 1st Pennsylvania Regiment, was sent on the 28th day of August 1778 from the hospital at Lititz to the one at Yellow Springs under my care; he having a wound in his left leg. By examining the wound, I found that it would require a long time before it could be healed, if ever, and he, having friends in the neighborhood, begged for a furlough, which was granted. He returned sometime afterwards and begged for another furlough, which was also granted. In the meantime, the hospital was broken up in September 1781.

"Given under my hand in Reading, the 15th day of October, 1785.

"Bodo Otto

"Late Senior Surgeon and Physician of the Middle Department."

The archives of the American Philosophical Society contain a paper that reflects the transfer of the army to other fields and records by omission, the closing of many hospitals that existed near Valley Forge the year before.

An imperfect return of established hospitals, officers, horses, and wagons necessary for the Medical Department. (The Southern department is not included.

Hospitals	Officers at Each	Sick at Each	Horses at Each	Wagons at Each
Fort Pitt (Pa.)	5	30	2	1
Philadelphia	12	130	14	10
Sunbury (Pa.)	4	40	3	1
Pluckemin (N. J.)	10	15	5	1
Basking Ridge (N. J.)	5	55	4	1
Albany (N. Y.)	12	140	6	3
FishKill (N.Y)	10	80	6	1
Trenton (N. J.)	4	20	3	1
New England	25	200	19	4
Flying Camp	10	136	14	2
Yellow Springs (Pa.)	6	65	3	1
	103	911	79	26

"The magazine of stores and medicines is at Philadelphia for the Middle and at Danbury and Springfield for the Eastern Department.

"December 31, 1779.

William Shippen, Jr. Director General"

The winter of 1777-78 was believed to have been unusually severe, but the diary of the Chaplain, Reverend James Sproat, records:

"January 11, 1780. Set out this morning for the hospital at Yellow Springs extremely cold riding against the wind. Stopped at the 'Sign of the Buck' then rode on to Mr. Todd's and lodged.

"January 12, 1780. This morning there were snow squalls with extreme cold. Mr. Todd accompanied me to the Springs. The lanes were filled with snow-traveling bad indeed. The weather thought to be colder than it has been for the past twenty years."

By this time, the Yellow Springs Hospital had been organized solely for the reception of those suffering from lingering illnesses and for treatment and rehabilitation of the badly wounded. Finding himself critically short of supplies on May 19, 1780, Bodo Otto sent an appeal for relief:

"To the Honorable, the Committee of Congress for Conducting the Medical Department:

"The memorial of Bodo Otto, surgeon of the hospital at Yellow Springs, showeth,

"That the hospital at the Yellow Springs now, and for some time past, has been maintained for the reception of those afflicted chiefly with chronic disorders, and our necessary stores for the sick are entirely exhausted. There is no money in the hands of the Commissary to purchase fresh provisions, so the sick have been obliged these several past days to eat salt provisions. There is but six days supply of bread on hand, and the gentlemen who have furnished us that article as well as meat for the past two years now refuse to supply us any longer. "Can it be supposed that a physician or surgeon can gain credit for perfect cures under these circumstances?

"The assistant physicians complain daily that they have not received any money for their services these past seven months; neither are they furnished with clothing, so it is uncertain how long they will be able to continue in their several capacities. The nurses and orderlies refuse to serve any longer, as they have received no pay. This being the de plorable situation of the hospital at Yellow Springs, your Memorialist entreats your Honors to take the matter into consideration and order some speedy relief, or the sick and wounded must unavoidably suffer. He is loath to complain without cause, but as the hospital has been under his direction for these past two years, supported with credit hitherto, he should be sorry to see it rendered useless and of no importance, His Excellency, General Washington, ordered the officers that if in case the sick are likely to suffer and not be relieved by the department they are to report the same to him."

Bodo Otto once again found himself in great need, and he, therefore, addressed:

"General Pickering. Honorable Sir:

"After my best respects, I think it proper to give you the earliest advice of the wants of this hospital for fire wood and straw, which I think are to be supplied through the channels of your department [Quar ter Master's], particularly fire wood, of which we are entirely destitute, and unless very shortly furnished we must inevitably greatly suffer. Neither have we had any straw lately nor can I obtain any for my patients' beds and must do without, though straw is essential for their comfort. Major Howell, Q. M. in Downingtown, has lately directed these supplies, but the adjacent inhabitants, who have hitherto assisted in their carriage and the furnishing of such necessities, having received no consideration for same in cash for upwards of nine months past, are discouraged. It is, therefore, impossible for my commissary to keep us sup plied therewith when he has no expectation of receiving the money to pay for his former contracts (at any reasonable time) nor promises for the future.

"I flatter myself. Your Honor will be pleased to forward my requisitions and adopt effectual means for our relief, which I hope and trust will be in a short time.

"August 26, 1780,"

Many claims of inhuman treatment of captives were made by both the British and Americans and were the subject of frequent letters between the respective Commanders-in-Chief. The English maintained a prison in New York Bay on board a condemned sixty-four-gun man-of-war, and the infection and disease, always present, were responsible for more American deaths than all the bullets of His Majesty's Army. "Old Jersey, the Hell," as the prison ship was known, became so unseaworthy because of worms, that she eventually sank at her anchorage. The names of 8,000 of 11,000 Americans there confined during the war have been preserved, and among them are Peter and Henry Hinch, Henry Hallman, three Chester County, Pennsylvania, boys whose families lived in the neighborhood of the Yellow Springs. News of their capture reached the parents in January 1781, and a petition was drawn immediately and sent to the President of the Pennsylvania Assembly.

"May it please your Excellency,

"We beg leave to lay before you the situation of Peter Hinch and Henry Hinch, sons of John Hinch and Henry Hallman, the son of Michael Hallman, all of the Township of Pikeland in the County of Chester, whom the Fortune of War has thrown into the hands of the Enemy.

"The fathers of these young men have, by their willingness on every occasion, shown their patriotism and fidelity to their country and being desirous to support their children during their captivity with every necessity, they now by the hands of their sons, George Hinch and Michael Hallman, the younger, do send them some money, etc., to relieve their necessities.

"We hope that your Excellency will be pleased to afford them such assistance as you may think most proper that these brothers may be successful, they being young persons of known integrity, during the present contest. "We are your Excellency's most obedient and obliged humble Servants.

"January 23, 1781. Yellow Springs.

"Bodo Otto

William Evans Peter Hartman, Major Frederick Otto John Reily, Captain, S. G. H.

Alexander M. Careche

John Heyl"

The existence and value of the hospital at Yellow Springs were again threatened by a shortage of supplies and medicines, and once more, Bodo Otto addressed the Continental Congress. The Journal of February 8, 1781, records:

"A letter of the 7th from Bodo Otto, physician and surgeon, was read; whereupon it was ordered that the letter from Dr. Otto be referred to the Board of War to take measures for preventing any interruption being given to the hospital at Yellow Springs; the same being maintained solely for the reception of proper hospital subjects."

Eight months later, in September 1781, a committee of Congress decreed that the three most important military hospitals, located in Boston, Albany, and Yellow Springs, should be abandoned. Dr. John Cochran, the then Director General, strenuously opposed this order, even soliciting the aid and influence of General Washington to have reconsidered, but without success. False economy and lack of appreciation of their need and importance was the explanation given to Dr. Otto when Dr. Cochran directed him to send his patients to Philadelphia and hold himself in readiness to report to some other hospital where his services would be most needed.

The last official evidence of the Valley Forge encampment thus disappeared from the neighborhood. Once more, the country thereabouts resumed a peaceful appearance, and the inhabitants returned to their everyday pursuits. Many of the soldiers who expired in the hospitals of the Yellow Springs group lie sleeping in unmarked graves on hillside farms, and local historians point out the places where they rest.

It would be a fitting tribute to the memory of these neglected heroes of the Republic, for whose independence and future they suffered and died, should take title to these hallowed spots and thereon erect

"Monuments to the Unknown
Soldiers of the American
Revolution."

CHAPTER FIFTEEN

PROFESSIONAL FEUD • Rush • Morgan Shippen- Correspondence and Criticisms Otto's Opinions Evidence

IT WAS NATURAL that Shippen, Morgan, and Rush, educated at the same University in Edinburgh, should unite their efforts to establish and develop a medical college for the American Colonies. Shippen probably had visualized such an institution growing out of the lecture school he proposed starting on his return to Philadelphia. Morgan's conception of the same hope was better and more thoughtfully planned, for he dreamed of a medical department within the College of Philadelphia and discussed the idea with several retired trustees then living in England.

Immediately on his arrival home in 1762, Shippen publicly announced his intent to give a course of instruction in midwifery and shortly afterwards supplemented this subject with a series of anatomical lectures.

Dr. John Fothergill, the English physician, evidently believed Morgan would be associated with Shippen in the proposed lecture school, for in commanding the plan to professional friends in Philadelphia, he wrote that an able assistant would join Shippen in Dr. Morgan.

Shippen's school had been in existence for three years when Morgan returned and presented his plan to the trustees of the College of Philadelphia. This undoubtedly was the reason for raising a question of precedence, in which both Rush and Adam Kuhn supported Shippen's claim of teaching seniority. It also caused the beginning of an undercurrent of resentment and jealousy between the two men.

It is true that to Morgan belongs the honor of being the first appointed professor in the Philadelphia Medical School by virtue of an action taken on May 3, 1765, when the trustees adopted the Morgan plan, but four months later, when Shippen applied for the Chair of Anatomy and Surgery, he wrote:

"I should long since have sought the patronage of the Trustees of the College but waited to be joined by Dr. Morgan, to whom I first communicated my plans in England and who promised to unite with me in every scheme we might think necessary for the execution of so important a point."

In the newspaper announcement of the Medical School on September 26, 1765, over the signature of Wm. Shippen, Jr., Professor of Anatomy and Surgery, and John Morgan, Professor of Medicine, Shippen's name appears first, as well as the details of his lecture course, thereby suggesting a public recognition of seniority.

Rush, a younger man by nine and ten years than either of the principal members of the Medical College staff, carried on an extensive correspondence from Edinburgh with Morgan and urged his own qualifications and claim to a professorship. Anticipating installation in the chair of chemistry, he suggested and submitted an inaugural address in which he stressed the importance of chemistry in its relation to medicine. Unfortunately, this paper gave recognition of Shippen's seniority over Morgan in the faculty and brought a protest in such strong language that Rush retorted with an ill-timed angry letter. Morgan's reply to this epistle, a strong and wordy one, follows:

Rush's Manuscript 25-1

Ridgeway Library

"Philadelphia, May 10th, 1769.

"Sir:

"When a misunderstanding once creeps in betwixt those who have lived on terms of friendship and professed regard for each other, it is generally productive of such animosity as persons between whom there has never subsisted any like degree of intimacy, seldom know. To prevent, if possible, the evil consequences that would ensue both from a breach of good understanding and to prepare the way for an amicable explanation and adjustment of some points not rightfully understood by one or another of us so as to maintain an uninterrupted harmony for the future, is the design of this letter.

"I shall be glad, therefore, whenever you are at leisure to return the visit of congratulation which I intend to make upon your arrival [in Philadelphia] that we may discuss matters amicably.

"Could disputes be prevented? It would afford me much pleasure. Should they happen notwithstanding my inclination to avoid them, I am determined to give no handle to censure for hastily yielding to that resentment which your offending letter intended to inspire.

"If there were any honesty in those eulogies you have in all your former letters bestowed on the friendly offices I have without ceasing done for you ever since I knew you and the very confidence which you acknowledged I gave you, I deserved a more generous and polite treatment at your hands than those attempts of wit and those ebullitions of an angry temper to which you have given vent in your last letter. What was the cause of this behavior? Why, I informed you, could I not have known of your having placed my name in the manner you had done in the designation of your thesis? For this, indeed, you could have made some sort of an apology, which I might have thought sufficient if I could be persuaded that the offense was accidental and that you gave me no room for charging you with having designedly and knowingly paid a compliment to another at my expense.

"In no letter that I ever received did you declare it to be accidental or undesigned, as your last asserted. All that you wrote to the purpose was that you did not think I would have taken it amiss or it should have been otherwise. But how you could imagine I would take it in good part is beyond my comprehension, especially as I was informed by a person whose veracity I do not think you would call in the question of a conversation you had on this subject with a gentleman at Edinburgh previous to the publication of your thesis, who knowing from yourself what was the order in which you designed to place the respective names, told you I was the oldest medical Professor but you maintained a contrary opinion and gave it to him as a reason for your placing.

"I mention this circumstance, which I otherwise would have chosen to suppress lest you should impute my punctilious exactness to a wrong cause.

"When a person has singled out from the number of his acquaintances one whom he would serve and patronize to the utmost of his power, it is natural to suppose if he finds anything which denotes the least suspicion of doubtful conduct or unfriendly return that he has a right to question that man and to expect the satisfaction of positive assurance that the information or suspicion was ill-grounded and to declare if this is not given, he shall esteem it no injustice to alter his conduct or continue to serve one that he deems ungrateful. Nor is it a breach of either honor or friendship to set forth the acts of kindness he has shown in hopes that what he has done and suffered for the person may induce that person to more readily give the satisfaction he demands. But that the mention of them with that view should be considered as upbraiding the person whom he had obliged and cancelling all former obligations is a doctrine wholly new to me.

"I always imagined, so foolish was I, that a man without some fault of his own may reap a lasting benefit both in reputation and fortune as long as he lives from obligations conferred where the good effects are permanent. I say I was so ignorant as think such obligation tion perpetually to binding and that when I have received such I was in duty and conscience compelled to make a due return or rashly disown the force of them. Had it once come into my head before hand that you entertained different sentiments from these, believe me, you never should have accused me of upbraiding you with the favors I have done you.

"When a man is fundamentally wrong in any grand article of belief, he commonly falls into a series of errors. This seems to be my case. I, whimsically conceited, wrote in confidence to you who pretends obligations or friendship for me to prevail on you to do me justice in a point of honor as of a sacred nature and to go no farther without my permission. But I find I was quite in the wrong here again and that men are released from all obligations of trust and confidence if it suits their convenience or inclination.

"Whatever you may suppose were the motives, the true and only reasons I had for insisting upon your not divulging the contents of that letter without permission were that it was not written for the perusal of any one but yourself and the fear that over hastiness of temper would tempt you to make a wrong use of it. Besides, should any misunderstanding arise betwixt you and me, I did not mean that other persons should be involved. But particularly I conceived Dr. Kuhn's behavior to me as being very unfriendly in a certain affair and that yours now appears very similar. I thought it not amiss, therefore, to acquaint you in what manner such conduct wounded me expecting that you would be the more ready to satisfy me in regard to your own behavior on the point of such delicacy, but did not mean you should trumpet it to others. Nor did I think the freedom I took with Dr. Kuhn gave you any right by disclosing the letter or bringing him into the dispute. A too great sensibility of injuries may have carried me further then my cooler judgment would approve in what I said of Dr. Kuhn. But as he and I have adjusted our differences, I hope we shall not renew them. Your declaration that out of tenderness for me, you had not shown my letter to my friends on the other side of the water but that you would keep it however and make proper use of it on your return, I despise. Now you know the reasons for my former prohibitions, make what use of that letter you please. I well know that unguarded expressions, while inoffensive when uttered to a man of honour, may prove a firebrand to kindle coals of contention in the hand of one who suffers himself to be governed by passions or who is defective in the principles of honour.

"Had you, instead of writing such a letter as your last, cleared up matters, it would have been more to the purpose. Had you simply declared that you thought me a younger professor in the college or that the dispute of seniority and precedency had never entered your head, I should have entertained regard for your candor and been satisfied; judging my information to the contrary arose from some mistake. But instead of this, you fly into a passion for seeming to dispute your word that it was a mere accident and not design, which by the by I never heard before, and to turn the tables by accusing me of cancelling all obligations for dealing plainly with you. It appears to me more like an act of evasion than an ingenuous behavior to one whom you still acknowledge to have conferred the highest favors upon you.

"I remove the misconstruction you seem to have put on my words. I find myself under the necessity of referring to some passages in your letter that contain strange insinuations.

"I had written to Cap't. Russel, among other things, that the dispute of seniority and precedency which had existed between Dr. Shippen and myself was at a full meeting of the Trustees of the College, determined in my favor. I told you that Dr. Kuhn's behavior, which had so sensibly affected me, tended to support Dr. Shippen's pretension to precedency although determined as above and further that the order in which you had placed our names had the like tendency as far as anything you could do, to support a claim already declared to be groundless. I urged that on this account. It was most necessary I should be made acquainted with the motives of your conduct whose cause I had so warmly espoused, for if you still thought yourself right, I was exerting myself for one, who instead of subscribing to the suffrage of the Trustees might do all he could to weaken their authority and to break through the established order of the college; for if you interested yourself in favor of any junior professor you would do the same for yourself although you acknowledge yourself to be chiefly indebted to me for the professorship of chemistry if you do obtain it. "In return, you insult me thus:

"Pray don't suffer the resentment of and his friends on my account. But before you make the choice of him, let me beg of you... that your reasons for it were because I had unhappily, for want of thought, placed Dr. Shippen's name before yours in my inauguration dissertation and that you were afraid if I was elected a professor I should dispute precedency with you. These are the very words of your letter; words are not easily to be forgotten.

"Can you really imagine that if you are elected a professor, you would have any grounds for disputing precedency with me or if you were to entertain any thought of such a thing that I am afraid you would meet with any success? If this is the meaning of your letter, let me tell you that such an apprehension was as far from my thought as the pole is distant from the pole.

"If you do not force my words to speak foreign to easy construction of them, I do not expect them to make such an impression on your memory as to obliterate the favors you have received from me. Remember that if you do not satisfy me of the integrity of your conduct, I declare you had no reason to expect the same vigorous exertion of my interest in your favor, but I in no wise intimate, however, that I would do the least thing to oppose what has already been done in your behalf or obstruct your way to the professorship of chemistry. So that the force of your irony, like an engine recoiling back on him that uses it, can injure none but yourself.

"I wish I knew your intentions in bringing Dr. Redman likewise so malapropos into your letter or could reconcile the sentiments which you have so often communicated to me concerning him with the observance of that divine precept you mention of 'speaking evil of no man.' I can not declare, your letters say, 'I ever received a single idea from Dr. Redman. I owe him no obligation; he never conferred a favor on me of any kind, but such as he was bound to do by the common rules of decency and good manners, though I pounded his mortars and posted his books six long years to deserve them. May he live to see the base ingratitude for his conduct to me.'

"This last pious wish of yours may throw some light on what you mean by the pleasure it would afford you to soothe the infirmities of his approaching old age and rock the cradle of his declining life.

"All I need to say further at present is that I shall be glad to have done with disputes and, if possible, live in peace with all men. Disputes are ever odious, especially among men of science, as they lay themselves open to the censure and abuse of even the lowest set of mankind.

"During the present misunderstanding between us, my lips have been hitherto sealed, nor has aught escaped my pen to make it known to others. If you had observed a similar conduct it would have been well.

"Differences between acquaintances are more easily remedied when they are unknown to the world and not widened by frequent discussions of them. I shall be glad to set you right and to be set right myself in what is amiss and then to forget what is past. In the meanwhile, I remain.

"Sincerely,

"Your most obedient and very humble servant,

"To Dr. Benj. Rush"

"John Morgan

The grammatical construction of this letter is so involved that it is difficult to understand and impossible to parse. In order that it might be more easily read, some liberty has been taken with the arrangement, but it in no way changes the subject matter.

The cause of this early difference with Dr. Shippen must have cut very deep into the memory of Dr. Morgan for, fourteen years after its occurrence, he dragged the story again into the light. It had little relation to his grievance over being removed as Director General, but in the summer of 1779, Dr. Morgan related the incident in The Pennsylvania Packet as proof that Dr. Shippen's grasping for rank and recognition was no new failing. He wrote:

"On the 20th of May 1765, about a month after my arrival from England at a public commencement of the College of the City, I had the honor of laying before the Trustees a plan for ingrafting a School of Physics on the original design of the Institution.

"I was already elected Professor of the Theory and Practice of the Physics and recommended Dr. Shippen to the Trustees for an appointment to the Professorship of Anatomy, and he was chosen to fill that place. Depending upon the influence he supposed he had among the Trustees, to degrade me from my rank as eldest Professor, which he pretended to claim, and to usurp precedence over me, he made an attempt but was foiled in it.

"The Trustees, at a full meeting, confirmed me in the rank of Senior Professor, of which fact the Hon. Edward Shippen, Esq., and Dr. Redman, two of the Trustees, were appointed to give us notice respectfully.

"Nothing but his envy then produced a contest for preeminence, which he called a misunderstanding."

Temperamentally, there was a great difference between Rush, Morgan, and Shippen. Shippen possessed a pleasing, easygoing, appealing personality; was excellent company and made loyal and lasting friends.

Morgan was more direct and serious in all his dealings but very jealous of his rights and dignity, while Rush was irascible, frequently changing his opinions and continually quarreling with friends and foes alike. John Adams' estimate of Rush, entered in his 1775 diary when Rush was 30 years of age, was: "Rush, I think, is too much of a talker to be a deep thinker-elegant, not great."

These outstanding figures in the medical life of Philadelphia worked harmoniously together for a number of years in spite of characteristic differences until the Revolutionary War was well advanced when the break came that resulted in attacks of great bitterness.

A number of historians have lightly touched upon the charges made by Doctors Rush and Morgan against Dr. William Shippen, Jr., Director General of the Continental Hospital. Usually, they expressed or implied a belief in Dr. Shippen's guilt of malpractice in office, regardless of official records to the contrary, viz.: first that a court martial organized by order of General Washington acquitted him on all counts; second, that Congress concurred in the verdict and reinstated him in office, and third, that when Dr. Shippen eventually retired, the Commander-in-Chief publicly commended him for the excellent service rendered in a most difficult task and during a time of great anxiety and trouble.

This vindication evidence would ordinarily seem to be most convincing, yet history has insinuated that Director General Shippen was lucky in escaping an adverse decision.

If a common belief of guilt were justified, why were the court martial charges not sustained? Surely, a miscarriage of justice could not have been due to an inability to collect evidence, for the Continental Congress and the Assemblies of Pennsylvania and New Jersey authorized Rush and Morgan to take dispositions where witnesses could not attend court.

Who were the principal witnesses summoned to appear at the trial, and what was the nature of the evidence offered to justify the indictment? What testimony was submitted by the defense in rebuttal? These are pertinent questions and the answers are very necessary to enable one to reach a correct opinion of the official decision.

Then follows another natural query of why, if the verdict were a proper one, hias Dr. Shippen's reputation been allowed to remain so long under a cloud when the minutes of the court might disperse it? Probably the answer to this question is that all such papers were stored in buildings burned by the British during the War of 1812. In any event, no pertinent documents can be found in the Revolutionary Archives in Washington.

Shippen always contended that Rush's intense hatred of him was the result of a belief that he had prevented Rush's obtaining army preferment or advancement and that he had finally forced Rush's resignation from the Medical Department; that Morgan's resentment and desire for revenge were due to an obsession that Shippen had schemed with friends in Congress to have him removed from the office of Director General, and that this was primarily that Shippen might have an opportunity to supplant him.

These were the grievances, real or imagined, that Shippen's friends thought inspired Rush and Morgan's attacks. Cruel charges, with and without sustaining proof, were sent to Congress as a whole, to selected groups of its members and to individual Delegates, to the Commander-in-Chief and even to the citizens through the newspapers until, after three and a half years of such intermittent bombardment, people and Congress were ready to believe the charges to be true. So, Dr. Shippen was eventually brought to trial.

In spite of the axiom in English law that a man should be considered innocent until proven guilty, it was only natural for the public to think that considerable proof must exist to warrant such serious accusations.

The fact that Bodo Otto, whose honesty, independence, and strength of character were universally recognized and whose humanity and sympathy for the sick and wounded soldiers had been so often manifested, appeared in court as a Shippen witness seemed a factor in the Director General's favor.

But the real question of guilt or innocence still remained unanswered, and with a desire to learn whether Bodo Otto was justified in his good opinion of Dr. Shippen or had been influenced by sympathy, the search for the missing proof was diligently made. The chance finding of a letter from James Lovell, a member of Congress, to his friend Samuel Holten, dated December 1780, supplied the long-sought clue for the court martial evidence. It said in part:

"You may amuse yourself, as one of the Medical Class, by reading the epistles of Rush to Shippen, in which you will find the writer has relieved himself a little upon me.

"Shenstone's benevolence made him wish he could afford to have his pockets picked frequently. I feel a portion of his spirit operating upon me at this time when I see poor Rush swelled near unto bursting, and I cannot doubt but that he finds some relief by throwing about his Slaver and Froth; therefore, when it falls upon my cloth, I slight the injury because he finds so much ease in his terrible case."

The letters referred to by the Hon. James Lovell were found in The Pennsylvania Packet, and here in editions between September 1780 and January 1781, appeared a recital of the testimony submitted by the principal actors and their friends.

The available evidence, as presented in the newspapers, will be restated throughout the next several chapters in their proper relation and sequence to the charges and to the trial. Considerable data, which has a bearing on the case but which may not have been available at the time of the court-martial, will also be offered.

It seems necessary to relate some well-known Revolutionary War history to understand the animosity between Rush, Morgan and Shippen and enable the reader to reach an independent opinion of the justice or injustice of the charges and the guilt or innocence of the accused.

CHAPTER SIXTEEN

SHIPPEN BECOMES DIRECTOR • Flying Camp Hospitals • Transfer from Field to Hospital Otto's

RESPONDING TO GENERAL WASHINGTON'S urgent appeal for reinforcement to meet an expected British attack in New York, Congress resolved on June 3, 1776, that a Flying Camp of 10,000 men is immediately established and further, that these troops be engaged to serve until December 1, 1776, unless sooner discharged.

The command was given to General Hugh Mercer, and on July 16th, he informed General Washington:

"I have just received a letter from the Hon. Mr. Hancock containing the order of Congress that I should march the Troops which are to compose the Flying Camp, to wherever the service requires in subordination to your instructions."

Congress also selected Dr. William Shippen, Jr. to organize and command the Hospital Department of this new army, and on July 16th Shippen received a communication reading:

"I have it in charge from Congress to acquaint you that they have this day appointed you Surgeon General and Director of the Hospitals of the Flying Camp... Should you accept the appointment, on the signification of such acceptance to me, I will immediately send your commission."

Whether Dr. Shippen solicited this position or knew it would be offered to him is unknown. Morgan contended the office was sought as a part of Shippen's scheme to supplant him, but the wording of the notification does not suggest it is being written to one actively seeking the commission but rather reads as though there were official doubts of Shippen's willingness to accept. Congress possibly remembered that only nine months before, he had declined to take charge of Continental hospitals as desired by General Washington.

June and July 1776 were busy months in all of the provincial counties of the Middle Colonies. Recruits were being enrolled, officers were chosen, and arms and equipment were issued. But little time could be spared for training, and the troops soon marched to the rendezvous of the Flying Camp in New Jersey. Meanwhile the British reinforcement had arrived by sea.

Having accepted the Hospital Directorship, Dr. Shippen was assembling the necessary personnel and collecting equipment in anticipation of expected demands upon them.

The disastrous battle of Long Island, which occurred on the last of August 1776, was the beginning of a series of conflicts in New York, necessitating General Washington's abandonment of that city and his retreat across New Jersey.

The hospital situation in New York, under Dr. Morgan, had become very serious even before the demands of the wounded upon it increased the problems. Morgan's refusal to issue medicines and supplies to regimental surgeons, because he expected a great need of them when the campaign was further advanced was not a popular or acceptable action. Officers and men and the regimental surgeons filed protests, and Congress sent a committee to New York to investigate conditions. On October 3, 1776, it reported:

"That the sick have been greatly neglected and a number, to the prejudice of the service, have died from want of necessaries and attendance."

Several days later, on October 9, 1776, Congress decided:

"That John Morgan Esq. should provide and superintend a Hospital at a proper distance from the Camp, for the Army posted on the east side of the Hudson River.

"That Wm. Shippen Esq. provide and superintend a Hospital for the Army in the State of New Jersey.

"That each of the Hospitals be supplied by the respective Directors with a number of surgeons, apothecaries, surgeon's mates and other assistants; also with such quantities of medicines as they should judge expedient; that no regimental hospital be in future allowed in the neighborhood of the general hospital."

This Congressional action was taken without consulting General Washington and, in fact, without even informing him of their intent. The resolution that divided the responsibility for the sick and wounded between these two men did not provide a directing authority to reconcile differences. Shippen wrote several years after that the division of the hospitals had been kindly meant for Congress, hoped it would thus reduce the demand for Morgan's removal and with a smaller army requiring fewer hospitals, he might satisfy everyone, but Shippen added:

"That the expectation was not realized, and the clamor continued and increased so much that they were obliged to dismiss him entirely or have no Army."

Dr. Morgan declined to accept a literal interpretation of the resolution of October 9, 1776, and continued to direct his surgeons in caring for the New York Army sick after they had been transferred to the Jersey side of the Hudson river. Therefore, on October 29 of the same year, Dr. Shippen wrote to General Washington from Newark, saying:

"My dear and Honored Sir:

"The winter approaches; the sick will suffer; many will perish unless timely care is paid to provide them proper winter apartments.

"The Congress have desired me to attend to the sick that are on this side of the Hudson River, but Dr. Morgan has directed his officers to follow his directions till they receive written orders from him or your Excellency to the contrary.

"I pray you will release me from my present disagreeable suspense and direct whether I am to superintend and provide for all the sick on this side, as I think Congress intends, or only those of the Flying Camp and Militia in New Jersey for which I was first appointed."

To this communication, the Commander-in-Chief replied on November 3rd:

"Although by the resolution of Congress, you are appointed Director General of the Flying Camp in New Jersey and Dr. Morgan for that of the Continental Army, which has lain on this side of the North River, yet I never imagined it meant to exclude either of you from the power of establishing hospitals on whichever side of the river you thought most convenient for your respective sick.

"Under the circumstances in which we left New York, we found it impossible to remove our sick up the Country on this side of the river. Dr. Morgan was therefore directed to provide and prepare hospitals for them in New Jersey to be under control of him and his assistants."

This difference in interpretation of Congress's intent put Shippen in an embarrassing position, and in his dilemma, he appealed for advice to General Mercer, his own commanding officer. Mercer replied on November 4th, directing him to lay the situation before Congress and adding:

"If the speediest measures are not pursued for the comfortable accommodation of the sick, now that winter has set in, many lives must be lost in a way shocking to humanity. I am well satisfied that nothing of the kind will happen when you take the lead."

General Mercer, a physician and surgeon by training and practice, had a proper appreciation of the medical problems of his army.

Acting under General Mercer's advice, Dr. Shippen wrote on November 9th:

"I think it proper to inform the Hon. Congress that I have not taken any of the Continental sick on this side of the North River, under my direction agreeable to their last regulation, because Dr. Morgan differs in his opinion with me concerning the meaning of Congress and because General Washington desires they may remain under his care, as you will see from the enclosed letter [dated Nov. 3rd] from his Excellency.

"The General makes no distinction between my appointment in July and your resolve of October and in my opinion has not seen the latter, which expressly says: 'all the sick on this side of the North River shall be under my direction.'"

Shippen's communication was referred to the Medical Committee of the House, and on Nov. 28, 1776, its report was submitted, and Congress further resolved:

"That Dr. Morgan take care of sick and wounded of the Army of the United States as are on the east side of the Hudson River, and that Dr. Shippen take care of the sick and wounded as are on the west side of the Hudson River, and that both be directed to use the utmost diligence in superintending the sick and wounded of the Army so that they may be effectively provided with everything necessary for their recovery."

Needless to say, this ruling was not cheerfully received by Dr. Morgan, but it enabled Dr. Shippen to proceed with a clear knowledge of the extent of his authority.

The sick and wounded soldiers of General Washington's forces were sent ahead of the retreating army, and distributed throughout Eastern Pennsylvania and in Philadelphia. Shippen accompanied many to Bethlehem, and it was here he received the resolve of Congress which he conveyed to General Washington, very diplomatically buried in the body of a communication on another subject. It read:

"Sir:

"Bethlehem Pa., Dec. 8th, 1776.

"I must mention to your Excellency that the moving of Dr. Morgan's Stores that have not been used these three months, has cost the Continental, I verily believe, as much as their first cost. Would it not be well to have them opened here, and the useful ones employed for the many sick who want them, and the remainder stored up?

"You know, Sir, how particular some folks are in doing business; your orders will be necessary.

"The Congress has explained their resolve and ordered Dr. Morgan's duty to lay entirely East of the Hudson River!"

This reference to Dr. Morgan's husbanding a reserve of hospital supplies seems to confirm the claim of the regimental surgeons and of General Greene that the Director General was inclined to withhold much-needed medicines that an ample quantity might be available to meet an emergency.

To Dr. Shippen's communication, General Washington replied from Trenton Falls on Dec. 12, 1776:

"Your proposition of opening Dr. Morgan's stores, I entirely approve and you are authorized to do so immediately, as it is in every event my ardent wish that the sick be provided for in the most happy manner our circumstances will admit, and I know of no good reason why stores should be preserved for a future day when they are so much needed at present."

It was shortly after the Battle of Long Island, where Bodo Otto served as surgeon of Pennsylvania troops, that Dr. Shippen selected him as one of the surgeons for the Flying Camp hospitals. The Berks County contingent suffered great losses in New York, and in a memorial addressed to Congress after the war, Dr. Otto wrote of the sudden attack and retreat at Long Island, where he lost his medicine and instrument chests.

The transfer from field to hospital duty must have been a welcome change to Dr. Otto, who, being in his 65th year, probably preferred the possibility of a more permanent location to the constant movement with the Army. Just when the promotion occurred or in what New Jersey hospital Bodo Otto served in 1776 is not a matter of record. A nurse's receipt, found in the Adjutant General's archives in Washington, indicates that he had charge of the commandeered Bettering House in Philadelphia, which was taken over in December 1776. Here, it is believed he remained until February 1777, when Congress directed that all troops be inoculated, and General Washington ordered that Dr. Otto be sent to Jersey to establish a hospital for that purpose.

The "Flying Camp" was conceived as an emergency measure, and those who enrolled were only obliged to enlist for a period of less than five months. No documents have been found that tell whether Shippen was answering an emergency call or planning to make a permanent position for himself, but when Morgan's troubles increased, and those in authority admitted that a radical change of hospital personnel was necessary, we find Shippen expressing a willingness to receive consideration in any contemplated change. If this were a change of heart after entering the medical service, it might have been due to a number of reasons. Someone with tact and prestige was needed to bring harmony and order into a department that was seething with discontent. Perhaps Shippen felt that he had the required qualifications and that it was his duty to try if those in authority wished, or maybe Shippen had enjoyed a taste of power as Director of the Flying Camp and decided he would take advantage of an opportunity to go higher.

In 1776, Dr. Benjamin Rush was on friendly and intimate terms with Dr. Shippen, and in a letter dated September 1776, wrote:

"The satisfaction you have given in your department will induce Congress to continue you if possible. I wish the same simplicity and economy were used in prescribing everywhere as we hear are used on the Hospitals under your care."

Again, on November 28, 1776, he said:

"I am bound in justice to good fidelity, to inform you that every person who comes from the camp speaks in the most respectful terms of your consideration toward the sick and wounded under your care."

In another letter, Rush expressed a belief that Shippen might continue in the service as Director without interfering with his private practice or lecture work.

Rush's letters surely indicated an unusual friendship for Shippen and suggested a willingness to promote Shippen's interest in Congress at the expense of Morgan, or perhaps it was because he believed that Shippen was the proper man to supplant Morgan. One also is curious as to whether the differences between them, indicated by Morgan's letter of May 10, 1769, still rankled with Rush and if there had not been more or less additional friction in the interval of time.

When General Washington crossed the Delaware into Pennsylvania early in December 1776, with the British following close behind, it was a grave question whether Philadelphia could be protected if the enemy crossed the river. Congress hastily removed to Baltimore, and Government stores and equipment in Philadelphia were transferred to points of safety.

John Morgan's removal from his position as Director General on January 9, 1777, was an act of Congress sitting in Baltimore, Maryland, and Rush, a member but absent in Philadelphia, addressed a letter to Richard Henry Lee as follows:

"Since my letter of this morning, I have heard of the removal of Dr. Morgan and Stringer from the Medical Department. I beg you would suspend the filling of their places till I have the pleasure of seeing you."

What did this letter signify? Was Dr. Rush seeking the position for himself, or did he wish to help promote Shippen to the vacant post? It must be remembered that one year later, Rush blamed Shippen for his own lack of advancement in the Medical Department, and Shippen's promotion may have been in spite of Rush's opposition or with his help.

Shortly after Morgan's dismissal, General Washington wrote Congress:

"It is in vain, however, to look back upon past misfortunes. I will not pretend to point out the cause, but I know matters have been strangely conducted in the Medical line. I hope your new appointment, when it is made, will make the necessary reform in the Hospitals and that 1 shall not, in the next campaign, have my ears and eyes shocked with the complaints and looks of the poor creatures perishing for want of proper care, either in the Regimental or Hospital Surgeons."

The only evidence indicating Shippen's participation in Morgan's removal is a letter written to his brother-in-law on January 17, 1777. It says:

"The sick soldiers are suffering for want of some new arrangement. I am pleased that you have adopted mine, so far as to dismiss the two Directors.

"We want assistant Directors. The Army and the sick are so scattered; and the pay must be augmented to 20 shillings or 3 dollars, or no men of education will engage. These things must be done immediately."

Then follows a comprehensive bid for consideration.

"Would it not answer good purpose and save the Congress much trouble, if I were called 'Inspector General' of the whole? I would then have a right to look into the conduct of all the Hospitals, and receive returns from them and order what proportion should go to each, etc."

At some earlier date in 1776, he also wrote:

"I saw Directors but no directing. Physicians and Surgeons, but too much above their business, and the care of the sick committed to young boys in the character of mates, quite ignorant and as I was informed, hired for half price, etc. Some I found honestly doing the duty of their station.

"How my own Department has been better filled does not become me to say, and I am not ashamed to own that I am conscious of many imperfections, but flatter myself none of them have arisen from want of care and integrity in Ye Director, or skill and industry in his physicians, surgeons and mates. All of the latter, he can with pleasure declare, have done more than their duty, cheerfully. Some imperfections have arisen from my own inexperience; some from a scarcity of many articles necessary for the sick, and more from the distracted flying state of our army, All these causes, I persuade myself, will in a great measure be removed in the next campaign."

Shippen always felt free to write frankly to his brother-in-law, and in one of these letters, presumably writer from Bethlehem in December 1776, he told of the feeling against Morgan among the medical men of the Army and repeated some of the gossip of Morgan's own men. This letter contains the statement from which it is naturally concluded that Shippen recommended Morgan in 1775 for the Director-Generalship over the hospitals of the Continental Army. Shippen wrote:

"I have my information [regarding Morgan] from the united voice of his own officers-methinks I hear you say:-'Yet this is the man you had chosen' but good God, did you or I believe he would be so damned a rogue?"

In another letter, Shippen wrote:

"I know I shall have your interest for my proper place, and when you find me tripping, turn me out."

Morgan soon importuned Congress to make an investigation of his hospital administration, but Congress was too busy to give much attention to matters that were past.

CHAPTER SEVENTEEN

RUSH-SHIPPEN CONTROVERSY • Rush's Fault-Finding Committee Appointed for Hearing Correspondence

IT WAS ON APRIL 11TH, 1777, that Congress chose Dr. William Shippen Jr. as Director General of the Continental hospitals. At the same time, the Medical Department of the Continental Army was ordered reorganized in an effort to correct some of the weaknesses made apparent under the previous Director. Dr. Benjamin Rush was likewise elected Surgeon General for the hospitals of the Middle Division, the third-ranking position under the Director General, but on the refusal of Dr. Walter Jones to accept the appointment of Physician General, Rush was advanced to that post and became second in importance to Shippen, with only the Assistant Deputy General between them.

The Physician General's duties, under the resolution of Congress, were superintending the physicians and practice of physics, and in the absence of the Director or his Deputy, he had all authority over the Middle Department hospital physicians and their subordinate officers, with power to order them to do such things as he thought proper. He was also required to report weekly to the Director General on the number and conditions of the hospital sick. The Surgeon General had similar authority over all surgeons and wounded cases. Rush's station was in the hospital at Princeton, but he was expected to visit the various units of the Middle Division in his official capacity.

Director General Shippen's headquarters at the time of his appointment was in Philadelphia, but after the British took possession of that city, he was removed to Bethlehem and later was constantly on the move, as indicated by many official communications from him, dated at different hospitals besides Revolutionary letters and diaries telling of meeting him at various places. Accepting these records as proof that Dr. Shippen exercised his office's visiting duties as he interpreted them, they tend to contradict Rush's claim that Shippen was seldom seen at any of the hospitals for which he was responsible. It was probably true that Shippen did not assume the inspection details that were supposed to belong to his deputies and the Surgeon General and Physician General, but it must be remembered that there were, at times, as many as twenty active hospitals in the Middle Division, and executive responsibilities would have given Shippen little time for the things that Rush cited as being neglected. Dr. Morgan wrote with pride that he had personally dressed the wounds of every casualty of the Battle of Long Island, which was undoubtedly a laudable undertaking, but it seems an admission of poor organization and misplaced efforts.

It would appear from the definition of his duties that the Physician General had the authority, in the absence of the Director, to have personally corrected many of the faults and abuses of which he so bitterly complained and, if an improvement in such vital matters were as simple to effect as Rush claimed, that he was negligent in his duty not to have initiated the reform, at least insofar as the hospital at Princeton was concerned.

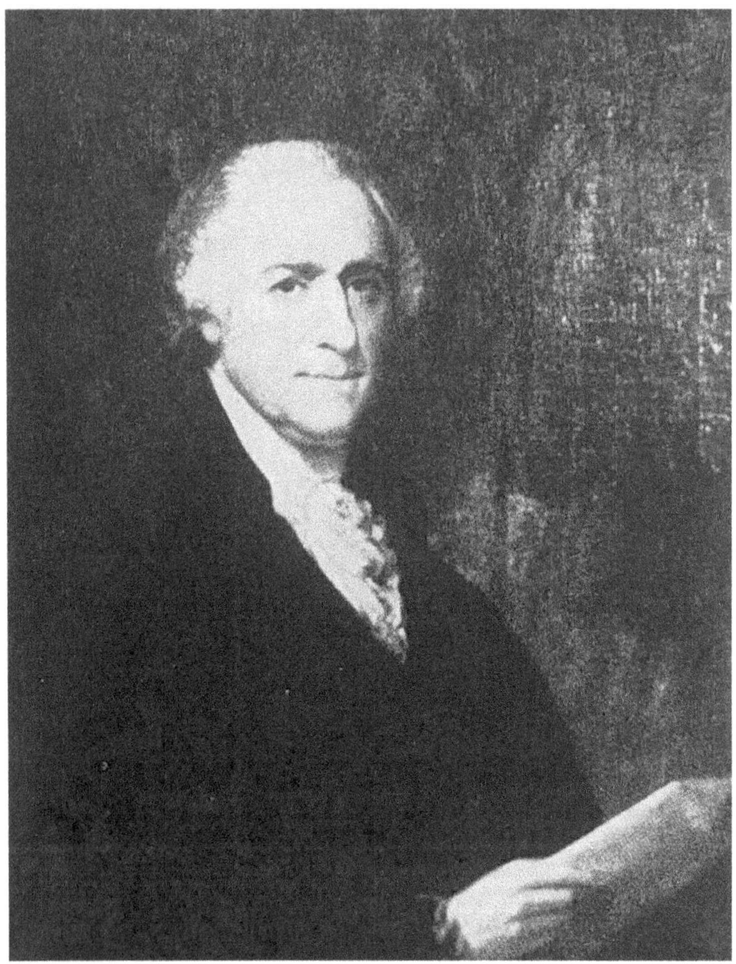

WILLIAM SHIPPEN, JR.

Director General of the Military Hospitals and Chief Physician of the Continental Army, 1777. (Portrait in the College of Physicians, Philadelphia).

Rush's whole life is a story of fault-finding and Don Quixote's experiences, with the difference that besides fighting for a principle and against men, his opponents usually aroused in him an intense hatred, and he pursued them relentlessly. It was in midsummer of 1777 that Rush began tilting at windmills and finding fault with the Continental hospital organization and management through letters addressed to John Adams. Then began a collection of stories and documents to be later used, first by himself and then by Dr. Morgan, against Dr. Shippen. It was late in August or early in September 1777, while on one of his inspection trips to the hospital in the old Barracks at Trenton, that Rush obtained a letter from the Senior Physician and Surgeon, Dr. Bodo Otto, addressed to Dr. Shippen, reciting an urgent need of medicines and stores for the sick. This letter was innocently given at Dr. Rush's suggestion and personally inscribed by him for Dr. Otto's signature. Rush's evident purpose in obtaining this communication was to possess written proof that the Trenton Hospital was not properly supplied with necessities, while Dr. Otto believed he had simply conveyed a list of his requirements to the Director General through the Physician General. The proof of this assertion lies in the fact that the letter was never delivered to Dr. Shippen but was saved by Dr. Rush and offered as evidence nearly two years later at the court-martial trial of the Director General. But the details and consequences of this situation will be told later.

Rush evidently had a definite plan in mind to build up a case against Shippen, and many of the hospital physicians and surgeons, with their mates, unknowingly lent themselves to that end. Quite a few furnished verbal and written complaints to the Physician General, believing that in reciting their difficulties of obtaining supplies, they were appealing to one who might help them. Undoubtedly, every hospital chief exaggerated conditions, and surely no physician or surgeon could be criticized for such attempts at deception that he might better serve the sick and wounded under his care. They saw nothing wrong in claiming they were entirely without a certain medicine or necessity when, in truth, they had a small supply in reserve. Neither did they hesitate to state that they needed fifty pounds of some specified drug when twenty-five pounds would have been ample and as much as they really hoped would be sent, or possibly they requisitioned two pipes of wine when one was all they required. It was well known that shortages existed in all hospital supplies and that no quantity ordered, however small, would be delivered in the amount specified.

This psychology of the hospital physicians and surgeons helped Rush to collect proofs, and furnished much evidence on which to later base his charge that Shippen disregarded hospital requisitions. But when this evidence was offered by Rush to sustain his charge, many of these complaining physicians and surgeons took the stand and testified to the truth as they believed it, repudiating their own earlier statements. Exaggerating complaints and misstating conditions for the purpose of benefiting their own patients were, in their opinion, quite excusable, but repeating careless and untrue statements under oath and injuring a man who, they considered, had done his best under difficult circumstances, was quite a different matter.

On December 8, 1777, Dr. Rush opened fire on the entire hospital system in a letter addressed to Mr. Duer for the information of Congress. It contained no serious charge against any official or individual but rather compared American methods of handling the sick and wounded with those of the British, which, he claimed, were less likely to be abused or exploited. In this communication, Rush recommended certain changes involving:

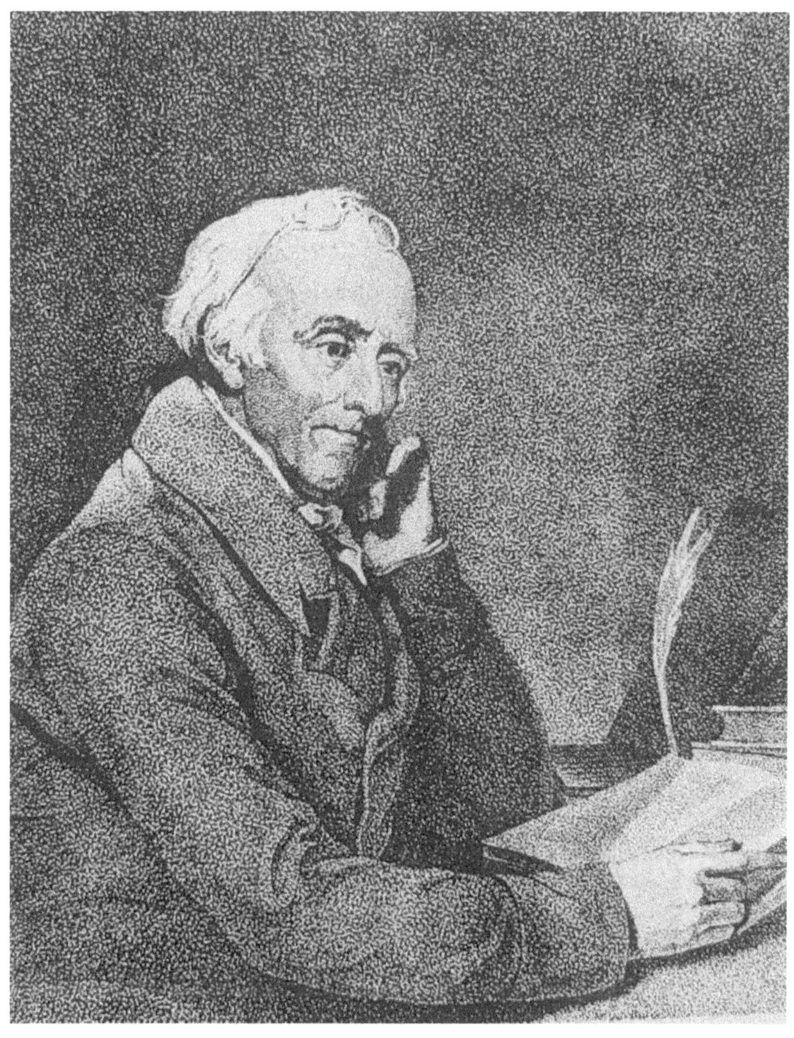

BENJAMIN RUSH

Physician General of the Hospitals of the Middle Department of the Continental Hospitals Army, 1777. Portrait by Sully. The engraving by Edwin. From American Medical Biography by James Thacher, Boston, 1828.

1st-The appointment of an Inspector General and Chief Physician whose only business would be visiting the hospitals to examine the quantity and quality of the medicines, stores, and instruments and to receive and deliver reports of the number of sick and wounded to the Commander-in-Chief.

2nd-That a Purveyor General be selected to provide the hospitals

with all necessities.

3rd-That Physician General and Surgeon General advance the stores to the hospitals and provide the Purveyor General with lists of necessities, as well as direct everything required for the recovery of the patients.

These were all constructive suggestions and especially opportune at a time when the hospital activities and needs were being augmented. Had Rush confined his efforts to a reorganization of the department along these lines, he might have had the cooperation of every right-thinking man in Congress and the Army, but unfortunately, he immediately followed this first communication to Congress with a second and wrote two similar letters of criticism to General Washington, in which he injected his personal attacks against Dr. Shippen and showed an animosity that caused the Director's friends in all departments to rally to his support.

The Medical Department had so increased in the number of hospitals that it had outgrown the organization plan adopted early in 1777, and Rush's timely suggestion might have produced much good, but then came the accusing letter of December 13, 1777:

"Dear Sir:

"In my letter to you a few days ago, I informed you that we had 3,000 patients in our hospitals. Since the dating of that letter

I have discovered that they now amount to 5,000. They consist chiefly of the Southern Army, and amount to near one-half of the number of troops which composed that Army during the last campaign.

"I have heard with great pleasure that you are about to new-model the army. For God's sake do not forget to take the medical system under your consideration.

"It is a mass of corruption by tyranny, and has wholly disappointed the benevolence and munificence of the Congress. It would take up a volume to unfold all the disorders and miseries of the hospitals.

"What do you think of 5,000 being supported with stores, hospital furniture sufficient for only 1,500 men? What do you think of 500 men in a village without a single officer to mount a guard over them or to punish irregularities? This is the case at this time in Princeton-and the consequences are old disorders are prolonged, new ones are contracted -the discipline of the soldiers (contracted at camp) destroyed-inhabitants are plundered-and the blankets, clothes, shoes, etc. of the soldiers are stolen or exchanged in every tavern and hut for liquors. I have witnessed these things for these six months and have complained of them to the Dir. Gen'l. to the Congress and to the generals of the army, to no effect. What do you think of 200 sick being crowded into a house large enough for only 150? This has been done in our place and the consequence of it is a putrid fever was generated which carried off 12 soldiers in three days (who all came in to the hospital with other diseases) and many more in the space of two weeks. Upon my complaining to the Dir. Gen'l. that he had crowded too many sick into one house he told me he was the only judge of that and that my only business was to take care of all he sent there. Your system justified his making me this answer altho' it does not oblige him to go inside a hospital, or expose himself to the least danger of being infected by a fever. Six surgeons have died since last Spring of fevers contracted in our hospitals and there is scarcely one who had not been ill in a greater or lesser degree with it. Nothing like this has happened in the Northern Department. The reasons of which are these: Dr. Potts has confined himself solely to the purveying business and Dr. Treat, who served as a surgeon in the British hospitals last war, has introduced the British system in its most minute parts into the hospitals under his direction.

"I wish some members of Congress (not related to Dr. Shippen) would visit our hospitals, and converse with the principal surgeons in it. Altho' Dr. Shippen has taken great pains to extort the power of ap pointing them out of the physician general and surgeon general's hands and has made some of them dependent upon his will, yet I believe you will not find more than one man among them who does not reprobate our system and who will not ring peals of distress and villainy in your ears much louder than anything you have heard from me.

"I bequeath you these broken hints as a legacy, being determined as

soon as I with honor and can a clear conscience leave my present charge, to send you my commission. I beg leave to repeat my solicitation in favor of Dr. Jones (of New York) being appointed Inspector General of your hospitals. He will save you millions of dollars and what is more estimable, thousands of lives in a year. I would rather serve as a mate in a hospital under him with the British system than those with the present Dir. Gen'l, in all his power and glory.

"I am bound in justice before I quit this subject, to speak with gratitude of Dr. Craik, and Dr. Bond, the Dir. Gen'l's principal assistants. We owe a great deal to their humanity and I cannot tell how much worse our situation would have been had it not been for them.

"The Dir. General has found out at last that none but a physician should have any hand in directing the hospital he attends and, to remedy the defect of his directing by proxy, he has lately given 100 of our Seniors, warrants to assist under him. That is:-I commissioned them to give the sick physic, but he commissioned them to prescribe what and how much they shall eat and drink-how much pure air they shall breathe and in what hospital they shall be attended, as if all those things were not properly the business of a physician and were not of a thousand times more consequence than Doses of Jalap or Ipecac.

"You may make any use you please of this letter, and my name with it. I know what it is to be a generous friend-and am equally tenacious of the character of a generous enemy.

"I am, Dear Sir, with compliments to my Colleague, Mr. Duane, your "Most humble Servant

"Princeton, December 13, 1777"

"B. Rush

Let us analyze the subject matter of this letter. It must be remembered that the Continental hospitals were usually located in small towns where there were no proper buildings for the purpose and that churches, barns and any other available structures were appropriated that would least inconvenience the inhabitants. It must also be recalled that Continental credit was questionable and pay slow, and it was not long before every community with troops or hospital quartered upon it found itself possessed of many bills of indebtedness they were unable to cash; consequently, local credit would be curtailed. The number of sick or wounded soldiers in the Army was not a matter within the control of the Hospital Department, so the claim that 5,000 patients were sustained with stores and necessities intended for only 1,500 could not be justly blamed on the Director General unless he had or could have obtained additional equipment from reserves or through appropriations of Congress.

The Government was not over-generous in its allotments to Dr. Shippen for hospital use, though both Rush and Morgan claimed the contrary, but official figures will later be given to disprove this assertion.

Five hundred men quartered on the inhabitants of Princeton must have more than doubled the normal population of the town. It is difficult to believe that these 500 men would be stationed there without officers. Perhaps Rush meant there were no soldiers and officers assigned to guard and maintain military discipline in the hospital. It even seems strange that this condition could have existed six months prior to December 13th, when on June 16, 1777, General Washington had recognized the need and issued a general order from headquarters directing:

"The commanding officer nearest any hospital to furnish a prudent officer to assist in the government of it so far as it relates to keeping the convalescent soldiers in order; having proper guard and the like; to see that justice is done to the sick; reporting any neglect or abuses they may observe, to the chief director of the hospital and then if not remedied, to the commanding officer of the post from which he was sent who, if he thinks the presentation just, is to communicate them to the Commander-in-Chief."

The Director General had no authority over troops of the neighborhood and how could he be rightfully blamed for the absence of a guard? For Rush to hold Shippen responsible for this condition, especially after admitting he had unsuccessfully appealed to Congress and the Commander-in-Chief to correct the trouble, seems rather unreasonable.

Nor could Shippen be justly blamed for the crowded condition of the Princeton Hospital in the largest available building—the College Hall. The village was overpopulated by reason of troops and the hospital, and no unoccupied buildings existed. Had not Dr. Rush similarly offended in October 1777 when he sent 100 additional patients to the Bethlehem Hospital with orders that they be accommodated, when he knew that all available space was occupied and that sick and wounded soldiers were being diverted to Easton? It is easy to complain and criticize others and point out a proper solution to a difficult problem, but when confronted with the responsibility of a similar one, the only immediate action often lies in repeating the very method criticized. How else were the patients to be attended, with space restricted and hospital staff so limited that the patients had to be concentrated to give the necessary attention? Undoubtedly the results were a high mortality rate, and from our more advanced point of view, ignorance played a big part in the great losses that followed, but were they avoidable under the conditions that then existed?

Dr. Rush's statements regarding Dr. Potts' system of organization are not borne out by the records among the Potts' mss. for Potts did combine the duties of Hospital Physician and Surgeon with those of a Director and, with only three or four hospitals under his care, he was able to give them unusual personal attention and supervision. The hospital problems in the North as well as the manner of handling them, were the same as Shippen later encountered in the middle division. One thing that Dr. Potts accomplished earlier in the North was the eradication of smallpox as a major disease, and this he did by a system of group inoculation long before the soldiers of the Army of the middle division were so treated, for it was not until February 1777, that Congress permitted General Washington to inoculate all his troops. Rush's favorable criticism of Dr. Bond was used to plague him when he attacked Bond after the Assistant Deputy Director testified for Shippen at the court-martial trial. The minutes of the Journal of Congress for January 1, 1778, records that:

"A letter of the 8th and one of the 13th Dec. from Dr. B. Rush to Mr. Wm. Duer, were laid before Congress and read.

"Resolved, that the said committee (Medical) be fully authorized to take every measure which they shall deem necessary for the immediate relief of the sick and report such alterations in the medical department as they shall deem best adapted to answer the end of its institution."

On January 6, 1778, another entry read:

"The committee to whom the letters of Governor Livingston and Dr. Rush were referred brought in a report which was taken into consideration, whereupon resolved; "That Dr. Shippen and Dr. Rush be directed to attend Congress on the 26th of Jan, to be examined touching certain abuses said to prevail in the hospital; "That the clothier general be directed to deliver to the order of the Director General as much linen and as many blankets as can be spared, the sick; to be retained in the hospital for the use of "That the clothier general be directed to supply the convalescent with necessary clothing in order that when properly recovered they may join the Army;

"That a member of Congress be forthwith appointed to visit the hospitals in the middle department; the member chosen Mr. John Penn."

A request was also sent to the clergy of all denominations that they solicit donations of woolens and linens for the sick soldiers in the hospitals.

These resolutions were all the result of requests made by the Director General himself and surely indicate a common shortage in the Army and the hospitals, not just a scarcity in the Medical Department. Another order that indicated the general situation directed Dr. Shippen to purchase stoves and the Quarter Master General to collect firewood so that sufficient warmth might be generated in the hospitals so that the scarcity of blankets and clothing would be less noticed. Officers of Pennsylvania troops were also detailed to travel throughout the Colony to collect bed coverings and wearing apparel, and orders were issued that in their distribution, preference should be given to the hospitals; yet Shippen was personally blamed for the shortage of such necessities for the sick and wounded soldiers.

Can any convincing evidence be deduced from all this that the privation and suffering in the hospitals were due to Shippen's indifference, ignorance of the requirements of his job, or desire to swell or retain the number of patients that he might have larger appropriations to spend in his department? But this was part of Rush's accusation against the Director General. Shippen undoubtedly had his faults and weaknesses, but his life record refutes every charge of inhumanity and indifference to the sufferings of the Revolutionary soldiers.

On January 18, 1778, Dr. Shippen addressed a letter to Congress in answer to the summons of January 6th, saying:

"General Hospital, Lancaster, 18th Jan. 1778.

"Sir:

"I am informed many complaints are made to the honorable Congress and General Washington against the hospital establishment, by Dr. Rush and by Governor Livingston, who has been imposed on by the Doctor's misrepresentation. Justice to my own and the character of my good officers calls loudly on me as the Head of that department to wait on Congress to show them that there is not the least cause for these complaints, as far as the establishment or officers of it are concerned. If the Physician and

Surgeon General is of any use, there may arise some cause of complaint at Princeton from his long absence from his duty without leave at this important period. I think it my duty rather to run the risk of suffering in my reputation, than that the sick soldiers should suffer by my absence. Next week I shall do myself the honor of sending or carrying a return of all the sick and wounded by which I flatter myself it will appear that our sick are not crowded in any hospital, that their number is not much if any larger than in my last return that very few die that no fatal disease prevails and that the hospitals are in very good order. These things being so, I rest satisfied that this honorable body will not make any alteration in the Medical Department, or suffer measures to be adopted that may reflect on my own or any of my officers' reputations, till I can be heard. I must add, some amendments to our system may be made but Dr. Rush, from his ignorance of the state of our Hospitals and not knowing his duty, has not hit upon any of them. If the Congress will give me leave I will point them out for their consideration next week.

"I have the honor to be Dear Sir, with the most perfect respect, Your and the Congress' most devoted and faithful servant, W. Shippen, Jr."

Dr. Rush also acknowledged the order to appear and replied to it with:

"Sir:

"Yorktown, Jan. 25th, 1778.

"I have taken the liberty of informing you that in conformity to an order of Congress to attend at this place on the 26th of this instant, I have obeyed the summons and am now ready to enter upon the business they have assigned for that day.

"As the Director General of the military hospitals has contradicted the aspersions contained in my letter to General Washington, in a public letter addressed to the whole body of the

Congress, I shall esteem it a particular favor if Congress will indulge me with the privilege of a public hearing in order that I may support the complaints I have made of the abuses which prevailed in our hospitals.

"I have the honor to be, with most respect, "Your most obedient and humble servant,

"B. Rush."

The committee of the House appointed to hear Rush and Shippen was composed of five members, of whom the Reverend Dr. John Witherspoon, President of Princeton College, was one. It was Rush who had been largely responsible for influencing Dr. Witherspoon's coming to the New Jersey institution from Scotland, and they were close friends, but Witherspoon's sympathy was apparently with Shippen, resulting in Rush's attacking him as biased. On the 27th (January 1778), Witherspoon wrote an absent member of Congress:

"Doctors Rush and Shippen are here just now and, even yesternight and afternoon, were examined before a Committee of which I am chairman, as to the abuses in the hospital. No pains will be spared to rectify what is amiss as far as is practical."

The committee appeared to accept Dr. Shippen's opinion of the conditions and the proper solution. Rush resigned, and on the following day, he wrote to a friend:

"To avoid the fate of Dr. Morgan as well as to gratify my own inclination, I have sent in my resignation."

In the fall of 1780, however, Rush enlarged the version of his reasons in an open letter addressed to Dr. Shippen, saying:

"The Chairman of the committee Witherspoon appointed to hear us, merits your thanks for the fidelity with which he executed the scheme you had conceived for driving me out of the Hospital Department; he informed me that I had lost ground in Congress and obligingly hinted to me that I should be dismissed unless I resigned my office of Physician General of the Hospitals."

Rush's communication to Congress was presented through Dr. Witherspoon, who, acknowledging it on February 2, 1778, wrote:

"I am favored with your letter covering your two forms of resignation. There was nothing exceptionable in either of them. I however gave in that which says you found you could not discharge your duty as you would, etc., which was accepted without a word from any person upon the subject.

"I am sorry for the necessity of this measure and yet I question whether you could have done anything more proper, for Dr. Shippen was fully determined to bring the matter to a contest between you, refusing positively to serve with you, which would have occasioned an examination and judgment troublesome to us, hurtful probably to both of you and uncertain in its issue.

"I have mentioned to some members what you proposed to me about the expedition [doubtless the projected expedition to Canada] you know of, but they seem to be at a loss what station or character you could sustain. Some difficulties are likely to arise in that expedition; if however it goes on and I can find any opening I shall remember your proposal."

It would be interesting to know the construction of the alternative form of resignation which Dr. Witherspoon rejected. It possibly contained an attack on the Director General, which Witherspoon thought better to suppress. The resignation filed read:

"January 30, 1778

"Sir:

"Finding it impossible to do my duty any longer in the department you have assigned me in your hospitals in the manner

I would wish, I beg the favor of you to accept the resignation of my Commission.

"I have the honor to be, with great respect.

"Your most obedient humble servant

"Benj. Rush."

Richard Peters, Secretary of the Board of War, writing to Robert Morris on February 3, 1778, commented:

"Rush has resigned. There is so much on both sides that I fancy both are wrong at least in some degree."

One hospital surgeon, writing to another, said:

"Rush has quarreled himself out of all his Posts."

On February 1, 1778, Rush wrote Shippen as follows:

"Sir:

"Lancaster, Pa.

"Before I received your message by Dr. Fallon, I had sent in my resignation. I think it proper to mention this circumstance lest you should attribute that step to any fear I entertained of suffering by a Court Martial. You know I have nothing to dread from that quarter and 1 take this opportunity of informing you that nothing but the remembrance of an early connection with you, a tenderness for your worthy family and in particular an affection for your amiable and promising son, have prevented my collecting and producing vouchers of the abuses of our hospitals which would ultimately have ended in your dishonor.

"To Dr. Shippen."

(Rush MSS. Ridgway Library)

"Benj. Rush."

More will be told later of the probable reason for Rush's reference to a fear of court-martial. The Gates Cabal had just been exposed, and though it is not believed Rush was actively involved, he was known to be sympathetic and had written an anonymous letter to Patrick Henry on the subject. Rush also relieved his feelings in a letter addressed to some unknown correspondent, of which he retained a copy found among the Rush MSS.

R.W. 29-120B.

No name was given to whom addressed.

"Dear Sir:

"Lancaster, Feb. 1st, 1778

"I set down in the name of our unfortunate countrymen to acknowledge the obligations of the hospitals to His Excellency Gen'l. Washington and to the Gen'l. officers of the army, for sending military Inspectors to see that the sick are properly attended and provided with everything necessary for them. The advantages resulting from having gentlemen independent of the officers of the hospitals constantly in their neighborhood, are so obvious that I wonder it has been so long neglected; especially as the Director General informed a Committee of Congress that he had repeatedly applied for them together with a small body of guards but to no purpose. I was happy in being able to inform the same committee that I had been much more successful in my application to the General Officers of the Army for, that my first letters to the Commander in Chief and to yourself had immediately procured a field officer to visit all the hospitals and a determination to keep guards and the discipline of the army among them.

"I find from examining Dr. Shippen's return of the number who die in the hospitals that I was mistaken in the amounts I gave of that matter in my letter to you. From his return of December last I find very few died in proportion to the number I have mentioned. All I can say in apology for this mistake is, that I was deceived by counting the number of coffins that were daily put under the ground. From their weight and funeral, I am persuaded they contained hospital patients and if they were not dead, I hope some steps will be taken for the future to prevent and punish the crime of burying the Continental soldiers alive. It is a new evil under the sun and I hope a new punishment will be discovered for it.

"As most all the abuses which have prevailed in the hospitals during the last campaign have been ascribed to a want of harmony between the Director General and myself, I have (to prevent the future operation of that apology for murder) resigned my commission. I sacrificed my feelings and judgment to harmony till my conscience grew uneasy with my silence. I complained with delicacy. I laid nothing to the direct charge of Dr. Shippen in my letter to Gen'l. Washington. I have always blamed his officers and the system for the principal abuses which prevailed in the department and, if I was forced into any personal charges of ignorance and negligence in Dr. Shippen, they were extorted in defending myself from his charges against me. I am so much absorbed in the great object of the war and in the means of carrying it on that I have not a moment's leisure to be angry or dispute with anything but putrid fever or with anybody but Gen'l. Howe.

"Apropos have made a great discovery! A sure and certain method of destroying Howe's whole army without powder or ball or without any of the common implements of death! Lead them through any of the Villages in Lancaster County where we have a hospital and I will assure you that in six weeks there shall not be a man of them alive or fit for duty.

"I am not disgusted or distressed with the opinion of our Superiors concerning the cause of my complaints or of my resignation. My dear country's freedom and independence are words as big with charm to me as ever. I shall therefore join the army in the spring as a volunteer and while there are 500 men in the armies of America, I shall never keep back the mite of my labor and life from the service of my country and posterity.

"With great esteem I have the honor to be, etc.

"Benj. Rush."

The first paragraph of this letter is a direct contradiction of his previous statement, contained in the letter of December 13, 1777, to Mr. Duer, in which he related complaining to "the Director General-the Congress and the Commander in Chief" about the absence of guards for a period of six months, with no effect. After resigning from the service, Rush retired to Princeton, the home of his wife's family, as the British were in possession of Philadelphia. Here, he brooded over his grievances and even contemplated giving up the profession of medicine and studying law. But his fighting spirit soon revived, and he began organizing his evidence against Dr. Shippen. On March 9, 1778, Rush addressed a letter to Mr. Daniel Roberdeau in which, returning to the attack, he outlined the testimony he offered to produce.

"Princeton, March 9, 1778.

"Dear Sir:

"I was so fully convinced that all the distresses and mortality of the military hospitals arose from the Purveying business being lodged in Dr. Shippen's hands, that in my complaints of the abuses which prevailed in the hospitals, I aimed chiefly to have that part of the system changed which gave Dr. Shippen the powers of a purveyor. I had no personal resentment against him and therefore took no pains to collect vouchers of his ignorance-negligence or injustice. A change in the system (such as I wish for) I was sure would place the sick and the public beyond the reach of suffering from those vices. The patience with which Dr. Shippen heard the hints I gave of his speculation and his declining to call upon me for public or private satisfaction for what I said of him before the Committee of Congress, were sufficient to convince any man that my insinuations were well grounded. I expected the Committee would have obliged me to prosecute him in a court martial. The task would have been disagreeable, unless I had been compelled to it. It is now too late to force me into that measure but a regard to the honor of the Congress and to my own character require that I should trouble you with the following facts to judge, after you have them, whether my charges against Dr. Shippen were founded on facts or whether a 'want of harmony was the cause of the extraordinary distress and mortality which had prevailed in the hospitals under his direction."

(Exhibits) "Bethlehem February 17, 1778

"This is to certify that the wine allowed to the hospital at Bethlehem under the name of Madeira, was adulterated in such a degree as to have none of the qualities or the effects of Madeira.

"That it was a common practice with the Commissary General to deduct one-third, sometimes more, sometimes less, from the orders for the wine sugar-molasses and other stores ordered for the sick by the surgeons.

"That none of the patients in the hospital under our care eat of venison-poultry or wild fowl (unless purchased by themselves) and that large quantities of those articles were purchased by Mr. Hape, the Assistant Commissary of the Hospital, by order of the Director General. That the Director General never entered the hospital but once during about six weeks residence at the village of Bethlehem although the utmost distress and mortality prevailed in the hospital at that time.

"That a putrid fever raged for three months in the hospital and was greatly increased by the sick being too much crowded and by their wanting blankets shirts straw and other necessities for sick people. "That so violent was the putrid fever that nine out of eleven surgeons were seized with it, one of whom died. That out of three stewards, two died with it and the third narrowly escaped with his life and that many of the inhabitants of the village caught and died with the said putrid fever.

"That there have died, 200 soldiers (in the hospital at Bethlehem), eight-tenths of them with a putrid fever caught in the hospital within the space of four months.

"Subscribed

"William W. Smith

"Samuel Finley

"James Finley

"Robert R. Henry."

"This is to certify that the return of the hospital at Bethlehem for the month of December was 420 patients and that there have died in the said month above forty patients." (Signed) Samuel Finley. (note)

"The return of the Director General to the Congress for December was only 320 patients in the Bethlehem hospital and the return of the Director General of the dead in the above hospital for December was only 21." (Rush)

"Lancaster-Feb. 12, 1778 "This is to certify that I delivered to the hospital in Lancaster, 120 coffins from October 6, 1777, to February 9, 1778; 32 in December and 33 in January, 1778." (Signed) George Burckhert.

The return of the dead in the Lancaster hospital by the Director General to the Congress for December only, 12." (Rush's note.)

"Similar vouchers with the above might be obtained from every hospital in the department if stronger testimony will be required of the negligence injustice and falsehood of the Director Gen'l.

"I hinted to the Committee of Congress that Dr. Shippen had sold six pipes of wine at Reading as his private property while the sick were dying from want of it. The Doctor's confession of his having that number of pipes upon his own account was received by the committee as a justification of that act. I said that I was not without my suspicions and many other acts of the same nature which had I mentioned, would not have admitted of the same apology. I shall mention a few of them. Dr. Fred Kuhn, a Senior Surgeon of the Hospital, informed me that he sold two pipes of Madeira from among the hospital stores in Lancaster by Dr. Shippen's order early last Spring. In the Fall, when Dr. Kuhn came to Lancaster to take charge of the hospital in that place, Dr. Shippen ordered him to make use of one of the pipes of Madeira for the sick in the hospital under his care. But to Dr. Kuhn's great surprise when he went and demanded the wine, a friend of Dr. Shippen's came with an order from the doctor and demanded the wine as the doctor's private property and sold the two pipes for the doctor at 400 pounds apiece.

"Dr. Potts informed me that he knew of Dr. Shippen's having sold several hogsheads of brown sugar to a person in Reading. William Bryan the Vice Pres. of Pa, asked me if loaf sugar was a useless article in our hospitals; I told him 'no' but that we could never get any amount of it to use either in diet or medicine. He then informed me that the Director General of the Hospital had sent 46 loaves of it from Manheim to a shopkeeper in Lancaster to be sold upon his account.

"These facts are known to thousands in Penn. and New Jersey. The tale of private property will not go down with honest thinking men. What would you think of a Colonel of a Regiment or a Commissary of Provisions who traded largely in fire-arms or bullets at a time when his soldiers suffered from want of them? The sick of the army died from scanty allowance of those very articles from the sale of which Dr. Shippen has made a fortune.

"I have not been able to collect an exact account of the deaths in all the hospitals in the Department from the first of November to the first of March. In Lancaster there have died 120 and in Reading 170-in Bethlehem 200-in Princeton above 100 and from comparing general accounts of the deaths in other hospitals, I think at the lowest computation they cannot amount to less than 700 or 800 more. Not more than 200 of these perished with disorders brought from the camp. The rest perished from want or died of a putrid fever caught in the hospital.

"Dr. Potts lost only 203 soldiers (inclusive of his wounded) between the first of March and the 10th of Dec. last. His sick who were at one time numerous, abounded in everything and no putrid fever ever found its way into any one of his hospitals.

"What would be the fate of a general officer who would throw away a thousand continental troops in a drunken frolic or sell them to an enemy? He would expiate his crime with his life. And shall 1,000 of your brave soldiers be lost ignobly in a hospital? Shall the cry of murder resound through every graveyard in the villages of Penn.? And shall no inquiry be made into these things? Is there a court in Europe so far gone in the system of favoritism as to suffer such things to pass with impunity? I am sure there is not and I have too high an idea of the integrity and disinterestedness of the Congress to believe that when the facts which have been enumerated are known to them they will suffer the affairs of the hospital the medical system. to be ended by few resolutions to amend Peculation is the only rock on which our country can be shipwrecked but if gigantic criminals escape, who will complain hereafter or who will not fear to offend impunity? Integrity are the only basis on which a republican government can be erected or maintained. Should a philosopher in Europe hear that the Director General of all the hospitals of the U.S. was a man who had been absorbed for the last fifteen years of his life wholly in pleasure that he was wholly ignorant of the method of governing and directing military hospitals as practiced in old European armies, that he entered his hospitals but once in six weeks, that he spent whole nights and days in reveling and debauchery, that he was universally suspected of having robbed the sick and the public of many thousands and that he had made false reports of his hospitals to his masters, I am sure he would suspect that we were no longer a great republic but that we were advancing fast toward the depravity of manners of an European country. "I must not omit to add here that Dr. Morgan cannot long be a stranger to the history of Dr. Shippen's directorship. Suppose he should charge him with some of his misconduct in print the Doctor as usual would probably be silent under it, but would not the honor of the Congress require that this officer should vindicate his innocence or suffer for his crime?

"In the British hospitals no purveyor's account can be passed unless it is certified by the physicians and surgeons of the hospital. Suppose a physician and surgeon of the hospital should be called upon to declare what stores have been appropriated for the use of the sick and charged to them in Dr. Shippen's accounts. I fear the Doctor's account would never pass the Commissioners. Dr. Brown (my late colleague) assured me that in no case had he seen for these several months, barrels of wine sugar-molasses, etc., come to the hospital without detecting upon an examination that a third and half and sometimes two thirds had been stolen from them.

"I beg that this letter may be shown to Messrs. Penn, Geary, and Lovell, likewise to Mr. Clingham.

"With great regards,

"Your friend and humble servant

"B. Rush."

This same collection of evidence submitted to Mr. Roberdeau had already been sent to General Washington several weeks before and was accompanied by an explanatory letter reading:

"Sir:

"Princeton, Feb. 25th, 1778,

I should think myself inexcusable in leaving the Army by resigning my commission without informing your Excellency that I was compelled to that measure by the prevalence of an opinion among some people that the distresses and mismanagement of the Hospitals arose from a want of harmony between Dr. Shippen and myself. Next to a conviction of my own soul that this was not the case, I wish to have it known to your Excellency that none of them originated in that cause.

"I beg your Excellency's acceptance of the enclosed pamphlet and am with the warmest sentiments of regard and attachment, your Excellency's most affectionate humble Servant,

"B. Rush."

This epistle, by reason of the date it was written, enters into an accusation of General Washington's that Rush had addressed him in terms of respect and honor shortly after attacking him anonymously. General Washington forwarded Rush's communication and evidence with a letter saying:

"Headquarters Valley Forge 21 March-1778

"To the President of Congress.

"Sir:

Enclosed you have a copy of a letter, which I received a few days ago from Dr. Rush. As the letter contains charges of a very heinous nature against D. G. Dr. Shippen, for malpractice and neglect in his department, I would not but look upon it as meant for a public accusation and have therefore thought it incumbent upon me to lay it before Congress. I have showed it to Dr. Shippen that he may be prepared to vindicate his character, if called upon.

"He tells me that Dr. Rush made charges of a private nature before a Committee of Congress, appointed to hear them, which he could not support; if so Congress will not have further occasion to trouble themselves in the matter."

On April 3, 1778, both of Dr. Rush's letters were laid before Congress, and it was resolved:

"That the committee be authorized to send for such persons and papers as they may judge necessary and allow reasonable and necessary expenses of the witnesses attending the business."

The Committee then wrote to Dr. Rush:

"Your letter of the 25th of Feb. to General Washington and of the 9th of March to Mr. Roberdeau, of which we presume you have draughts, having been laid before Congress, produced an order of which the enclosed is an authenticated copy.

"We wish to proceed in this business so as to obtain the most perfect information of the malpractices, if there are any, of the Director General and to this end we desire that you will be pleased to ascertain the procedure and transmit to us the charge and upon oath, the evidence you have or can procure against him; also the names of the witnesses and places of residence.

"If there are any difficulties in the way of collecting the evidence upon the subject, you will be pleased to point them out with, if in your power to do so, the means of removing them.

"We are Sir

"Your very humble and obedient servant

"Wm. Henry Drayton

"Samuel Huntington

"W. H. D. for Mr. Banister"

"Yorktown April 7th, 1778"

To this communication, Dr. Rush replied:

"Princeton, April 20, 1778. "Messrs. Wm. H. Drayton, Samuel Huntington and John Banister, members of special Committee of the Congress:

"Gentlemen:

"I was favoured with your letter a few days ago enclosing a copy of a resolution of Congress of the 3rd instant.

"I foresee many difficulties in the way of a Committee of Congress coming at a knowledge of facts with respect to Dr. Shippen in maladministration of the military hospitals. Should the evidence be listed at Yorktown, the sick in the hospitals would suffer from want of Surgeons to attend them, for there are nearly as many witnesses against him as there are Surgeons in the hospitals.

"I expected that the mode of trying him would have been by a Court Martial and for that reason I transmitted an account of his conduct to the Commander in Chief of the Army before I wrote to a member of Congress upon the subject.

"The Army has written laws for the government of all its members Dr. Shippen belongs to the army and most of the surgeons who are to be witnesses against him are in its neighborhood and can attend without much expense to themselves or the public. Besides there is a possible resolution of Congress for this purpose in the regulations of the hospital on the 11th of April, 1777. The words are

"That the Director, deputy directors, physicians and surgeon generals, and all other officers before enumerated shall be tried by a court martial for any misbehaviour or neglect of duty as the Commander in Chief shall direct.

"If the Congress should agree to this mode of enquiring into Dr. Shippen's malpractices, I shall give in a list, of the 'names' of the witnesses with their 'respective places of residence,' to the officer appointed to receive them and shall esteem myself bound by the duty I owe to my country, to appear at the court as his prosecutor.

"I am, gentlemen, with all due respect, your most

Obedient

Humble

Servant

"Benj. Rush."

A long lapse of time follows the receipt of this letter before any notice of it is recorded, but on June 4, 1778, the Journal noted that:

"A letter of the 20th of April from Dr. Rush to Messrs. Wm. H. Drayton, Samuel Huntington, and John Banister, the committee appointed on 3rd of that month to inquire into Dr. Rush's charge against Dr. Shippen, was read."

No comment, no action, and the matter is no longer a subject of any public record. Rush contended that Shippen's friends in Congress killed the investigation or suppressed the report, but the acceptance of such a conclusion casts a reflection on an honorable body of men, and if Rush's charges were justified, it would have made them a party to the crime of concealment.

Is it possible that the Committee of Congress checked Rush's charges against evidence and information in their possession and found discrepancies that cast doubt on Rush's sincerity? Let us follow this thought and see what it develops. It will be recalled that the disastrous Battle of Brandywine and the result of the fight at Germantown, had sealed the fate of Philadelphia and that a removal of the hospitals from the neighborhood became necessary.

On September 19, 1777, Dr. Shippen addressed the Moravian authorities at Bethlehem, informing them of his need for accommodation for 2,000 patients in that immediate neighborhood. The sick and wounded from Mt. Holly, Bordentown, and Trenton, N.J., including those at Bristol, Pottsgrove, Buckingham and the Philadelphia district, were removed as fast as possible, and new hospitals were established in Lancaster, Lititz, Ephrata, Reading, Easton, and Northampton. Great confusion existed and little thought or system was shown in the distribution of patients and necessary supplies. The sick and wounded were transported in open springless wagons without any special protection, often in freezing and inclement weather, and many died from exposure. To further complicate the situation, reserve Army equipment, personal effects of withdrawing citizens and Government records were rushed out of the danger zone over the same highways and to identical destinations. It was among these disorganized hospitals that Dr. Rush soon appeared in an effort to gather evidence to sustain his accusations against Dr. Shippen, and he undoubtedly found some disgruntled medical men who were sympathetic to him and willing to add their complaints to his. Dr. Samuel Finley, one of these, later qualified his statement made to Dr. Rush with a letter saying:

"I do certify that in the certificate that I signed at Dr. Rush's request, I did not mean in the least to cast any reflection on the Director General.

"The weak Madeira wine mentioned there was served for only about two weeks, being, as the Commissary told me, the bottom of the pipe; before that time and afterwards we had good wine and plenty of it. As to the quantity not being issued (in amounts) as ordered, Dr. Shippen knew nothing of it.

"Although the sick did not get venison, poultry or wild fowl, yet the Doctors of the Hospitals had these things sometimes in lieu of beef, they being so cheap. What the Director had, he paid for himself and I am assured by the gentlemen who bought these things that all the Director had, did not cost more than sixteen dollars. (signed)

"Samuel Finley."

"Bethlehem, March 30th, 1778."

At the court-martial trial two years later, where most of Dr. Rush's exhibits were combined with Dr. Morgan's evidence, John Scott, a Steward at the Bethlehem Hospital, was asked:

"Do you know any thing of a certificate signed by W. W. Smith, Samuel Finley and Mr. Henry?"

To which he replied:

"Dr. Rush proposed a paper in the Commissary room at Bethlehem-s what it was I don't remember now, though I heard it read; but it was against Dr. Shippen. The two Juniors signed it in my presence-viz., W. W. Smith and Samuel Finley, but I left the room when Dr. Henry was going to sign. When the gentlemen were preparing to sign Dr. Rush said:

"'We will bring the Shippens down; they are too powerful and have reigned long enough,'" to which Dr. Smith replied:

"I will join you with all my heart."

Scott further affirmed that he spoke to Dr. S. Finley, telling him to consider well what he was about, for in all probability, he would repent it, to which Scott said the Doctor answered he would not, for Dr. Shippen's directorship would be short.

To another hospital physician and surgeon, Dr. Shippen put the question, referring to Dr. Rush's assertion:

"Do you know of 1000 men having died from my fraud, want of humanity or industry and preference for pleasure to discharge of duty? Or do you even know of any one man having died from those causes?"

To both these questions the Doctor answered in the negative.

Dr. Brown, the Physician General who succeeded Dr. Rush, stated that the period between the months of December 1777 and January 1778 was the time of greatest mortality as well as confusion in the hospitals, for patients were being transported from one place to another with many actually dying on the road or in the wagons while en route as well as at places where they halted. He further admitted it was impossible to accurately record the number or causes of deaths. He also said he believed that had they possessed more accommodation, fully one-half of the hospital patients who died might have been saved. Rush always claimed that more hospital space could have been readily obtained had Shippen so ordered, and there were those who agreed and joined Rush in his statement, but it is a significant fact that the few who did were all men who might have profited by Shippen's downfall.

Several hospital physicians and surgeons wrote during the winter of 1777-78 that it was almost impossible to accurately return the number of the sick and wounded, so is it any wonder that many of the hospital reports disagree? General McIntosh, whom General Washington ordered to direct the transfer of the Bethlehem Hospital when it was abandoned in the spring of 1778, reported to the Commander-in-Chief that only 81 soldiers had died between January 1 and April 12, 1778, and that 122 had been discharged to rejoin the Army. These figures, of course, could have only represented a portion of the total losses, and though there were many who submitted lists of hospital patients and casualties, no two of them agreed.

To help counteract the effect of Rush's letter and exhibits sent to Congress, Shippen solicited statements from a number of officers in the Medical Department, and among those responding was Dr. John Augustus Otto, the youngest son of Dr. Bodo Otto, who wrote:

"I do hereby certify as a surgeon mate in sundry hospitals, that I have seen Dr. Shippen at them all; inquiring about their condition and giving directions concerning them; that they have been well supplied with all necessities the county afforded; including sugar, molasses, wine and other hospital stores; that I came to act at Reading in Jan. 1778 and continued until the hospital was broken up; that while I was there the sick did not suffer for want of care in Surgeons or a proper supply of Hospital Stores."

Francis Allison, Jr., writing from the Lititz Hospital on April 14, 1778, said in brief:

"I have supplied the place of a Senior Surgeon in the middle division since Aug. 1st and during that time I have never known sick or wounded to be served with adulterated wine; neither did they lack stores and much attention was paid them by Dr. Shippen."

Nicholas Garrison, a Senior Surgeon, wrote that the sick soldiers at Bethlehem did not greatly suffer for want of care, as Dr. Shippen had well supplied them with essential necessities.

Dr. Moses Scott, writing from the hospital at Ephrata on April 10, 1778, said:

"I attended the Hospital in Bethlehem 3 months and upwards. No wine delivered was found adulterated except one flask of Port when the wagoner was suspected of drinking part and filling the container with water."

David Cowell, a senior surgeon, wrote from Manheim on April 15, 1778, that he had been in the service since September 18, 1776, and he had not experienced any adulteration of wine or shortage of stores and that Dr. Shippen had supplied him with everything needful.

Opportunities for the peculation of hospital stores, adulteration of wine to cover illicit withdrawals from barrels, and the stealing of supplies from the wagons en route from storehouses to the many stations scattered throughout the county were constantly present. Roads were bad, travel slow and distances comparatively great, and often several days would be consumed in the journey; but to lay the blame for the shortages and irregularities that resulted against the honor of the Director General seems to savor of persecution; yet Rush made the insinuation of personal responsibility and participation against Shippen when he quoted Dr. Brown as saying that one-third to one-half and sometimes two-thirds of the wine, sugar and molasses arriving at the hospitals were missing. Wine, sugar and other edible commodities, which Rush charged Shippen sold out of Government-owned supplies for his own benefit, were found on every gentleman's table. Newspaper advertisements throughout the period of the war prove that all these articles were constantly offered for sale in every market, so anyone possessed of the price and inclination could purchase for his own consumption or buy for a profit. Had Shippen not been tempted to embrace opportunities of this nature, the other charges made against him might have had an early death.

Unfortunately, Congressional parsimony, or probably a real difficulty in financing all departments of the Army, resulted in a constant shortage of the very necessities in which Dr. Shippen did limited speculation. The fact that he had wine and sugar to sell and that the hospitals were in need of them gave a handle to Shippen's accusers.

Dr. Rush's comparison of hospitals in the Northern Department under Potts with those responsible to Shippen was cleverly conceived and presented to make the Director General appear at a disadvantage. The facts and figures as written by Rush were approximately correct for a limited period, but there was no more fairness in so using them than there would be in our day in selecting a city's most favorable week of vital statistics to base a claim for an annual health and death rate. The chapter on "The Northern Campaign" and the quotations from Dr. Lewis Beebe's "Journal" reflect a truer picture of the general condition in Dr. Potts' hospital. The campaign in Canada and New York State covered a period of time from the spring of 1775 until the winter of 1777-78, and Dr. Potts held the responsible Northern Hospital position from June 1776 until December 1777. During the early days of the Northern expedition, the sick and wounded of the Army suffered from every hospital disorganization and privation imaginable, and on May 10, 1776, Dr. Stringer wrote General Washington they had neither medicine nor instruments, with no possibility of obtaining a supply. On June 10, 1776, General Arnold reported 3,000 sick, and Col. Trumbull wrote:

"I did not look into a tent or hut in which I did not see either a dead or dying man."

While a physician said:

"I wept until I had no more power to weep."

John Adams, one of the Congressional Committee sent North, reported on July 4, 1776, that:

"The Army was diseased, eaten with vermin, and had no medicine."

Dr. Potts, writing shortly after his arrival at Fort George, mentioned the cruel diseases present, which he included smallpox, dysentery, bilious and putrid fevers. Colonel Wigglesworth, reporting from Fort Ticonderoga on September 27, 1776, stated there were no medicines of any account in the Continental chests. On September 22, 1776, the official records noted only 5,247 of the Northern Army fit for duty, 3,917 sick in camp, and 915 absentee convalescents. Dr. Beebe, surgeon of a New Hampshire regiment, wrote in his journal on July 28, 1776, that he "visited the hospital at Fort George and counted upwards of 300 graves, all of which had been opened in about five weeks."

Every Northern hospital return found among the Potts' collection of papers reports a number of fever cases, and Dr. Potts himself, when submitting his resignation, claimed disability due to two attacks of putrid fever.

But to return to Dr. Rush's favorite statement regarding the hospital under Potts administration.

In the late winter of 1777, an army was gathered for Northern Nein York that operated under the very conditions Dr. Rush had observed were conducive to good health. They had been inoculated and were immune to smallpox; had been recruited wholly in New England and were therefore of similar habits and less liable to disease than mixed troops from different sections; they were living in open country and were frequently on the move, with constant changes to new and unpolluted camping grounds. The result of all these favorable conditions was an unusually healthy body of men. It also so happened that the New England Colonies had intimated they would not send any more soldiers into Northern service unless Congress protected them against negligence and privations when sick by providing more and better hospital facilities. The consequences were that four great wagon-loads of medical necessities were sent to the

Northern Army, and Dr. Potts was granted the large sum of $870,000 within the period between January and November of 1777.

The New York State Army returns of July 20, 1777, reported 6,023 officers and men assembled, with only 459 sick and hospitals well-staffed with fifteen surgeons and seven mates. On October 4, 1777, a total of 7,969 officers and men were recorded as enrolled, including 885 patients under the care of 25 hospital surgeons and 15 mates.

These reports registered the best condition of the healthiest American Army found in service during the entire war, and Rush picked them out for comparison with the worst period of Shippen's hospital directorship.

The few sick of the Northern Army sent to the Continental hospitals found ideal conditions for excellent care and quick recovery: good log buildings, designed and erected for the special purpose; an ample supply of medicines and necessities sent by Congress; a large hospital organization in relation to the number of patients and a reserve of cash to purchase anything needful. Sheep and beef were delivered on the hoof to the hospitals to supply meat, and gardens were maintained to raise fresh vegetables.

The conditions in the Middle Department were quite different. The Army under General Washington's command was different, as large as that assembled in the North. It had suffered several defeats, and the morale was low. At times, it was without food and cold and wet weather and lacked clothing for protection. The result of all this was a weakened army subject to much sickness. Money might have corrected many of the troubles that followed, but during the same relative time, when Shippen needed large appropriations of cash to purchase medicines and supplies, including an increase in hospital staff, Congress allowed the Middle Department just one half the amount given to Dr. Potts.

Morgan claimed to have spent only $33,870 in the period of his eighteen months' directorship and charged that in a comparable period of twenty months, Shippen's expenses were nearly $2,000,000. It so happens, however, that Shippen handled the expenditures of the hospital department for only ten months, and official records show that in that period, the sum of $430,000 passed through his hands. It should also be noted that in the year 1777 Continental money was worth only about half in purchasing value of what it was during the year and a half of Morgan's administration.

Furthermore, no proper comparison between the expenses of the Continental hospitals under the two directors was possible because prior to Morgan's dismissal, regimental hospitals existed throughout the Army, and these were largely maintained by the Colonies to which the regiment belonged. It was in January 1777 that Congress forbade such hospitals, and the Army reorganized into a body of Continental troops, so the cost and care of the sick were then transferred from the Provincial to the Central Government.

Rush's statement regarding Shippen's expenditures is even more foolish than Morgan's, for in a letter written to John Adams long after the war, he said:

"Mr. Morris informed me that the expenses of the hospital department one years informed merge of the finances, were reduced from five to one million dollar, estimated value took chanting the value of paper money in gold and silver coin for both years."

Since Government records show that Dr. Shippen's allotments were less than half a million and the Purveyor General, who handled the purchasing after February 1778, was allowed but little over two million dollars in depreciated currency for practically all of 1778 and 1779, it is apparent that Dr. Rush's statement has no value.

It is probable that much of the foregoing information was within the knowledge of the Committee of Congress appointed to investigate Rush's charges or that such evidence was collected and presented by Shippen, and, if so, it may account for the fact that Rush's accusations were no longer officially noted in the Journal of Congress.

Rush was further handicapped at this time by the embarrassment resulting from General Washington's identifying him as the author of an anonymous letter sent to Patrick Henry, saying:

"York Town, January 12th, 1778 "Dear Sir: The common danger of our country first brought you and me together. I recollect with pleasure the influence of your conversation and eloquence upon the opinions of this country. You first taught us to shake off idolatrous attachments to royalty and to oppose its encroachments upon our liberties, with our very lives. By these means you saved us from ruin. The independence of America is the offspring of that liberal spirit of thinking and acting which follows the destruction of the scepters of kings and the mighty power of Great Britain, but, Sir, we have only passed the Red Sea; a dreary wilderness is still before us, and unless a Moses or a Joshua is raised up in our behalf, we must perish before we reach the Promised Land. We have nothing to fear from our enemies on the way. Gen. Howe, it is true, has taken Philadelphia; but he has only changed his prison; his dominions are bound on all sides by his own sentries. America can only be undone by herself. She looks up to her counsels and arms for protection; but, alas! what are they?

"Her representatives in Congress dwindled to only twenty-one members-her Wilson, her Henry, her Adams, are no more among them. Her counsels weak and partial remedies applied constantly for universal disease. Her army, what is it? A Major General belonging to it called it a few days ago in my hearing 'a mob.'

"Discipline unknown or wholly neglected. The Quartermaster and Commissary Department still filled with idleness, ignorance and peculation; our hospitals crowded with 6,000 sick; but half provided with necessities and accommodations, and more dying in them in one month than perished in the field during the whole of the last campaign. The money depreciated; without any effective measures being taken to raise it. The country distracted with Don Quixote attempts to regulate the price of provisions; an artificial famine created by it and a real one dreaded from it; the spirit of the people failing through a more intimate acquaintance with the cause of our misfortunes; many submitting to Gen. Howe, more wishing to do it, only to avoid the calamities which and threaten our country. But is our case desperate? By no means; we have wisdom, virtue, and strength enough to save us, if they could be called into action.

"The Northern Army has shown us what Americans are capable of doing with a General at their head. The spirit of the Southern Army is in no way inferior to the spirit of the Northern. A Gates, a Lee, or a Conway, would in a few weeks render them an irresistible body of men. The last of the above named officers has accepted the new office of Inspector General of our Army, in order to reform abuses; but the remedy is only a palliative one. In one of his letters to a friend he says: 'A great and good God has decreed America to be free or the best counselors would have ruined her long ago.'

"You may rest assured of each of the facts related in this letter. The author of it is one of your Philadelphia friends. A hint of his name if found out by the handwriting, must not be mentioned to your most intimate friends. Even the letter must be thrown in the fire. But some of its contents ought to be made public, in order to awaken, enlighten and alarm the country. I rely upon your prudence, and am, dear Sir, with my usual attachment to you and to our beloved independence,

"Yours sincerely

"To His Excellency Patrick Henry"

Governor Henry immediately enclosed the letter to General Washington and wrote him as follows:

"Williamstown, February 20th, 1778

"Dear Sir: You will no doubt be surprised at seeing the enclosed letter in which the encomiums bestowed on me are as undeserved as the censures aimed at you are unjust. I am sorry there should be one man, who counts himself my friend, who is not yours.

"Perhaps I give you needless trouble in handing you this paper. The writer of it may be too insignificant to deserve any notice. If I knew this to be the case, I should not have intruded on your time, which is so precious.

"But there may possibly be some scheme or a party forming to your Prejudice. The enclosed leads to such a suspicion. Believe me, Sir, I have too high a sense of the obligation America has to you, to abet or countenance so unworthy a proceeding. The most exalted merits have ever been found to attract envy, but I please myself with the hope that the same fortitude and greatness of mind which has hitherto braved all difficulties and dangers inseparable from your station, will rise superior to every attempt of the envious partisan.

"I cannot tell who is the writer of this letter, which not a little perplexes me. The handwriting is altogether strange."

Not getting a prompt reply, Patrick Henry again wrote to the Commander-in-Chief on March 5, 1778:

"By an express I enclosed you an anonymous letter which I hope got safe to hand. I am anxious to hear something which will explain the strange affair which I am now informed is taken up respecting you. Mr. Curtis has just paid me a visit and by him I learned sundry particulars concerning Gen. Miflin, which much surprised me."

Before getting Patrick Henry's second letter, General Washington had written him from Valley Forge under date of the 27th of March, 1778:

"About eight days past I was honored with your favor of the 20th ult. Your friendship, Sir, in transmitting to me the anonymous letter you had received, lays me under the most grateful obligation.... However, being intimately acquainted with the man I conceive to be the author of the letter transmitted and having always received from him the strongest profession of attachment and regard, I am constrained to consider him as not possessing at least, a great degree of candor and sincerity, though his views in addressing you should have been the result of conviction and founded in motives of public good. This is not the only secret insidious attempt that has been made to ruin my reputation. There have been others equally base, cruel and ungenerous, because conducted with as little frankness and proceeding from views perhaps as personally interested.

Before closing this letter, General Washington received Governor Henry's second epistle, which touched him even more than the first, so with less restraint, he wrote:

"Camp, 28th of March, 1778

"Just as I was about to close my letter of yesterday, your favor of the 5th inst. came to hand. I can only thank you again in language of the most undissembled gratitude for your friendship. The anonymous letter with which you were pleased to favor me, was written by Dr. Rush, so far as I can judge from a similitude of hands. This man has been elaborate and studied in his profession of regard for me; and long since the letter sent to you. My caution to avoid anything which would injure the service, prevented from communicating but to a very few friends, the intrigues of a faction which I know was formed against me, since it might serve to publish our internal dissensions; but their own restless zeal to advance their own views has so clearly betrayed them and makes concealment on my part fruitless. I cannot precisely march the extent of their views but it appears in general that Gen. Gates was to be exalted in the ruin of my reputation and influence.

"This I am authorized to say from undeniable facts in my possession and from publications the evident scope of which could not be mistaken, and from private detractions industriously circulated. Gen. Miflin, it is commonly supposed, bore the second part in the cabal; and Gen. Conway, I know, was a very active and malignant partisan; but I have good reason to believe that their machinations have recoiled most sensibly upon themselves."

Rush had early knowledge of Washington's recognition of his handwriting, and it was undoubtedly known among the friends of the Commander-in-Chief in Congress and the Army.

Not many years after the death of the great Revolutionary leader, Chief Justice John Marshall began writing a story of his life in collaboration with the General's nephew, Judge Bushrod Washington.

Learning that the manuscript contained an objectionable reference to him, Dr. Benjamin Rush wrote to Judge Washington on August 29, 1804:

"I have this day heard that a letter from me to Governor [Patrick] Henry of Virginia, which was sent by him to General Washington, with the General's answer to it, are to be published in the history of his life.... I shall mention one paragraph only, in this letter [dated March 27th, 1778]"

"This man (alluding to me) has been elaborate and studious in his profession of regard for me, and that long since his letter to you.

"The letter written to Mr. Henry was dated the 12th of January, 1778. I resigned my charge of the Military Hospital on the 30th of the same month. All official intercourse ceased from that day between General Washington and me. I retired to private life, remote from the Army, immediately, nor did I ever see General Washington until fourteen months after the date of my letter to Mr. Henry, and then, first at Morristown in New Jersey.

"In the month of December 1777, I addressed two letters to the General as Commander-in-Chief of the Army, dated from Princeton. The first, stating the errors, abuses and distresses which prevailed in the Military hospitals, the second, containing complaints of the administration of the hospitals by the Director General. The mistake on the part of General Washington, in reference to time in which those letters were received is a natural one especially by a person daily occupied receiving and writing letters.

"After this statement of fact, I submit to your judgment whether it would be proper not to publish the letters alluded to, or to erase the passage objected to, in General Washington's letter to Governor Henry as well as the inference he has drawn from it."

Under the date of September 5, 1804, Dr. Rush wrote a similar letter to John Marshall, in which he said:

"I assure you, Sir, no expression or comment of mine between the 12th of January and 27th of March 1778 [the day General Washington's letter is dated], would warrant the injurious reflections upon me that are contained in it.

"After this statement of facts, permit me to request as an act of justice as well as a favor to me, that you erase the passage objected to, from the General's letter. I repeat again, they are founded upon a mistake."

Judge Washington graciously granted Dr. Rush's request, and in acknowledging the courtesy, Rush wrote:

"I take the liberty of suggesting to you that the erasure of the two sentences formerly mentioned that reflect upon me will be satisfactory. I wish it done so as not to leave a suspicion of a chasm in the letter, in the public mind. As the erasure will not make more than ten or twelve lines, the new sheet may be composed so that those erasures will not be perceptible."

That Benjamin Rush was greatly disturbed at the thought of General Washington's reflections upon him being published was very apparent. But whose recollection of facts and dates was in error? Did Dr. Rush really address General Washington between January 12 and March 27 (1778) with the deference and respect claimed, or was the Commander-in-Chief mistaken in believing that he had received a letter so inscribed within the specified time?

Unfortunately for Dr. Rush, his memory had failed him, for he completely overlooked his letter to General Washington from Princeton, dated February 25, 1778, saying he could not separate himself from the service without informing the General of the real reason for his resignation and closing with the convicting salutation:

"With the warmest sentiments of regard and attachment, your Excellency's most affectionate humble servant,

"B. Rush."

So General Washington was apparently justified in his belief that Dr. Rush had greatly violated the code of honor by expressing consideration and affection but a short time after making an anonymous attack. It was a time when the Commander-in-Chief rightfully expected his friends and enemies to come out into the open and show their true colors, but General Washington harbored no resentment, and Rush later wrote of an unexpected courtesy extended to him at the Morristown headquarters, saying:

"In consequence of my knowledge that he [General Washington] was in possession of my letter to Governor Henry, I did not call upon him at that place, but a card was sent me by the General asking me to dine with him. I went and was treated with great politeness and attention. I believe from that time, he had generously dismissed from his mind the remembrance of my letter."

That night at Morristown, Benjamin Rush entered in his journal: "March 20th, 1780-Dined with General Washington; the General uncommonly cheerful; talked chiefly of affairs in Ireland."

John Marshall's "Life of Washington" contains the correspondence of Patrick Henry and the Commander-in-Chief, with the part objected to by Dr. Rush expunged and the omission indicated by a series of *. Had not Dr. Rush kept copies of his correspondence with Judge Bushrod Washington and Chief Justice Marshall, this part of our story could not have been told.

CHAPTER EIGHTEEN

MORGAN'S ACCUSATIONS • Shippen-Stands • Trial Formal Accusations • Presented Acquittal by Court Martial

DR. JOHN MORGAN'S REMOVAL as Director General of the Continental Hospitals, coupled with Dr. Stringer's separation from the Northern Department, surprised them both as well as the Army. Stringer promptly sought an explanation from his commanding officer, General Schuyler, who sent a protest to Congress, resulting in an official rebuke through resolutions, saying:

"That as Congress proceeded to the dismission of Dr. Stringer upon reasons satisfactory to themselves, Genl. Schuyler ought to have known it to be his duty to have acquiesced therein."

"Furthermore; that the suggestion in Gen. Schuyler's letter to Congress that it was a compliment due to him to have been advised of the reasons of Dr. Stringer's dismissal, is highly derogatory to the honor of Congress; and the President is desired to acquaint Gen. Schuyler that it is expected his letters for the future, shall be written in a style more suitable to the dignity of the representative body of these free and independent States and his own character as their officer."

Dr. Morgan was quite stunned by his unexpected discharge and made a formal protest through General Washington, who, forwarding it to the President of Congress, wrote:

"A few days ago, Dr. Morgan sent me the enclosed manuscript which is a vindication of his conduct upon which he desires a court of inquiry may be held. I transmit it to you by his direction. As I do not know what particular charge was alleged against him, I can say nothing to it or about it.

"You will find a plan of his also enclosed, for the better regulation of the hospital, but I think all his hints are included in Dr. Shippen's."

Included in the package of dispatches (February 14, 1778) from Headquarters with Morgan's protest, the Commander-in-Chief submitted an approved plan for a hospital reorganization drawn up by Dr. Shippen in collaboration with Dr. John Cochran. It is interesting to note that Morgan's and Shippen's suggestions were quite similar, so the outline must have appeared good and workable to both and not so full of faults as Morgan later charged.

Congress was too busy with necessary and important business to give serious thought to Dr. Morgan's personal grievances and request for an official investigation. Becoming impatient, he submitted another voluminous memorial on July 31, 1777, which was referred to a committee of the House. Nine days later

"Congress took into consideration the report of the Medical Committee on the memorial submitted by Dr. John Morgan which recited that Dr. Morgan had been dismissed, though no cause was assigned for his discharge. Yet your committee, on inquiry, finds that general complaints of persons of all ranks of the Army and not any particular charge against him, together with the critical state of affairs at that time, rendered it necessary for the public good and safety of the United States, that he should be displaced; which were the reasons for his dismissal; that the Doctor's memorial appears to be a hasty and intemperate production; notwithstanding which, as he conceived himself injured and requested an inquiry into his conduct, your committee are of the opinion that a committee of Congress should be appointed for that purpose."

Morgan made the same mistake in his procedure, as did Rush. Instead of confining his efforts to a justification of his own administration and ridding himself of insinuations of serious personal faults, he made the important feature, an attack on Shippen: attempting to prove that all accusations against himself had originated with his successor whose purpose, he alleged, was to discredit him. This allegation was quite outside the real question involved and resulted in a definite censure being included against Morgan, in the committee's report. Morgan began his "Vindication" with a statement:

"That a mean and individious set of men have looked upon my elevation to the rank of Director General and Physician-in-Chief with evil eye and have long been concerting my removal, is a matter of which I have too substantial proof to doubt."

Then he wrote:

"Had Congress supposed that I had too much and he, [Shippen], too little to do, I would cheerfully have transferred to him the superintendence and management of as many as his heart desired, only reserving my rank and the command of my own officers, hospital and stores. But I have good reason to believe that his underhanded attempts to interfere with me in my department, and his interests with a particular set which has been employed to effect my removal with a view to promote his design of succeeding me, have operated more powerfully to accomplish it than all others that have been held up as the ostensible cause of my removal.

"Is it not manifest that the Director [Shippen] and his attachments have from his first coming into the service, pursued such measures as they conceived were best calculated to raise him over the shoulders of every man who stood in his way?

"I am persuaded that both he and his adherents have not only watched for but made occasion to serve as a plausible pretext for displacing me.

"I had intimations given me more than once that pains would be taken to deprive me of my rank and distinction to make room for a rising competitor.

"The ears of the honorable Congress were abused and I fell a sacrifice."

The Congressional minutes contained no further reference to the Morgan investigation until September 18, 1778, when it was recorded that Dr. Morgan had filed still another communication. The House Committee did not submit the Morgan report until March 13, 1779, when, upon being read to Congress, it was

"Ordered to lie on the table for the perusal of the members, to be taken into consideration on Thursday next."

No other notice, however, is recorded until June 12, 1779, but in the interval some irregularities were found which are noted in a statement made by Henry Laurens and preserved in Burnett's "Letters of the Continental Congress."

"When Dr. Morgan's memorial and the report were given in at the Table on March 13th [1779], Mr. Drayton (Chairman) pressed for a day for a consideration, saying:

"'Perhaps I may not be here; therefore I wish for a short [near] day.' "Three or four days after, Dr. Morgan called upon me and sought my aid to bring on the consideration. I assured him of my good will toward him (with great sincerity) and added:

"I was sorry he had been so very severe upon particular characters; that it did not in the least degree help his cause; that a plain of what appeared to him to be facts, would have left Congress unbiased judges, whereas such language as he had adopted would at least, seem to have been calculated to prejudice the mind of the members of Congress. Dr. Morgan replied he had struck out those parts to which he supposed I alluded. I was amazed but gave no answer.

"About two weeks afterwards, I saw Mr. Drayton at the Table in Congress, take up the Committee's report of which Dr. Morgan's memorial was a part and having a paper in his left hand as a director, obliterate several parts of the memorial, to which I called the attention of two members of Congress."

Mr. Laurens' recollection of the incident was then continued in the third person.

"On the third of June [1779], Mr. Searle moved in very affecting terms, for consideration of the aforementioned Morgan report. Mr. Drayton warmly seconded him.

"Mr. Laurens rose and said he knew of no report respecting Dr. Morgan that was before the House; that there had been one but it had undergone such alterations and obliterations since it had been delivered to the House, as, in his opinion, destroyed its original character.

"The President expressed surprise and asked:

"'The report of the Committee since it was delivered into the House?'"

"Mr. Laurens replied:

"'Yes, Sir, since; and some parts long since.'

"Mr. M. Smith and Mr. Penn said, Dr. Morgan, with permission of the Committee, had struck out some parts of his memorial which had been thought to contain too severe a reflection against particular persons.

"Mr. Laurens replied he knew Dr. Morgan had done so, but he would ask his honorable colleague, Mr. Drayton, if he also had not obliterated several parts?

"Mr. Drayton arose and admitted that he had; that there were some severe epithets which had been struck out or expunged in order to make it go down the better.

"These were his very (foolish) words and the President said to him: "'After the paper was delivered to the House, you had no right to strike out or alter a single iota.'"

Nine days later (June 12, 1779), Congress reviewed the Morgan report as submitted, and after reciting the various steps taken in the investigation,

"Resolved: that the said Dr. John Morgan hath in a most satisfactory manner vindicated his conduct in every respect as Director General and Physician-in-Chief, upon the testimony of the Commander-in-Chief, general officers, physicians in the General Hospital Department, and other officers in the Army; showing that the said Director General did conduct himself ably and faithfully in the discharge of his duties. Therefore it was: "Resolved: that Congress are satisfied with the conduct of Dr. John Morgan while acting as Director General and Physician-in-Chief in the hospitals of the United States and that this resolution be published."

Just three days after his Congressional vindication, John Morgan addressed a letter to John Jay, President, saying that he was very appreciative of the action of Congress in restoring to him his unsullied reputation and expressing the belief that it was the duty of all good citizens to bring to the attention of the public the dereliction of any person in office as well as to furnish proof of his guilt. He then continued:

"I do hereby charge Dr. William Shippen, Jr., in the service of the United States, with malpractice and misconduct in office. And whereas, Congress by a resolve of the House has subjected a director of the General Hospital on any accusation of misconduct, to be tried by court martial, I therefore now declare my readiness to give before the proper court having jurisdiction, the necessary evidence in the premises, against the said Dr. William Shippen."

This letter was written from Philadelphia and dated June 15, 1779. On the day of its receipt, Congress

"Resolved: that a copy of the said letter be transmitted to the Commander-in-Chief and that he be directed to cause such proceedings to be had thereon, that the charges alluded to in it be speedily inquired into and justice done."

It was also ordered that an extract of the letter with a copy of the resolution be transmitted to Dr. Shippen. Meanwhile, Dr. Morgan had appealed to Dr. Rush, who, replying on July 17, 1779, wrote:

"You desire to know what matters I am willing to testify on oath, respecting Dr. Shippen's conduct in the Military hospitals while I was with him. To this request I shall answer in a few words.

"(1) That he discovered a total ignorance of his duties as the Di rector General of the hospitals. This ignorance appeared in every part of his conduct but more especially in his manner of laying out the public money, which rendered the expenses of the Department four times greater than necessary.

"(2) I shall declare upon oath that he discovered [displayed] the greatest negligence of his business. During the space of nine months I never saw him but twice in any hospital. All my letters and petitions to him for necessities for the sick, were treated with neglect. Many hundreds of our brave countrymen died in the hospitals for this cause; whose lives might have been saved if they had had the use of those necessary and comfortable things which the Congress allowed.

"(3) I shall prove upon oath that Dr. Shippen traded largely in hospital stores; that he transported large quantities of wine, loaf and brown sugar, in public wagons through different villages of Pennsylvania, and afterwards sold them as private property. That our soldiers suffered and died for want of these stores, at the very time he disposed of them, and that the continent had been obliged to replace them at immense expense.

"(4) I shall prove upon oath that he deceived the Congress with false reports of the number of sick and deaths in the hospitals, and with false accounts of the diseases that prevailed in the hospitals, and the state of the hospitals in general.

"I wish you better success in your attempt to serve your country and the interest of humanity by bringing Dr. Shippen to justice, than I met when I impeached him in March, 1778, and specified most of the crimes I mentioned in this letter.

"I have no personal resentment to gratify against him and I was satisfied that my charges would appear well grounded, and that justice would certainly take place when his accounts were called. For I have good reasons to think that he cannot produce vouchers for a quarter of the money that has passed through his hands."

With apparent impatience because of the inactivity of Congress but at the same time encouraged by the prompt action on his June 15 accusation, Morgan again wrote:

"To His Excellency, John Jay, Esq., President of Congress.

"Phila., July 19th, 1779.

"In obedience to the invitation and command of Congress, I step forth on the principle of love of my country and public good, and charge Dr. William Shippen, Jr., with malpractice and misconduct in office; and pledge myself to appear in support of the charges when called upon, before the proper court having jurisdiction in the premises. I expected that on such declaration, Dr. Shippen would have been immediately brought to trial. More than a month however has since elapsed and the movements of the enemy have made it impractical for the General to appoint an early court martial for that purpose. How long the state of affairs may occasion this trial to be postponed, is not known. Perhaps it may be during the whole of the ensuing campaign. I there. fore deem it my duty, to present to Congress that these charges which 1 mean to bring against Dr. Shippen, appear to be of such a nature that for the honor of Congress and service to these States, the putting in arrest and immediate suspension of Dr. Shippen from office is absolutely necessary.

"John Morgan."

Shippen's effort to obtain some commitment from General Washington was met with a postponement. He addressed Congress:

"Sirs:

"West Point, July 28th, 1779.

"I have earnestly solicited His Excellency, Gen. Washington, to grant me a court martial but he says the circumstances of the Army are such as to make it very inconvenient now... I have only to pray the Honorable Congress to order Dr. Morgan to furnish the Judge Advocate with a copy of the crimes of which he proposes to prove me guilty, that I may know how to prepare my defense and be ready at the first moment that I can be indulged with a trial, to acquit myself with honor and bring my accuser to shame and disgrace."

Dr. Bodo Otto did not wait to learn the sentiments of the Army or the Medical Department regarding Morgan's attack on Shippen but immediately declared himself in association with another hospital chief of a neighboring station.

"Dr. William Shippen, Jr.,

"Yellow Springs, June 18th, 1779.

Director General,

"Dear Sir:

"We, the undersigned, having occasionally met together at this post, were not less alarmed than incensed when told that Drs. Rush and Morgan still pursued you with their relentless spirit of revenge and defamation. Our information is that from the complaints of these gentlemen to Congress, you are arraigned on the charge of neglect of duty and infidelity in your office as Director General.

"We make no doubt, Sir, but that the whole body of your surgeons throughout the continent (whom you well know to be the eyes of inspection and arms of execution within the Hospital Department) will exhibit virtue, honor and truth enough, to support you on this occasion with their honest and united testimony against every effort of vindictive spleen and calumny, originating not from public, but partial, views; not to comfort but to confound our present happy arrangement of hospital government we must acknowledge is principally derived which from the modern, combi combined endeavor of you and your subaltern officers, to promote hospital interests.

"We further assert as our opinion (and we believe the opinion is pretty general) that since the date of Dr. Rush's exit from among us, our hospitals have improved and hospital government has become uniform. Dr. Morgan's service was before our time but the unanimous testimony of many officers who acted under him and you, is to the effect that his dismissal proved another lucky era of change in the Hospital Department.

"Unsought and unsolicited by you or any man; uninfluenced by any views of partial or partisan influence, we however on our part do hereby avow and declare to the world that from the date of our respective commissions on the hospital staff, through all the posts and hospitals in which we have exercised command, we never had cause to complain of your directorship, either in the purveying or prescriptive lines, and we think the charges exhibited against you, of neglect of duty and infidelity in office, are as malicious as they are false and unfounded.

"We remain, dear Sir,

"Your obedient humble servants, "Bodo Otto, Senior Physician and Surgeon,

"James Fallon, Senior Physician and Surgeon."

Officially, the Shippen matter dragged, though Dr. Morgan personally was very busy preparing for the expected trial. On October 25, 1779, he wrote another letter:

"To His Excellency, Samuel Huntington, Esq., President and The Honorable Congress of the United States of America.

"Sir:

"I think it proper to inform Congress that after collecting the necessary evidence on the certificates and depositions of numerous witnesses in Pennsylvania and Jersey, I had a conference with His Excellency, Gen, Washington, on the subject of Dr. Shippen's trial, and he was pleased to declare that after the operation of the present campaign he would immediately order a court martial for the purpose of trying Dr. William Shippen, Director General of the Hospital; to be composed of officers of suitable rank, and this is all that can be done on the part of His Excellency.

"I have also conferred with the Judge Advocate General and laid before him a statement of the charges and the evidence and he advised, considering the nature of the charges and that witnesses reside some distance from the Army, to pray Congress that it be pleased to recommend to Pennsylvania and New Jersey an Act to empower proper officers to issue writs of subpoena to oblige necessary witnesses to attend court and give in their evidence.

"I persuade myself that Congress readily perceives that unless some mode is adopted to require attendance of witnesses, in vain will be every attempt in the future to bring public delinquents to justice, not with. standing the loud cause of the good people of these States to inquire into and reform those abuses from whence have proceeded many of the calamities they now experience.

"Submitting these matters to the wisdom of Congress and relying wholly on their justice for a candid interpretation of these efforts of mine to serve my country, I remain

"Your Excellency's most obedient and humble servant.

"John Morgan."

Morgan followed this letter of October 25 with still another, dated Philadelphia, November 22, 1779. Again, it was addressed to Congress:

"In my letter of July 19th last, after having impeached Dr. Shippen, Jr., with malpractice and misconduct in office, I demanded his suspension as the constant practice of other nations, of our own Army and as a necessary rule of war. I showed on sufficient evidence that attempts were made to bribe and corrupt witnesses, to put it out of my power to appear against him. The following September, finding him still in office unsuspended, I undertook the journey to camp with the intention among others of charging him in person with crimes in office, and to confront him before witnesses. He knew of my coming and withdrew to Philadelphia. On returning to the city, I solicited Congress to pass the necessary resolve compelling witnesses to attend court martial or to fall on some measure to give evidence on facts a due force, and prayed that the charges of the trial might be at the expense of the United States.

"Congress was pleased to resolve that in cases not capital, depositions might be given in evidence provided the prosecutor and person accused were present at the taking of same but no provision was made to receive depositions as evidence, if the adverse party had reasonable notice of the time and place and should neglect to attend.... And I further beg leave to observe that no sooner had the above resolve of the 16th passed the House, than Dr. Shippen again withdrew himself to the city so as to render abortive, every attempt to serve him with notice for taking the depositions of evidence. I am sorry that the resolutions of Congress for "that purpose, have been so easily and immediately evaded. I formerly attempted to remove any objections to putting Dr. Shippen under arrest, such as leaving the Department without a head. Dr. Brown was then present on whom, if I am rightly informed, the care of the hospital would naturally devolve during Dr. Shippen's suspension and trial. I now understand that Dr. Brown will go to Virginia to spend the winter which will deprive me of material evidence and may be given as a reason by Dr. Shippen's friends, why he ought not to be tried in the meanwhile. While he continues in the exercise of his office, other evidence may in like manner be removed; and thus one excuse after another may be perpetually assigned as a reason why he shall not be compelled to prepare for his trial or attend to the taking of evidence, necessary for same, and thus delays framed in an endless circle.

"If it is urged as a reason against his being dealt with on this occasion as has been usual for a General and other officers, because there is no one of the same rank to supply his place, I beg leave to remark... that there are deputies, assistant Director Generals, Physician and Surgeon Generals, to supply the place, and they are now numerous in the present establishment. Should there now be a reduction of officers as is said to be contemplated, other evidence which I can now call upon may be removed. Should a trial be now ordered, the examination of his books and accounts may be a necessary measure to detect fraud. He may plead the want of leisure for settling his books. Did not Congress order two years ago that he immediately settle his accounts? Has he ever done so; or will it be done, or evidence be examined to convict him of guilt till he is suspended? Or must these matters be left till the trial is appointed to the increase of expense and difficulties so that the whole ensuing winter may be consumed in fresh delays.

"I have already informed Congress that my charges against Dr. Shippen are no trivial complaints. No man in Dr. Shippen's place can be charged with blacker crime, or that more concerns the dignity and honor of the United States to take cognizance of them and to pursue such steps that justice may not be eluded through delay, or neglect to secure and establish the necessary evidence to prove the facts. It is in cumbent on me therefore to inform Congress, that since I first called upon this honorable house for justice upon the accused, some persons who then offered to testify to facts necessary to prove particular parts of his criminality, have since gone from the continent. Others have, and some are about to remove to such a distance that objections may be made to the expense of summoning them to attend. Their testimony could now be taken without difficulty were Dr. Shippen suspended, so that he could be called upon immediately, to attend the taking of evidence "Perhaps it becomes me to specify some of the charges which I shall undertake to prove against him, to induce Congress to suspend and oblige him to prepare for trial. I shall now do so.

"I charge Dr. Shippen among other things, with behaving in a scandalous manner unbecoming an officer and a gentleman; with fraud; dealing in hospital stores on his own account; selling wine and sugar to hunters and tavern-keepers while sick and wounded soldiers suffered miserably for want of them; and in lack of due care in attending and providing for them; and that they died in great number under circumstances disgraceful to the United States and shocking to humanity. I charge him with having refused to pay debts, contracted by hospital commissaries and forage masters, for the use of the sick, though he did not dispute the justice of the account; till it cost the creditors the whole amount or a great part of the money to recover same or till it fell far below the value due because of the rapid increase of prices of hospital stores and depreciation of money. And I charge him with employing public wagons in transporting his stores from place to place. When I acquaint you, Sir, that a number of people to whom these facts are known are distressed by them and dissatisfied at every appearance of delayed justice and are ready to prove the facts whenever Dr. Shippen is ordered to attend an examination, I cannot suppose that this honorable house which till now has been unacquainted with the matter, will hesitate to put a stop to Dr. Shippen's career until he has undergone a trial and is acquitted.

"His Excellency, Gen. Gen. Washington, informed me when at camp, that had he known the campaign would pass as it did, the trial might have taken place before now without injury to the service. And I am therefore convinced that if Congress will but signify its pleasure that Dr. Shippen be suspended, the reason for deferring it being removed, His Excellency will immediately give orders for that purpose. Gen. Washington was pleased to assure me that it did not lie with him, but with Congress to give the necessary orders for rendering testimony binding when given by witnesses out of the Army. Should Congress think it proper to appoint a committee to examine into the number and nature of the evidence, I am ready to attend.

"I only pray for measures calculated to promote the welfare and interests of the United States; to remove every bar to a fair and speedy trial; to deprive even the prosecutor himself, of all manner of excuse should he fail in what he has undertaken, for no other motive than public justice and service of these States.

"I have so long and fatally experienced the wits of Dr. Shippen to baffle and elude justice, that I cannot but be anxiously watchful when naked, defenseless and unsupported but by the righteousness of my motives, I find myself a prosecutor; opposed to a man holding in his hands the means to bribe and seduce witnesses and some of those under his influence has actually proceeded to bribe and seduce. I daily see so many difficulties arising from the influences of his office, that if he is not shortly suspended and if I fail in making good my charges. I shall in conscience believe that my failure is only to be imputed to obstructions in the way of a speedy trial; to his remaining so long unsuspended after accusations were brought and to his continuing to hold in his hands the charms and terrors of office, contrary to the usual customs of war. I speak freely from a sense of duty that if Dr. Ship pen's trial be long deferred, evidences removed, no effectual method called upon to secure testimony, and Dr. Shippen not be convicted, I may stand acquitted to my conscience, of the charges made by Congress to the public on May 1st, that the honorable House was not convinced there had been as much diligence used in detecting and reforming abuses as in complaining of them.

"But I submit to the wisdom and uprightness of Congress, and am, your Excellency's most obedient servant,

"John Morgan."

This communication, which likewise stressed the need for authority to obtain depositions, with Morgan's earlier letter, was submitted to the committee of the House, which reported on November 16, 1779. Congress then

"Resolved; that it be recommended to the executive authority of the respective States, upon application of the Judge Advocate for that purpose, to grant proper writs, requiring and compelling any person or persons whose attendance shall be requested by the said Judge, to appear and give testimony in any case depending before a court martial; and that it be recommended to the legislatures of the several States, to vest the necessary power for the purpose aforesaid, in their respective authorities, if the same be not already done."

Morgan was apparently fearful that the action outlined by Congress did not adequately cover all possible situations, for on December 20, 1779, he again recited his difficulties in a letter addressed to Samuel Huntington, Esq., President of Congress:

"Sir:

"I beg leave to inform Congress that when the resolution of November 16th was sent to the Assembly of Pennsylvania, it was so near the close of the session that they lacked time to pass any law obliging witnesses to attend a court-martial; nor is there any law in this State that can oblige anyone to leave his boundaries to give evidence in another State. But a committee reporting upon it, stated that the expenses in such cases ought to be borne by the United States. I observe by a vote of Congress, dated April 3rd ('78), that in the case of Dr. Rush's bringing charges against Dr. Shippen, that Congress resolved to appoint a committee to send for such persons and papers that they might judge necessary and allow reasonable and necessary expenses to the witnesses attending that business. I humbly pray that a similar resolve may now pass to enable me to induce witnesses to attend the trial of Dr. Shippen. One resolve in Congress, dated Nov. 16th is, that in cases not capital, depositions may be given in evidence provided the prosecutor and person accused are present at the taking of the same. In many States, depositions are deemed good evidence in courts of law if the person accused has had reasonable notice of the time and place and then neglects to attend. Unless that is the meaning of Congress by the said resolve, it is in the power of the accused person to evade the force of evidence by absenting himself, though he received due notice. As an instance of this, I enclose Peter O. Beas deposition No. 3 taken this day before William Rush, Esq., Justice of the Peace. The prosecutor and deponent waited from 9:00 until 10:00 o'clock for the accused person, who had due notice, to attend as appears by copy of the summons sent him for that purpose; he then failing to appear, the deposition was taken. I have also given him notice of my intention to take depositions at Reading and Lancaster but he has failed to inform me whether or not be will attend. If I should proceed [on the journey] and he not attend, and the depositions on that account be considered as ex parte evidence, I had better save myself any further trouble unless Congress, in its wisdom, will point out a mode of rendering testimony of witnesses effectual and obtainable.

"My proceeding to Lancaster, Dunkers Town, Reams Town, and Reading, and afterwards to Allen Town and Bethlehem, etc., was to take depositions in order to save the expense of summoning great numbers of witnesses at an inclement season far from home, and where comfortable accommodations and subsistence for man and horse may be difficult to procure; also in order to get over the difficulty of obliging them to attend (though the nature of the case will require that some shall attend in person) though this greatly depends on the resolutions and directions of Congress.

"Phila., Dec. 20th, 1779."

The last two letters from Dr. Morgan to Congress seem to contain a note of irritation as though he felt others were not taking Dr. Shippen's prosecution as seriously as they should and even suggests he believed he was not receiving proper cooperation.

Morgan overlooked no detail in his preparation for the coming trial and even anticipated difficulty of obtaining lodgings and other necessary accommodations at Morristown; for on January 30, 1780, a month and a half before the date designated, he wrote Major a General Greene:

Phila, January 30th, 1780.

"Dear Sir:

"I fear he shall be at some loss to obtain convenient quarters for attending the courts martial of Dr. Shippen's approaching trial, unless some of my friends who have power and sufficient interest, will se so good as to put me in a way of engaging them. Col. Wadsworth promised to look out and let me know where it was most likely I could be provided, but I understand he has proceeded on his journey and I have not heard from him.

I shall take it as a favor if you can in any way assist Col. Biddle, in pointing out how and where I can be accommodated. One piece of kindness often serves as a foundation on which to build the hope of another; your politeness to me, when I was last in camp, of which I retain a grateful sense, is the reason of my presuming now to trouble you with this application."

Court convened on March 15, 1780, and Dr. Rush's prompt attendance is recorded in his diary:

"March 14th-Set off to attend as a witness at Dr. Shippen's trial at Morristown, N.J.

"March 16th-Arrived-Trial postponed until the 20th.

"March 20th-Returned to Morristown-Spent one hour giving in my evidence.

"March 21st—spent five hours in giving evidence-dined with Dr.

Cochran. "March 22nd Spent five and a half hours giving evidence and answering questions.

"March 24th-Returned to Philadelphia."

Morgan maintained constant communication with Rush during the trial through letters giving many details of the evidence submitted with the names of the witnesses examined. Many of these epistles are among the Rush manuscripts in Philadelphia.

The trial was soon interrupted and postponed, which Morgan explained in a letter, saying:

"To His Excellency Samuel Huntington, Esq.,

"Morris Town, March 28, 1780.

"President of Congress.

"Sir:

"On the 16th inst. the court martial met for trial of Dr. William Shippen, Jr.

"The Resolution of Congress, of Dec. 24th last relative to admitting depositions of persons not in the line of staff of the Army to be read as evidence in trial not capital before court martial, was laid before the court and Dr. Shippen then made no objection to that resolve; where-upon some depositions were read in support of the first charge. Next day finding he could not stand before the force of such evidence and the testimony in other depositions which I was prepared to produce, Dr. Shippen moved the court that no more depositions be read against him, pleading that he not only was not present at the taking of same, although he could not deny having had sufficient notice beforehand of the time and place of their taking, had he chosen to attend, but he alleged that I was never named or recognized; by Congress as his prosecutor; that he was not under arrest at the time, nor served with the charges.

"On this, were produced the resolutions of Congress of November 16th as well as December 24th, and shown to be passed in answer to my letters and setting forth the permission of Congress that I act as his prosecutor. It was set forth that on my visit to Camp in October last, that I had urged Gen. Washington to suspend his power of acting, on purpose to give him an opportunity and to oblige him to prepare for his defense; that the General declined putting him under arrest at the time was on account of the then situation in the Army with respect to the enemy, which might be attended with ill consequences to the Hospital Department at so critical a period, by being deprived of the assistance of its principal officer; also in consideration of the hardships that might attend the long arrest, before it would be possible to appoint a court martial; but that the General must have considered him amenable to the resolves of Congress, after the charges against him, the same as if he were under formal arrest. In answer to his objection of not having been served with the charges, I referred to his letter of July 20th, 1779, addressed to the President of Congress, desiring he might be furnished with the charges against him, and my letters of July 19th and November 28th specifying the charges which are substantially the same as those on which he is now tried, including a resolve of Congress dated November 24th ordering Dr. Shippen be served with a copy of said letter and charges.

"The court however complied with his request as well as set aside those depositions for the present, so as to allow Dr. Shippen further time to prepare evidence in his defense.

"On this occasion I am compelled once more to address Congress; to refer them to my former letters and their resolutions on this subject, earnestly entreating to know whether all former resolutions on this subject are annulled; and whether the fruits of my labor and expenses of near twelve months, devoted to this service and executed agreeable to the direction of Congress are to be thrown away as of no account, or what new measures are to be pursued to make testimony of more validity than repeated resolves of Congress appear to have been. "The Judge Advocate informed me in due time, that if depositions are to be taken over again it was not within his power to attend; his presence being required in camp, and he would therefore authorize me in his name and stead to cite Dr. Shippen to attend the taking of such depositions. I gave Dr. Shippen this information by letter, the receipt of which he neither acknowledged nor denied. In that letter I told him, that if he would be at pains to convince me that the resolves of Congress were not binding on him or that there was any informality in the notices I sent him, I would previous to the time appointed for trial, send him fresh citations to attend and examine the deponents over again in his presence, that both parties might come to trial fully prepared to bring matters to a speedy decision; but after the court was appointed, I would not if I could help it, beat the ground over again.

"I cannot but consider the conduct of Dr. Shippen to evade trial, as a temporizing expedient, unworthy of an innocent man and a man of honor to endeavor to wear out his prosecutor by obliging him to sacrifice that time which is necessary that he employ for the support of his family, in an irksome pursuit after justice and to weary him with expenses and delays.

"A sense of what I think owing to the dignity and honor of Congress and what I have undertaken from no other motive than love of my country and the demands of public justice in this dilemma, I submit myself to the wisdom and impartiality of Congress, and remain

"Your Excellency's most obedient and humble servant

"John Morgan."

Dr. Shippen's reasons for his action in asking an adjournment are told in a letter to Richard Henry Lee, dated Philadelphia., April 16, 1780:

"My dear Sir:

"I have been before the court martial three weeks but have not yet finished owing to a dispute over the evidence.

"The Congress resolves that in cases not capital, depositions taken from persons not belonging either to the line or staff of the Army before a magistrate, if the prosecutor and person accused are present, may be read in evidence.

"Morgan, supposing himself to be the prosecutor as well as the persecuted, cited me to attend [the taking of such depositions] through the deepest snow of the winter which he broke for two hundred miles and was one day dug out and once froze in his saddle. I did not attend And but when the weather was better, sent a friend around to interview the same persons and obtain certificates from nine-tenths of them, to the effect that they knew nothing against Dr. Shippen and did not mean to injure his character but that Dr. Morgan had earnestly and meanly importuned them to depose something or other.

"When I appeared before my judges, conscious of my innocence and not doubting but that in a court martial, my certificates would be received to counteract such depositions, I admitted them to be read. After we broke up, it was whispered among my friends that I was on slippery ground and that my certificates might be of no use and not legal testimony; in short that if I convinced their [the court's] honor and conscience that I was innocent, they could not acquit me because the testimony was not legal. Upon this, I thought I was running too great a risk, as some weak, wicked or angered person might have been persuaded to swear falsely (against me) and begged his [Morgan's] affidavits might not be admitted; urging five reasons against them and begged for time to [better] prepare my defense, and to take all these dearly earned oaths over again. This they granted; took seven or eight oral witnesses and adjourned until May 15th ('80).

"My persecutor is now made a Deputy Judge Advocate and we will set off in four or five days to go around the circuit and make the poor people again give their former attestation; this is the most curious piece of business ever undertaken. He [Morgan] gives me much trouble; the matters happened so long ago and at so many places, and he is so meanly industrious.

"There is hardly an action in two years that I am not obliged to explain. If you can recollect any P person who wrote or complained to Congress of his [Morgan's] malconduct and the suffering of the sick under his care, do write of them to me by the first post. He wants to prove that all the clamors were raised by me to obtain his place, which you know is not true. I know the force of his testimony but am very clear I can oppose it abundantly, if the court martial will allow anything for the distressing winter of 1777.

"It is very mortifying to have every boy, formerly my pupil, asked what he knows against the Director General; but I must go through with it...."

This letter has a note of weariness and discouragement that can be readily understood. The answer from R. H. Lee finally arrived from Richmond, Virginia, written on May 7, 1780:

"I arrived here six days ago to give attendance as a member of the present General Assembly, and here I received your favor of April 16th on the 5th inst.

"You ask, must the wicked enemies of our country prosper and go unpunished? I answer, they probably will until virtue learns to be as industrious as vice, and men in general come to prize the former more than the latter. The stimulated industry that marks your persecutor, strongly demonstrates that some other quality than virtue, influences his conduct. The bitterness of revenge, working on disappointed ambitions, is plainly perceptible at this distance of mine.

"I cannot recollect particular complaints against Dr. Morgan out of Congress, but I remember perfectly well that in Congress, Mr. Chase [of Maryland] did most warmly oppose Dr. Morgan's longer continuance in the directorship; saying repeatedly that not a soldier would be obtained from Maryland, if the Director were not changed. I remember his mentioning particular instances of Morgan's misconduct which appeared strong at the time. I make no doubt but that you may get the information you want from Mr. Chase and also be availed of his testimony. If there were any written complaints filed, they no doubt may be found among the records of Congress.

"Having had the pleasure of a great share of your confidence and correspondence, and having been a member of Congress at that time, it seems more than probable that had you excited clamors against the Director with a view of succeeding him, I should have heard or known something about it; and yet I can declare before God and man, that I neither knew or heard of any such thing. I well know, that before Dr. Morgan's appointment to the directorship, you expressed yourself against taking that office, and that it plainly appeared to Congress. I believe there is scarcely a gentleman who was then a member of Congress, who does not well remember how great and general was the dissatisfaction at that time, against the Director General; so much so that I soundly affirm it appeared to me, as I know it did to many others, that a change in the directorship was indispensable to collecting another army; the former having been chiefly disbanded in the Fall of 1776.

"It (your proposed proceedings) appears to me a new mode of judicial proceedings, for the prosecutor to be the evidence taken although the defendant be present because if they differ concerning the propriety of any insertion [evidence], who is to determine? Or is either of the parties to decide for himself against the other? In such a case, an individual whether he were able or otherwise, must be considered as an atom compared with North America, the safety of which depends absolutely on an army and one speedily obtained.

"I heartily wish you a successful discharge from persecution, for I do most firmly believe that your services have greatly availed the public..."

So once again the old hospital circuit of 1777 and 1778 was ridden; Yellow Springs, Lancaster, Ephrata, Reading, and Bethlehem were visited in an effort to revive memories and obtain statements regarding incidents that had become history. How unimportant these bygone things must have seemed to many of those interviewed; some of them were much more concerned with finding solutions for their then present problems rather than helping to place the blame for things that were past. Even while the court martial was getting underway, frantic appeals were again being sent out for drugs, supplies, and money needed by the hospitals of the Middle States. Only four days after the judges convened, Dr. John Cochran, Chief Physician and Surgeon of General Washington's Army, wrote pathetically to the Purveyor General:

"To Dr. Jonathan Potts:

"Morristown, N.J., March 18th, 1780.

"Dear Sir:

"I received your favor by Dr. Bond and am exceedingly sorry for the present situation of the hospital finances. Our stores have been expended for two weeks past and not less than six hundred regimental sick and lame are languishing, and must suffer.

"I flatter myself you have no blame in this matter, but curse on him by whom this evil is produced. The vengeance of an offended Deity must overtake the miscreants, sooner or later. It grieves my soul to see the poor, worthy fellows pine away for want of a few comforts which they have dearly earned.

"I shall wait on his Excellency, the Commander-in-Chief and present our situation, but am persuaded it can have little effect, for what can he do? He may refer the matter to Congress; they to the Medical Committee, who will probably pow-wow over it a while and no more is heard. The few stores sent on by Dr. Bond in your absence are not yet arrived; I suppose owing to the badness of the roads. If they come, they will give us some relief for a few weeks."

Dr. Jonathan Potts was still serving as Purveyor in the spring of 1780, but was without necessary appropriations from Congress to perform his regular duties.

Again in an effort to find a scapegoat to blame and censure for conditions, history was repeating itself, and ugly rumors were circulating with insinuating fingers pointing at the Purveyor General. It was being whispered that Dr. Potts had also profited from opportunities for personal gain and would be investigated.

No suggestion of irregularities could have been further from the truth, but it seems to have been the fate of nearly every officer in the Revolutionary Army who handled money to be accused or suspected of peculation.

Even Dr. Morgan had an unofficial charge of irregularity made against him in New England during the winter of 1775 and 1776, which he considered sufficiently important to demand an investigation that he might be cleared of all suspicion.

The medical personnel were now alert and jealous of the reputation and honor of their department, and one of them promptly informed Potts of the clouds that were gathering around him. He wrote from:

"Porto Bacco, Maryland, March 1, 1780. "My friendship and anxiety for your welfare will not permit me to conceal anything you ought to know, where your character might be injured by it; and I should think myself unworthy of the friendship which you have expressed for me, were I not to forewarn you of the danger which seems to threaten.

"You will excuse me, my friend, when I speak plainly and tell what I have heard; it is the part of a friend when he sees a storm arising against his friend, to give timely notice that he may prepare himself accordingly.

"Then let me tell you that there are stories industriously propagated in this part of the country, much to your disadvantage, and the same I feel sure, from letters I have had, prevail at camp; that you keep a hospital at Reading with two Seniors (Surgeons) by way of a pretext of sending wagon-load after wagon-load of stores when there are no sick in that place. It is likewise said you have a sham hospital at Chester for twelve Virginia soldiers with an immensity of stores and a new Senior Surgeon employed.

"These, with many other things, are said to be abuses, which Congress I daresay has had hints of, and which are given as a reason why they (Congress) don't do that justice to the Medical Department which they have done for the rest of the Army. I am told that a gentleman saw an account opened for the Reading hospital, when he knew there were no sick there. My dear Sir, these things are of a serious nature; how they are founded I am entirely ignorant, but I make no doubt of your being able to make it appear you have done nothing but what you had a right to do and can answer for.

"As a friend, I thought it my duty to acquaint you with these accusations for I have reason to think they will be made a handle against you.

"Our conduct at present cannot be too circumspect. Many are watching us and willing to make mountains out of mole hills. Our department lies under many scandalous aspersions and our enemies are watching for every opportunity to magnify them. Indeed I am afraid ambition among ourselves will draw many ills upon us.

"Keep Dr. Cochran and the Army well supplied; their wants are most noticed. It is said many changes are to take place in our department.

"James Craik."

Shortly afterwards, Potts answered many of these rumors, in his resignation letter sent to the President of Congress:

"Honored Sir:

"Having received information that an Act of Congress has taken place, respecting my department, which I have not yet seen, founded on an idea of abuses committed therein, especially as to a hospital being kept in Reading attended with a number of wagons, etc., I have to assure you that such a report is entirely groundless as there has been no hospital at Reading for nearly two years past.

"After the evacuation of Philadelphia by the enemy, there were three or four wagons employed in transporting hospital stores, from different parts of the country to the General Hospital at Philadelphia and when that was effected, they were discharged; as to fixing or establishing hospitals in any place, it comes not within the line of my duties. You well know, Sir, I have only to supply the hospitals with such necessities as may be required by the Director General, the Physicians and Surgeons Generals and the Senior Surgeons. As I wish you to be fully informed of the number of gentlemen employed in the purveying line of the Middle District and what horses they keep, I will enumerate them to the best of my knowledge.

"Dr. Potts, Deputy Director General, who acts only as Purveyor, resides in Reading, and for one year past has kept his own horse.

"Dr. Thomas Bond, Jr., Assistant Director General, acts in the Middle Department when not engaged in the hospital near the Army, and resides at or near Philadelphia. "Dr. Craik, A.D.G., who is constantly with the Army.

"Dr. Goodwin Wilson, who has acted as Paymaster and Secretary since the resignation of Mr. Joseph Shippen. "Mr. Hugh James, Commissary, who keeps the magazine of stores at Philadelphia.

"Jacob Parker, Assistant Commissary, located in the Bettering House (Philadelphia).

"Alexander McCaracher, Assistant Commissary at the Yellow Springs.

"There is also a steward at each hospital and James James, a clerk to the magazine at Philadelphia; two wagons and ten horses kept at Philadelphia are employed to convey stores to the different hospitals and there are two horses for riding express.

"The Director General, the Assistant Directors, the Physician and Surgeon Generals, the Senior and Junior Surgeons and the Commissaries at the hospitals, occasionally keep horses belonging to themselves, at the place they reside. The principal officers, from one to three. There is also one or more wagons in proportion to the number of sick, to each hospital, employed in securing and transporting forage, etc., and these are either obtained from the Q.M.G. or hired in the neighborhood.

"It is now upward of four years since I had the honor of receiving my first commission. I am conscious I can with truth say I have served you with faithfulness and integrity; my health is so impaired by two putrid fever attacks, contracted in doing my duty, that at present 1 am incapable of it.

"Here give me leave to obviate a reflection thrown upon me by the wicked and malicious whose base insinuation I shall always despise; this that I made a fortune out of my commission. Sir, this is far from the truth. I was fortunate in some adventures at Sea otherwise I must have been reduced from a handsome little fortune to misery.

"I have a numerous family to maintain and it is my duty to take care of them which I cannot do on my present pay. For these and other reasons, I must beg you to appoint some other person to act in my place. Be assured, Sir, I mean not to forsake the general cause; nothing shall be left undone in my power to promote and assist, and when it pleases Heaven to give me health, I shall with alacrity, accept any place Congress may think me qualified for."

Congress had been comparatively generous to the hospitals during 1778 and 1779 following Potts' appointment as Purveyor General, and the results were reflected in a satisfactory supply of medicines and stores. Then, an esprit de corps was developed within the department. Many letters were found, exchanged between different hospital chiefs, commenting on the better results and telling of good conditions and contented spirits. A visiting chaplain, the Rev. Dr. James Sproat, who made the rounds of the hospital every two weeks, has left a journal in which he constantly wrote of the hospitals of 1778 and noted they were "clean and airy and the inmates well attended." Not once did he record witnessing suffering from want during that period. He wrote of Dr. Otto and his two sons' hospitals at Yellow Springs: "The hospitals are well provided for, and the gentlemen take good care of the sick."

A similar comment was made about the hospital at French Creek under Dr. Barnabas Binney. On May 15th, it was recorded:

"His Excellency went out to the Yellow Springs two days ago to visit the hospital themselves and found them in fine order; he spoke to every person in the bunks, which pleased the sick exceedingly."

But with the beginning of the year 1780, Congress again became neglectful of the hospitals and, during the ensuing twelve months, allowed only $431,000 in depreciated currency for hospital use, the same amount that Shippen had drawn during 1777 and with similar results. The sick and wounded were again in want, and the pitiful cry sent out by the physicians and surgeons for supplies was heartrending.

Congress became so parsimonious that it issued orders for small quantities of necessities instead of appropriating money for the Purveyor General's use. Once, on May 20, 1780, it authorized delivery of only two hogsheads of sugar and two of spirits. Suspicion and lack of confidence were in the air. Rush and Morgan's attacks on Dr. Shippen had so aroused Congress, the Army and the public that they all suspected the Medical

Department of being rotten to the core. Dr. Barnabas Binney well expressed his general feeling on the subject in a letter to his friend, Dr. Solomon Drowne, of Providence, R.I. He said:

"It can be no ways entertaining to observe the changes this unhappy war has produced. The most contemptible of the people are alternatively rising and deposing. A few good characters intermix but are suppressed by the majority of obtrusive, brazen pretenders. This is not more the case in politics than in medicine. The dirtiest and basest acts are every day depreciating the profession, while every third person is a doctor, till the very appellation has become the butt of satire, ridicule and contempt. For my own part, I have continued in the Army till this time, almost to my utter ruin; while parsimony and perfidy, with a hasty stride, have unremittingly continued to mark the vestiges of public conduct toward je data time too when their [Congress] resolutions, relative to the Medical Department, have plainly insinuated that surgeons and villains are synonymous terms.

"Thus, suffering with the Army in general, and doctors in particular, I have made a pretty hand of it."

Dr. Drowne, who had studied medicine in Philadelphia, wrote regarding the possibility of his receiving a belated college degree, and Dr. Binney, answering, said:

"I remember in one of your letters you expressed a desire of graduating. Since that time there has only been one commencement of any note, at which Crossby and Long Island Smith were graduated in Physics. This was in the height of the disputes between Morgan and Shippen. Crossby merited his degree but Smith was graduated more in opposition to poor Shippen who laid himself most shockingly open to Morgan, the most implacable, revengeful man under the Heavens.

"Rush retains his medical excellency but has made himself odious by political whims.

"The college here is now much as it was, I believe, at the commencement of the war."

Assuming that all the foregoing facts and rumors were common knowledge among the Medical Department personnel, what could have been the thoughts of the hospital officers who received visits from Dr. Morgan as Deputy Judge Advocate in connection with their chief, Dr. Shippen? What was their mental reaction to a request for a deposition or a summons to attend court? Did they look upon Dr. Morgan as an avenging angel, sent by an outraged people to see justice done and wickedness punished, or did they suspect Army laws were being enlisted and abused to enable Rush and Morgan to pay off personal grudges? Their own problems were too complicated, and their personal troubles too immediate and real to find them much interested in Morgan's stories of abuses; besides, their hospital patients needed all their attention. No wonder bad blood was eventually shown on the witness stand, and as might have been expected, the testimony became sharp and acrimonious.

Rush and Morgan constantly declared that their activity in prose- cuting Shippen was prompted by an obligation of public duty, but whatever their, the result was, the sick and wounded in the hospitals were most punished. A wonderful opportunity then existed for Shippen's prosecutors to render a great humane service to their country by offering their talents to the authorities, for hospital physicians and surgeons were by necessity leaving the Army to seek a living for themselves and their families, and those remaining were thoroughly discouraged.

The hospital situation was desperate, and Congress was finally forced to take action as a result of a letter from General Washington. The Medical Committee then reported to the House:

"That they have conversed with Dr. Cochran and other gentlemen of the hospital department, by whom and the many distressing accounts that the committee almost daily received from every quarter, it appeared that the department was in want of almost every article necessary for comfortably sustaining the sick and wounded soldiers. They are therefore clearly of the opinion that the sum of $200,000 is immediately necessary to put the department on such footing that what the General apprehends in his letter may be avoided."

How much of these hospital problems was made known to the officials of the court-martial is not a matter of record. If evidence were needed that lack of money had been the underlying cause of most of the past hospital sufferings and casualties, it was then present to be seen.

Had sufficient appropriation been made available in 1777, more physicians and surgeons could have been enrolled, additional hospitals established and officered, and all the necessities supplied. But hard money and credit were constantly limited throughout the war, and insufficient to properly finance the different departments of the Army.

It sometimes seems, in reviewing the conditions and the evidence, that many of the charges against Dr. Shippen were as far off the mark as would have been the case had General Washington been held accountable for shortages of Army food, clothing and ammunition, or lack of housing for protection of soldiers in camp or on the march.

Meanwhile Drs. Shippen and Morgan had returned to Morris town after collecting depositions and summoning witnesses a second time. Court was promptly resumed, and by June 27, 1780, all depositions and testimony had been formally presented.

"The court [then] met according to adjournment and the evidence produced being restated and compared, it proceeded to determine on the several charges exhibited against him [Shippen]; and having considered the first charge with the evidence; viz.

"Fraud in selling hospital stores for his own use and transporting them in public wagons,

"They are of the opinion that the evidence offered on that charge is insufficient to support it and they do therefore acquit him of it. "Having considered that part of the second charge which relates to Dr. Shippen's 'speculations in and selling hospital stores while the sick were perishing for want of them, they are of the opinion, that although that part of the charge taken connectedly is not sufficiently supported by evidence, on which account they do acquit Dr. Shippen, yet they are clearly of the opinion that Dr. Shippen did speculate in and sell hospital stores; that is, stores proper for hospitals, while he was Purveyor General. This conduct they consider highly improper and justly reprehensible.

"They do [also] acquit Dr. Shippen of the latter part of the charge to wit:

"peculation and adulteration of hospital wines at Bethlehem'

"as it appears to be entirely groundless.

"Having considered the third charge, they are of the opinion that no evidence has been produced with respect to the books and accounts Dr. Shippen kept; neither have the books been produced to show they were regular; and as no evidence has been shown they were irregular and no evidence.. to prove want of sufficient vouchers and checks in the department, and it does appear in evidence that vouchers have been taken for the expenditures of stores, they do therefore acquit Dr. Shippen of this part of the charge; and having considered the latter part of the same charge, they do fully acquit Dr. Shippen of it.

"Having considered the fourth charge, to wit: 'neglect of hospital duty whereby many soldiers died in a manner shocking to humanity, and to making false reports to the President of Congress, of the state of the hospitals under his care,

"the court has reviewed the evidence produced relative to it, and are of the opinion that Dr. Shippen is not guilty and they do acquit him of it.

"Having considered the fifth and last charge, to wit:

'scandalous practices unbecoming an officer and a gentleman, in calumniating and aspersing the character of his superior officer with a view to vilify and supplant him, and the evidence submitted, they are fully and clearly of the opinion that it is groundless and malicious; they do [therefore] honorably acquit Dr. Shippen of it.'

"Submitted by Edward Hand, Brigadier General and President."

The verdict of the court-martial was delivered to the Commander-in-Chief and promptly forwarded to Congress with the accompanying letter:

"Headquarters, Passaic Falls, July 15th, 1780.

"To His Excellency, Samuel Huntington, Esq., President of Congress.

"Sir:

"I have the honor to transmit to your Excellency in two packets, the proceedings of the court martial in the case of Dr. Shippen, Director General of the Hospitals, for the approbation or disapprobation of Congress. The trial having taken place in consequence of their orders, this circumstance and the Doctor stationed in the Army, have induced me to think it most proper to refer the matter to their decision. I would beg leave to observe however, that the Medical Department is in such disorder already, that it is of great importance that the affair should be brought to a conclusion in whatever way Congress may think proper, as soon as possible.

"Your most obedient and humble servant,

"George Washington."

Then came a month of interrupted consideration of the papers, and in the meanwhile, John Armstrong, a member of Congress, wrote to Gen. Horatio Gates:

"The court martial has clearly acquitted Dr. Shippen of all the charges exhibited against him, except speculation in some articles needed by the public in his own line, for which, says the court, he is reprehensible.

"The General having thrown the decision of that matter upon Congress, we are now tormented with reading the large bundle of rubbish and testimony but have not yet come to the Doctor's defense; it will probably end, indeed must end, in approving the sentence of the court martial."

Becoming anxious or impatient at the slow review of the evidence, Shippen addressed

"His Excellency, S. Huntington, Esq.,

"Sir:

"Allow me to beg the attention of the Honorable Congress to the deranged state of the Medical Department and to the suffering of the sick and wounded in our hospitals in consequence of no person having their direction; give me leave to humbly and earnestly entreat that I be relieved from my very distressing state of suspense.

"I have defended myself, Sir, and acquitted myself of all malicious charges made against me to Congress and trumpeted through every street of every State, with an unparalleled and malignant industry. Will Congress longer deny me an opportunity of informing my countrymen and fellow citizens of my innocence and acquittal by the court martial? Will they not hasten to join their approbation of my faithful Services? That I may maintain that unspotted character among my Countrymen, I have so constantly and to the best of my ability endeavored to deserve.

"I have the utmost confidence in the sense, justice and humanity of this honorable body and am with most perfect consideration, Sir, "Your and their most obedient and faithful servant,

"W. Shippen, Jr."

The Journals of Congress on August 16, 1780, record:

"Congress resumed the consideration of the proceedings of the court martial on the trial of Dr. Shippen, Director General, and having gone through the evidence, defense and judgment of the court, they continued on August 18th, when they resumed the consideration of the proceedings, and a motion was made by Mr. Timothy Matlack, seconded by Mr. William Churchill Huston, as follows;

"That the court martial having acquitted the said Dr. Shippen, the said acquittal be confirmed."

"A motion was [also] made by Mr. Abraham Clark, seconded by Mr. Nathaniel Folsom, to amend the motion by inserting after 'W. Shippen,' these words: 'except that part of the second charge relating to his speculation in hospital stores on which the court judged him highly reprehensible.'"

The final action of Congress was that: "The court martial having acquitted Dr. Shippen [it is] ordered that he be discharged from arrest."

Most writers agree in their belief that Congress considered Dr. Shippen subject to censure for dealing in supplies similar to those purchased for the hospital, but they have also expressed the opinion that most public men thought both Doctors Rush and Morgan had been actuated in their prosecution, by a spirit of revenge. Congress immediately took under consideration, another reorganization of the Medical Department with all its principal officers elected by them instead of appointed by others. In this plan, Dr. Bodo Otto was among the fifteen Senior Hospital Physicians and Surgeons chosen to direct the principal institutions for the care of the sick and wounded of the Continental Army.

Under this reorganization, Dr. William Shippen was again elected to the position of Director General but continued in office until January 3, 1781, when he asked leave to resign his commission. Dr. John Cochran was chosen to fill his place.

CHAPTER NINETEEN

COURT-MARTIAL POST-MORTEMS • Morgan's Appeal to Public • Shippen's Reply • Otto's Testimony

DR. MORGAN DEFINITELY STATED to Congress that if given the opportunity to bring Dr. Shippen before a court-martial, he would convict the Director General on the charges he would make or abide by the verdict.

The five indictments filed were:

1st: Fraud in selling hospital stores and transporting them in public wagons.

2nd: Speculation in hospital stores; adulteration of wine and diverting (Government) supplies to his own profit.

3rd: Keeping no regular set of books as vouchers for purchasing or disbursing (supplies).

4th: Neglect of hospital duties, whereby many soldiers died in a manner shocking to humanity, and making false reports to the President of Congress.

5th: Scandalous practices unbecoming an officer and a gentleman, in calumniating and aspersing the character of his superior officer.

Dr. Morgan fully expected to function as the prosecuting officer, though without an official position in the Army, as well as the chief witness; to this, Dr. Shippen took exception, and on May 27, 1780, Morgan wrote to Rush:

"On Tuesday I am to deliver in [to Court] the Dr. Shippen papers on which the charges are founded, which will be accompanied with an explanation of the circumstances by the Judge Advocate..... He [Shippen] objected to me as having acted in the place of the Judge Advocate [Morgan substituted as such in the gathering of depositions] and claimed that my evidence would tend toward a formal vindication of myself, which is the same thing as being a party interested in the event. The Court therefore determined against taking my evidence and I have prepared a statement of affairs in writing for the Judge Advocate, to enable him to lay it [the evidence] clearly before the Court. I am well satisfied with his [the Judge Advocate's] ability and integrity and apprehend that it [the accusation] will receive the prosecution I am not permitted [to give] and be examined upon.

"My idea of the matter is that if the Court finds him guilty, they will leave him as little room as possible to complain that he has not had fair play."

In another letter that Morgan wrote, taking exception to some method of procedure introduced by Shippen, he said:

"I do not think it will blind the Court in respect to the facts now before them."

But Morgan changed his position and opinion when the court-martial rendered its decision that Dr. Shippen was not guilty. Then, every action of the Court, from its method of handling the case down to its verdict, had been wrong; the trial officers had been biased and prejudiced; most of Shippen's witnesses were branded as liars and perjurers, and even the majority of Congress were accused of being a party to the crime, by reason of their approval of the verdict. In these opinions, Dr. Rush concurred, so they decided to appeal the court-martial decision to the American people in the hope of obtaining a moral conviction in order that Dr. Shippen should feel the disgrace of public condemnation.

The Pennsylvania Packet was the vehicle selected through which to present their case and, beginning with its edition of September 2, 1780, Dr. Morgan ably opened for the prosecution with the following introduction:

"Dr. John Morgan appeals to the free citizens of the United States of America on the subject of Dr. William Shippen, Jr.'s impeachment and trial by a Court Martial.

"Friends and Countrymen:

"I am sorry to be obliged to appear again before you in the character of an author, but my reputation and, what is more important, your interests have made it necessary.

"A Court Martial has passed a cold and unanimous sentence, by which Dr. Shippen is partially, and I may say, dishonorably acquitted of the charges preferred against him. Gen. Washington without approving, referred it to Congress and they after three days' debate, have put the strongest mark of disapprobation in its power, on the sentence of the Court, by refusing to approve. That Honorable Body having no power to alter the sentence, has left the praise or dispraise of his acquittal to the Court. Upon a motion to postpone the motion for discharging him from arrest, in order to bring in another which was read, for dismissing him from the service, five States voted for it, five against and one was divided, by which the motion was lost; and that because many were of the opinion should that motion pass, it would be acting counter to the principle adopted by the Congress; viz., not to set aside any sentence of a Court Martial. On that footing alone, my countrymen, unacquitted by Congress Dr. Shippen is discharged from arrest, yet by the sentence of the Court, he is held forth under the character of a speculator in hospital stores, while he acted in the high rank of Director General and Purveyor of the Hospitals.

"I know the pains I have taken to bring this man to justice, have been attributed to unworthy motives. But this has ever been the plea of guilt. Who can hear of a country robbed of soldiers enlisted in the cause of freedom and virtue, dying from want of necessities expended upon the schemes of pleasure or speculation, and not feel a glow of resentment against the author of such calamities; the reading of which called forth tears of distress from a sympathizing and compassionate Congress while they were sensible it was not within their power to dismiss him without a breach of the rights of a subject.

"I rejoice, my friends, that my exertions in the cause of civil liberty have been crowned with such a glorious effect, although it shelters Dr. Shippen. Yet, my countrymen, it is because we have felt too little resentment against public speculators, that we now fight over an exhausted treasury and bewail our country on the brink of ruin.

"As an acquittal, however disgraceful the circumstances attending it are to one not lost to all the finer feelings of sentiment, is a matter of triumph, when restored to a power, and may delude the ignorant into a belief that the charges were groundless, I think it my duty to lay before the Bar of the Public, the occasion of the impeachment and short extract of the proceedings of the trial; [this will serve] till Congress sees fit to publish them at length, by which every man will be able to judge whether the prosecution has been malicious and groundless, or whether it was virtuous, honorable and deserving the approbation of the community, to whose candid and impartial decision I shall willingly submit my own judgment.

"To state the grounds of this prosecution, it will be necessary to inform you of the following facts:

"Dr. Shippen was impeached [accused] before Congress for selling hospital stores as private property and neglecting his duty, by Dr. Benjamin Rush in April of 1778. The Congress ordered a committee to inquire into the charges, but Dr. Rush refused to bring his proof before the committee though he offered to appear before a Court Mar. tial, provided one was immediately appointed. The Congress, engaged in other matters, then overlooked this offer and Dr. Shippen continued in office with all its means of corruption. Had Dr. Shippen been arrested and tried, all his powers of seduction and intimidation of witnesses, could not have saved him. Hundreds who were then under the influence of resentment and pity for the suffering of the sick, then before their eyes, would have appeared as witnesses. He would have then had against him the evidence of many respectable gentlemen, the force of whose testimony he could not have eluded; men now removed to parts of the continent, too remote to be summoned as witnesses, as well as several more who perished from fever which his mismanagement generated and continued by crowding the sick too much together; and lastly, he would then have had two witnesses, who later appeared in his favor, testifying to facts that the same Court Martial might have found sufficient to have broken him. But a continuance in office for near two years after his impeachment, afforded great opportunities for a man of much less address than he, but possessed of the treasuries of the public, the power of creating lucrative fine sinecures and offices, to awe and seduce witnesses and dispose matters in his favor.

"Nor did the influence of Dr. Shippen's office only extend to his deputies and dependents in the Medical Department. He had been able to make his own place a very fine sinecure and the engine of corruption and power. He resided chiefly at Philadelphia, from June 1778 until the time of his trial, enjoying in pomp and pleasure the emoluments of his speculations.

"I blush to mention it, but while he was impeached of the highest crime of office, men of elevated station in public affairs, ate and drank at his table. Treats thus given are an American species of corruption. In entertainments to which they had been invited, choice Madeira wines from the hospitals, flowed plentifully to cheer his guests while distressed soldiers, applying for necessities for their sick and wounded companions, were driven away. "I could wish to pass over in silence, that the sweets of his office did not even desert him wholly at his trial. A wagon-load of stores, proper for hospitals, instead of his books, accompanied him to camp to relish himself and his friends. No one better understands the force and application of that form of argument than Dr. Shippen.

"Roused with a patriotic indignation, and not doubting of support from this State in so perilous, yet so important an undertaking as that of attempting the demolition of undue influence, venality and corruption, I stepped forth from a sense of duty and impeached Dr. William Shippen, Jr., Director General of the Hospitals, before Congress.

"I required two things, to render my attempts successful; first, agreeable to the practice of all old countries and the usages of war in our own, that he should be fortwith put under arrest that he might no longer be entrenched in power or guarded by the terrors and charms of office; secondly, that his books should be immediately inspected and a speedy trial take place so that he might not, if detected of one crime, that of fraud, have it in his power to conceal or cancel it by the commission of another, and sink it into that of simple speculation; and that no slips might be taken to defeat the prosecution, and that it might not suffer, from the death or removal of witness. Had these requirements been granted, willingly would I have submitted to the penalty of all charges I could bring against him, of which I should fail in the proof."

Dr. Morgan immediately followed this article with several others, resulting in the Director General's reply:

"Dr. Shippen begs leave to inform the respectable public, that while his persecutor is endeavoring to impose on them by partial testimony and misrepresentation of facts, he is earnestly soliciting Congress to publish the whole proceedings of the Court Martial, that the public can form some opinion with propriety, and which will prove to demonstrate the wickedness, malice and falsehood of Dr. Morgan; and prove that Dr. Shippen deserves the praise and not the censure of the country."

Morgan's attacks continued unabated, and Shippen, finally resorting to the newspaper in his own defense, wrote:

"To the Public:

"I have been called upon before a Court Martial by the malice of a displaced and angry man. After a long and full trial, in which every effort of malice and every low art was employed, I have been acquitted on every charge; that acquittal has been carefully examined in Congress; has been by them approved, and I have been reelected to the office from which it was the object of the prosecution to remove me.

"After so minute an investigation of my conduct and so honorable an acquittal, ought I not to appear in a fairer light than before to every. sensible and good man? My prosecutors, or rather my persecutors, not content with this, have now called me before you, and by publishing part of the testimony and misstating the facts, have endeavored to deceive you into being the instruments of their malevolence. However, they do not seem to be aware of the extent of their undertaking; because if you could believe what they alleged to be true, it must inevitably follow that the Court Martial which acquitted me, and the Congress that confirmed the acquittal, were blind or corrupt beyond all example. "I have no objection to being tried at your Bar, and although the duties of my office make it inconvenient, as my adversaries well know, yet I will devote as many leisure hours as will be sufficient, to introduce Dr. Morgan and Dr. Rush in their proper characters and convince you that every charge made against me is false and malicious.

"The malice and wickedness of these men will appear plain to you from the following, [evidence and depositions] declared on oath by sundry respectable witnesses, which I shall give in succeeding papers."

In the edition of the Packet one week later, Dr. Shippen continues:

"As some persons may be ignorant of the true motives which actuate Drs. Morgan and Rush in accusing and persecuting me with so much perseverance and virulence, and may think it impossible that any men could be at so much pains and expense to prove what has no existence, I persuaded myself to break a resolution to treat them and their rantings with silent contempt, but I will do so only so far as will be necessary to show their wicked designs and convince you of the propriety of my conduct.

"Dr. Morgan was appointed Director of the Hospitals in the year 1775, by a majority of one voice which I charitably obtained for him at his request. In January 1777, he was dismissed from the service with ignominy, in consequence of the clamors and complaints from officers of all ranks in the Army as appears [of record] in the journals of Congress.

"When my fellow citizens went out in the flying camp in the summer of 1776, I was called upon to attend them as Director and Chief Physician in their hospitals. A multitude of complaints of suffering of the sick under Dr. Morgan's care were made about this time and my conduct was much commended, as appears from the following extracts of letters received from Dr. Rush, then a member of Congress.

[Letters dated September and November of 1776, here quoted, have already been reproduced in a previous chapter.]

"And in April of 1777, I was appointed Director General by the unanimous vote of the Thirteen United States. The Doctor [Morgan] was greatly mortified by this appointment, and not willing to give credit to the true cause [of his discharge] assigned by Congress, chose rather to suppose, though very falsely, that his disgrace was effected by my means; and that I, as he represented in his fifth charge, reviled and calumniated my superior officer, in order to vilify and supplant him. Actuated by this opinion, he seeks revenge and has employed himself from that time to this in collecting by every means, material for accusations which have been carefully examined by a Court Martial and, notwithstanding every advantage given him during the trial of nearly three months, he was not able to support one of the charges made; therefore they were all rejected and I was acquitted.

"It is not surprising, my worthy fellow-citizens, that men actuated by such strong resentment and malevolent motives, should endeavor by byery imaginable means to gratify their malice, but is it not surprising that after having failed of success before a Court Martial and with Cong gress, they should attempt to impose upon the public by stating only one side of the evidence and by insidious assertions of which there is no supporting evidence?

"But the judgment of a disinterested and unimpeachable Court Martial on every charge, and the reasons they themselves give, will, I am persuaded, satisfy every candid man that there was no foundation for the charges made against me; that no motives but the deepest malice could have prompted a continuance of them, and that no men but such as were determined to gratify the worst of passions at every hazard of their own reputed time, could have been the author of them."

These articles of Shippen's were inspired by previous ones of Morgan's, which contain recitals of court-martial testimony and depositions in support of the prosecution. Shippen's replies also included his evidence submitted in rebuttal, but for the sake of a clearer judgment of their relative value and a better sequence, these exhibits have been deleted from many of the articles quoted and will be presented later in the chapter.

Dr. Morgan's response to Dr. Shippen's last publication was:

"I congratulate you, my fellow-citizens, upon the invaluable privilege of a free press which I consider a palladium of liberty, the scourge of knaves, the terror of despotism, and the refuge of the oppressed; by means of it, driven as I have been by an act of tyranny into exile with the enemy, as David was by the persecution of Saul, I have nevertheless been enabled to cite Dr. Shippen before your impartial Bar, and compel him to attend, however reluctantly. Although entrenched in power and guarded by the arts of bribery and seduction, he has long affected to treat your opinion of him with silence and contempt.

"False, sophistical, and consummately weak as Dr. Shippen's publication in the 'Packet' of Saturday last appears, with the yeas' of nine, against the 'nays' of two, staring him in the face and consigning him to a merited disgrace, he does with the same effrontery as his man, Dr. Cutting, did before him, assert that he is honorably acquitted. In what follows I should agree with him if the Court Martial had had acquitted with honor, which they have not done; 'that they would have been blind and corrupt beyond all example' (of the charges I have brought against him and the testimony I have advanced) the conclusion is no affair of mine. Blind, Dr. Shippen's Court Martial was not; though it acted inconsistently in pronouncing him guilty of speculation in public stores, and inflicting no punishment. Neither was Congress blind or corrupt in passing judgment on the proceedings of the Court, for it refused to ratify the acquittal. If, however, some of that body have shown themselves either blind or corrupt, we are not to wonder. Among only twelve Apostles, we read that one denied his Master through fear, and another, for the sake of speculation, betrayed him for thirty shekels of silver; this proves that Judas, who was the Purveyor General of the Apostolic Board, and carried the bag, was the father of all speculators, down to the Purveyor General of the American Hospitals. Happy would it be for America, if all Proto-Speculators were to experience his remorse and follow his example.

"After being stigmatized by the Court Martial as a speculator in hospital stores, and after Congress refused to acquit him, Dr. Shippen's appointment so far from being honorable to him, will, till it is effaced by an act of ample justice, be a lasting and dishonorable blot on the historic proceedings of that body [Congress] which dismissed his predecessor, who they declared discharged his duty ably and faithfully, on the clamor of Dr. Shippen and his friends. And yet contrary to the strong remonstrances of six virtuous States that voted for Dr. Shippen's dismissal, they reinstated him in office. This has given occasion for some to declare aloud, that Congress has appointed a monster to be the head of the Hospital Department.

"For my own part I rest assured that the Honorable body, paying a due deference to your opinion when it shall deliberately reflect on what it has done, will rectify its former proceedings and thereby, as it can in no other way, fully vindicate its own honor.

"November 21st, 1780."

"John Morgan."

Dr. Morgan's newspaper articles were addressed both to the public and to Dr. Shippen personally, and one indited to the Director General, published on December 12, 1780, said:

"By a singular concurrence of events, you appear to the world as a political paradox. While indolence, love of pleasure and dissipation were your cardinal qualities and you were an entire novice in the management of a military hospital, you were chosen the Chief Physician of that department in a separate district; a position that required personal industry, capacity, humanity and integrity, to govern it with success. With the single talent of what is called good-fellowship, you have balanced the want of every other quality and have kept an army and an infant republic in equilibrio betwixt exalting you to the pinnacle of honor and consigning you to a merited disgrace.

"You have been found guilty by a Court Martial, of speculating in hospital stores and escaped the smallest reprehension for it, while lesser bffenders have for smaller crimes, suffered exemplary punishment. Of other public charges against you, a Court Martial has given you a partial, cold, dishonorable acquittal; Congress has refused to ratify even that acquittal, and yet so paradoxical is everything that relates to you, you have again by a single ballot, which was no ballot, been re-elected Director General of the Hospitals.

"You are certainly the wonder of the public and ridicule of your department."

Dr. John B. Cutting, the Apothecary General, had engaged in a newspaper controversy with Dr. Morgan several months before the latter began these public attacks on Dr. Shippen. This exchange of open letters became very personal and bitter in character, and both parties passed the lie. Among the things that Cutting wrote was that he had been informed Morgan intended to leave the country and settle in the West Indies when the British evacuated Philadelphia and only changed his plans on receiving assurance from Dr. Rush of help in a contemplated attack on Dr. Shippen.

It became evident during the trial that considerable of the testimony submitted by the prosecution could not have been known or personally collected by Dr. Morgan, who presented it, and Shippen, commenting upon this, wrote:

"As Dr. Morgan remained in the city with the enemy, all the time (1777-78), he was quite ignorant of my conduct [during that period] and was obliged to obtain information and assistance from Dr. Rush before he could plan his prosecution."

Morgan gave great importance to a comparison between the relative size of the hospital organizations maintained by himself and by his successor but ignored two facts. First, that the classification of the medical staff, and to a certain extent, their number, we mandatory by Acts of Congress; and, secondly, that the general Directors were quite different and therefore not subject to the of caring for the sick and comparison as made. When Dr. Morgan was Director, Congress had decreed that an army of 20,000 men should have

A Director General and Chief Physician

4 Surgeons	1 Clerk
1 Apothecary	2 Storekeepers
20 Mates	1 Nurse to every 10 sick

Laborers, occasionally.

But after April 8, 1777, regimental hospitals were no longer maintained, and with an experience that proved the previous hospital facilities totally inadequate, Congress directed that the Continental Medical Department should be augmented to

1 Director General.

3 Deputy Directors General.

1 Intermediate Assistant Deputy Director.

4 Physicians General.

4 Surgeons General.

1 Physician and Surgeon General for each army.

Necessary number of Senior Surgeons to command and direct individual hospitals.

Junior Surgeons, as assistants to the Hospital Chiefs.

Surgeon Mates, as conditions required.

An Apothecary General for each district.

Apothecary Mates, as needed.

Commissaries for the different hospitals, as well as in all medical warehouses.

Clerks, Assistant Clerks and Paymasters are necessary for the hospitals and executive officers.

A Steward for every 100 patients and a Matron in the same proportion.

1 Nurse to each 10 sick or wounded soldiers.

Stablers, assigned to every hospital as well as at headquarters, that the horses of the physicians and those required to ride express, haul straw, firewood and supplies, should be attended.

Morgan totaled Shippen's organization under this set-up as 494 individuals, but an analysis of the listed personnel disclosed the fact that only 113 were of the medical profession proper, compared with 26 under Morgan's administration. Furthermore,

Shippen's lists included all those engaged in the Eastern and Northern Hospital Departments, while Morgan's activities were limited to General Washington's Army, then located either in New England or in New York.

These facts and figures seem to support Shippen's claim that instead of being overmanned, as Morgan and Rush stated, he was finally shorthanded during the critical days of the winter of 1777 and 1778 when charges were made against him of criminal negligence by overcrowding the sick and wounded; it was, therefore, impossible to establish more and smaller hospitals.

The evidence submitted by Dr. Morgan to sustain his first charge consisted largely of depositions; one from William Bennett, a tavernkeeper of Bucks County, Pennsylvania, related that he had bought one tierce (336 lbs.) of brown sugar and one-quarter cask (311/2 gallons) of Madeira wine from Dr. Shippen at a total cost of three hundred and ninety-three pounds and five shillings (the Pennsylvania Colonial pound was the equivalent of two dollars and forty-three cents Continental money). Another affidavit, made by Michael Bright of Reading, recited that he knew of a sale by Dr. Shippen of two pipes (126 gallons per pipe) of Madeira wine to John Hartman, a hotel man of Reading, and of a similar transaction with Henry Hoffa, who kept a tavern at White Horse, four miles from Potts Grove.

Allen Moore deposed that while in partnership with Morris Rodgers, he had bought and sold a cargo of wine, out of which Dr. Shippen acquired two lots; one of six pipes for 900 pounds sterling and the other of thirteen at 1,950 pounds sterling. Moore further stated that he urged Shippen to purchase the whole cargo, but the Director did not do so. This might either indicate that there was more wine available on the market than the hospitals needed or that Shippen lacked sufficient Congressional appropriations for the purpose. Other transactions with Shippen were reported by Moore as well as by the large wine dealers, Nesbitt & Company. Morgan's accusation charged that it was out of this first specified purchase that Shippen made deliveries to the different tavern-keepers and that he retained the proceeds of the sales of these Government-owned supplies, but on cross-examination, neither the men who sold the wine nor those who bought it could furnish any evidence to sustain the Prosecution.

A contract wagon master and driver deposed that a public conveyance and employee were engaged to deliver the sold wine and sugar, but Dr. Shippen swore, and was sustained by Dr. Bond, who examined his books, that the wine and sugar he disposed of, had been paid for with his own money as well as their transportation; Shippen further asserted that the public account records would disprove Morgan's accusation. Commenting on Morgan's charge of using hospital conveyance, Shippen wrote:

"As to employing public wagons to transport my immense [?] stores, and my cruel impressing of Rembelt's wagon for purpose of delivery, regarding which so much has been said, I will only observe that if I have used public conveyances and not given credit for them, the whole amount would not exceed Twenty pounds; furthermore, that as Director General, I was entitled to a wagon to transport my baggage, etc., but I did not put the Continent to that expense and thereby saved them Seven Hundred and Fifty pounds. It is moreover in proof before the Court, that credit was given for the wagon I employed for private use and my books will show it. Mr. Rembelt has later deposed that neither I nor any of my officers impressed his wagon and that I was ignorant of the whole matter; Mr. James has also testified that I was not in Bethlehem where the sugar and wine were stored, for ten days before the affair was transacted."

Morgan's comment on several of the acquittal items was:

"As the Court was so very complacent to Dr. Shippen as not to find him guilty of any particulars, however strongly supported by the oaths of honest and independent witnesses, it is not to be wondered at that it should acquit him of such parts of the charges as he was not obliged to confess."

It was upon the initial accusation of the indictment that Dr. Morgan laid the greatest stress, for it was his hope that by proving a charge that Dr. Shippen had appropriated Government-owned hospital stores, sold them for his own benefit, and delivered them at public expense, he would bring the Director General to everlasting disgrace.

"Speculation in hospital stores," the first part of the second charge, was not only frankly admitted by Shippen, but he called many witnesses to testify he had often mentioned it. Dr. Shippen contended that buying and selling articles of common trade for profit was not prohibited by law or army regulations, and the extent of his purchases was so ridiculously small that they could in no way have affected market prices. In fact, the evidence submitted by Morgan and Rush on this charge involved transactions of less than six pipes of wine and a few tierces of sugar. The court-martial, however, found "speculation" by Dr. Shippen, in his position, "reprehensible" and therefore censured him in the acquittal verdict, and it was on this point that Morgan built all his arguments of unpunished condemned guilt.

Morgan declared he had been informed that Shippen had admitted to a total profit of ten thousand pounds on his wines and sugar transactions ($24,200), but he did not produce a witness or deposition to sustain this statement. In the last part of the second indictment, "adulteration of wine," Shippen denied any knowledge. Several depositions were submitted by Morgan regarding suspected adulterations, with insinuations that they had been deliberately committed to cover up illicit withdrawals from wine barrels, but on examination, the witnesses admitted that they did not suspect Dr. Shippen of any part in them or believe that he had any knowledge they had occurred.

Thomas Stockton, a commissary at the Princeton Hospital, testified he once received sixteen or twenty gallons of wine from the warehouse, which he thought had been adulterated, and Dr. Jacob Hall remembered having wine at Bethlehem which had the name but not the quality of Modeira. A number of physicians told of receiving weak wine at different hospitals but, on cross-examination, admitted to a belief that the casks had been tampered with en route from the storehouse.

Morgan's third charge was that Shippen kept no regular books of account or proper checks and vouchers for all his transactions and no list of his obligations; that he refused or neglected to pay just and reasonable debts contracted for the hospitals.

That Dr. Shippen did keep adequate books of accounts was declared by the Director General himself and confirmed by Dr. Bond, who had examined them. Government records also show that Dr. Shippen submitted his records for auditing before receiving a final settlement when he left the service. Many hospital physicians and surgeons also told of their methods of making written requisitions for hospital necessities, and the commissaries testified to using such orders as their inventory vouchers. But someone planned to cast doubt on Shippen's testimony regarding his books, as late as December 23, 1780, for The Pennsylvania Packet of that date, carried a card addressed:

"To the Printer:

Having been informed that affidavits are to be published in your paper to the disadvantage of Dr. Shippen, Jr., in his absence, obtained from one Patrick Garvey, a criminal now in prison, you are desired to insert the enclosed certificate that the public may not be imposed upon by such a witness, and at the same time let it be known by authority from New Jersey, that it appears the said Patrick Garvey is there charged with being a spy; has changed his name and is expected to be sent to that State and tried for his life. Signed, 'A Friend to Truth.'"

The aforementioned certificate read:

"I do hereby certify that Patrick Garvey was committed to the gaol in the City and County of Philadelphia, on the 22nd of November last, being charged with treasonable and dangerous practices to the State and remains in custody this day as committed by His Excellency, Joseph Reed, Esq., President of the State of Pennsylvania.

"John Raynold, "Gaoler."

"Philadelphia Gaol, December 21st, 1780."

True to predictions, Garvey's affidavit appears in the paper but without being sponsored by either Dr. Morgan or Dr. Rush. It said:

"In January of 1780, Dr. William Shippen, Jr., Director General, applied indirectly to me to settle his books. The gentleman who made the application, informed me that Dr. Shippen made particular inquiries respecting my ability to settle accounts; my character, and asked him if I was a person in whom he might confide, remarking that he had neglected taking receipts, etc., and finally that the purpose for which he wanted me was to transcribe his books. For this service, he said Dr. Shippen would give One Hundred Guineas if I would undertake the task.

"The gentleman told me he was struck with astonishment at the proposal, yet was determined to inform me of it. I told him I detested Shippen and his money and would have nothing to do with him. The gentleman expressed his satisfaction at my determination and remarked that Shippen was an infamous character, corrupt beyond all description, etc., that there was no possibility of bringing him to punishment owing to the number of his friends and dependents in office.

"December 15th, 1780."

"Patrick Garvey."

To support the second part of the third charge, "Neglect or refusal to pay just and reasonable debts," Dr. Morgan offered a number of depositions. Philip Eppright, an ex-steward and commissary of Reams Town, deposed that he had expended quite a sum of his own money for hospital necessities but had been obliged to wait a long time for repayment. William Bawsman testified that four hundred pounds had been due him for supplies furnished by the Medical Department for so long a time that when paid in depreciated currency, the sum received represented only a portion of its original value. Susanna Babb, Hannah Lewis, and Elizabeth Meley, all of Reading, Pennsylvania, were deposed. They had housed, fed, and nursed a total of twelve wounded soldiers of the Germantown and Brandywine Battles, and though they had cared for and sustained them for many weeks and had demanded pay from Dr. Shippen, no money had ever been received for their services.

Shippen did not enter a denial or defense to these depositions here set forth, but it can be easily imagined he might have replied that he lacked sufficient money to pay all his hospital obligations, and some had, therefore, been neglected. Many people of the Revolutionary War period having business relations with the Government could have told similar stories of unpaid debts.

The fourth charge, "Neglect of hospital duties," was, in Morgan's and Rush's opinion, a very important accusation, for if it could be proved, Shippen would stand before the American people as a creature to be despised. Most of the evidence submitted by the prosecution on this point had been collected by Dr. Rush during the winter of 1777 and '78 when Morgan had resided within the British-occupied City of Philadelphia. Much of Shippen's defense on this charge consisted of letters and depositions gathered to counteract Rush's early accusations. Among those summoned to personally give testimony on this subject was Dr. William Brown, Physician General, who expressed an opinion that one-half the men lost in the hospitals might have been saved by means easily procurable with money.

Rush and Morgan always contended that Shippen had sufficient allowances from Congress for all humane purposes, but it was because of his ignorance and neglect that available money was not properly used. Another witness for the prosecution was Dr. James Hutchinson, Physician General of Pennsylvania and previously a Senior Surgeon of the Flying Camp. He testified to a general shortage and even being entirely without surgical instruments in the Lancaster Hospital. When bringing this point out as a reflection on Dr. Shippen, one might wonder whether Dr. Morgan remembered how he had sent Dr. Binney from New York to Philadelphia to purchase greatly needed surgical instruments and received a report that there were none to be had. Shippen's published comment on Dr. Hutchinson's testimony was:

"If Dr. Hutchinson, when answering all the meaningless questions Morgan could suggest for twelve hours, seemed to imply any neglect in me, he answered on cross-examination:

"That he did not know of any sick soldiers suffering or dying from my neglect."

It was a constant statement of both Morgan and Rush when one of the hospital organizations testified favorably for Shippen that he could not do otherwise and hold his position. Stories of inducements to testify for the prosecution were also related but not by Shippen. Of this same Dr. Hutchinson, Dr. Barnabas Binney wrote to a friend:

"Dr. Hutchinson has had his rise, progress, zenith, and now is declining fast. He ingrafted his medical greatness upon political factions and secured himself a lucrative post of idleness [Physician General of Pennsylvania] till the present day. But let factions go as they may; that locquacious, self-applauding impudence which we unhappily want, will ever be a fortune secured to him."

Another one that Dr. Binney intimated had been rewarded for his testimony against Dr. Shippen was a junior surgeon known in the service as "Long Island" Smith to distinguish him from another with the same name. Smith received an M.D. degree from the Medical School in Philadelphia through the endorsement of Morgan and Rush, and as Dr. Binney wrote, "to spite Shippen," for in Binney's opinion and "Long Island," Smith had served him as Junior Surgeon for one year-Smith's attainments did not merit the honor.

Dr. James Tilton, one of the outstanding medical men in the Revolutionary Army, whose ideas of military hospitals, had they been adopted, might have saved many lives, was another witness quoted against Dr. Shippen. Morgan reproduced his testimony as follows:

"Dr. Tilton, a Senior Surgeon in the General Hospital, testified before the Court that in November of 1777 he was directed to convey the wounded of the Battle of Brandywine from Philadelphia to Princeton; that he was detained for a time by bad weather at Bristol on his way to Trenton but that he sent word to Dr. Shippen that such of the sick as were not moved to Bethlehem, might be expected at Trenton, and considering that good quarters were necessary for such men, he had also written. Yet when he arrived, [he found] no quarters had been provided, except the very infectious barracks from which sick persons ill with putrid fever, had been removed for the admission of the wounded, who in other respects were healthy men; that Dr. Tilton remained there for three or four days and then continued the transfer to Princeton. Some days after their arrival, several wounded men developed fever of such putrid malignity, that he was obliged to consider the infected barracks at Trenton as the cause of the infection; [he further testified that] in the latter part of November the hospitals at Burlington and Trenton were removed to Princeton which then contained five hundred filthy, dirty, and lousy patients."

Dr. Shippen's response to Morgan's recital of Tilton's testimony follows:

"Dr. Tilton, who may be supposed to be a competent witness, is the only one who has ventured to give an instance of my actual neglect. He deposed that he sent me one written and two verbal messages to Trenton, asking to have proper quarters prepared for the wounded men from Brandywine and that the barracks were the only quarters he found ready, out of which putrid cases had just been removed. He said he assumed this, by reason of the fact that some of his men were taken with putrid symptoms, three or four days after they arrived at Princeton, where one died; therefore he was obliged to suspect the barracks as the chief cause. It fully appears, however, that even the suspicion was false, for Dr. Bodo Otto, Sr., and his son, Frederick who attended the barracks, had deposed there had not been a putrid case in their hospital for three weeks before Dr. Tilton arrived. Furthermore, Conrad Kotts, the commissary, has sworn that the barracks were emptied and well cleaned for the reception of the wounded from Bristol under Dr. Tilton‘s care."

Dr. Tilton‘s own testimony seems to shift the suspicion of contamination from the Trenton Hospital to his own permanent one at Princeton. "Five hundred filthy, dirty, and lousy patients" were certainly conducive to a putrid fever epidemic. It might also be again mentioned at this point that Dr. Benjamin Rush, the second-ranking medical man in all the Continental hospitals, was then maintaining his headquarters at Princeton and was, in a measure, responsible for its condition.

Commissary Kotts' deposition follows:

"I do certify that I acted as Assistant Commissary to the hospitals of Trenton from December 1776 until January 1778, during which time, Dr. Shippen's constant directions to me were to purchase everything necessary and comfortable for the sick, and he furnished me with money from time to time, for that purpose; that I always obeyed the instructions of the senior doctors and considered their orders as my vouchers; that in common, I was well supplied with sugar, molasses, wine, spirits, rice, and other hospital stores; that Dr. Shippen visited the hospitals several times, inquiring into their condition and giving repeated directions to supply them with every necessity, as well as to see they were kept clean. I seldom missed inspecting once or twice a day, to see they were so.

"Dr. Shippen always appeared to me as attentive and humane, to the sick under his care."

Dr. Shippen also published a résumé of Dr. Bodo Otto's testimony relating to this important fourth charge as follows:

"That all hospitals he [Dr. Otto] attended, were well supplied with wines, sugar and other hospital stores, medicines and instruments; that he had no reason to complain; that my [Shippen] orders by letter as well as verbally, were that everything he thought necessary for the sick and wounded, should be provided for them; that his orders to the commissaries were always obeyed and considered as their vouchers; that the hospitals he attended were as well supplied with necessities while I was Purveyor, as they have been since; that I performed the duties of Director General with humanity, frugality and skill."

Dr. Shippen consolidated the defence evidence on this accusation of neglect in a lengthy article, part of which follows:

"In the fourth charge, I am accused of neglect of duty whereby sick and wounded American soldiers suffered and died in a manner shocking to humanity. This accusation if true, I would look upon as a crime of the blackest dye and should not think myself worthy of existence, had I not acquitted myself of it before the Court Martial and proven that I exerted every nerve, devoted every hour, sacrificed every private interest and pleasure, to relieve the unavoidable distress of 1777 and make the sick comfortable. I have abundant testimony of this, as has and will appear hereafter.

"I have never denied, for it was unavoidable, that there were many sufferings in the hospitals after the Battles of Brandywine and Germantown, but the witnesses brought by my enemies proved when crossexamined, that they were not owing to my neglect, to a deficiency of stores or to a want of surgeons, commissaries, nurses, medicines, or other things that I ought and could supply. They arose partially from a want of clothing and the covering necessary to keep the soldiers clean and warm; articles that at that time were not procurable in the country; they were also partially due to the fact that our army was raw, unused to camp life, exposure, fatigue, discipline and great hardships; from their being obliged to fly before an enemy in a cold and inclement season and [under such circumstances] the sick and wounded were moved great distances in open wagons for I was ordered by General Washington in December 1777, to remove all the sick from New Jersey and vicinity of the camp, into Lancaster County. Notwithstanding all these distressing circumstances, the transfer was effected with little loss and by the uncommon care and attention of all the hospital officers, the consequences were not near as fatal as was feared or expected.

"If these sufferings were not unavoidable or had arisen from my neglect, why did not officers from all the ranks in the army complain of me? Why did they not apply to the Commander-in-Chief and to Congress for my dismissal, as they did of Dr. Morgan in 1776? His Excellency's attention and humanity to the sick and wounded soldiers were too great, not to have known of their sufferings, and had my neglect produced them, he would certainly have brought me to condign punishment. He saw the soldiers' distress and dropped a tear; he knew the situation was unavoidable; he saw us exerting ourselves for their relief to the utmost and could not say, as he did of the soldiers on the east side of the Hudson where my accuser presided, that his eyes and ears were shocked by the looks and complaints of the poor creatures, perishing for want of care.

"But it is pretended that there were scenes of distress at Reading, Pennsylvania, that would shock humanity. Lord Stirling, who was quartered there a considerable part of the time and General Mifflin, who was there all the winter, made no complaint, nor did the Selectmen of the Town. Is it creditable that such shocking treatment of the sick as is pretended, would have escaped their observation or knowledge? Or that if they saw or heard such things, they would not have been the first to speak to the author of them, if they arose from willful neglect? But neither from Lord Stirling, General Mifflin nor the Select men was there any complaint, certificate, or deposition offered, reciting these inhumane scenes, and much less of my neglect, cruel treatment or misconduct.

"It would be trifling with the patience of the public to enter into the incompetency of the witnesses Dr. Morgan produced or the low arts he employed to draw certificates and depositions from poor ignorant people; had they understood them, they would never have been given. I will take notice of one, Mr. Peter O'Zeas, who, when cross-examined, said:

"He did not know that any sick or wounded soldiers ever suffered or died from my refusing to relieve them, or through neglecting my duty as Director General; that he thought a great deal of the sufferings of the patients at Reading arose from want of blankets, change of linen and because of their coming in open wagons; that the time of the greatest suffering was in January."

Many other letters and depositions that were presented to the Court touching on this fourth charge were also reproduced by Shippen. One had been penned by Dr. Isaac Foster, the Deputy Director General of the Eastern Department, written from Danbury, Conn., on October 2, 1777:

"Everything in our department goes on smoothly and I can with truth assure you, that the hospitals are in such repute that the sick soldiers are as anxious this year, to be admitted into them, as they were last, to avoid them."

William Smith, a senior surgeon, had also written from Philadelphia under date of July 3, 1779:

"I do certify that during the space of two years in which I have acted as a Senior Surgeon in the Hospital Department under the direction of Dr. Shippen, no instance of the truth of any charge lately exhibited by Dr. Morgan has come to my knowledge; on the contrary, as far as I have had an opportunity of judging the duties of the Director General as they relate to the hospitals, they have been ably and faithfully fulfilled; the sick being amply provided with all kinds of stores as the times would permit and every necessary attention has been paid to render them as comfortable as possible.

"In the execution of his office, the Director without descending from the dignity of his station, has always used the power committed to him with that moderation which has merited the esteem of his officers, and in every respect within my knowledge, he has appeared humane, vigilant and solicitous for the comfortable accommodation of the sick."

The Rev. Peter Miller, head of the religious order at Ephrata, Pennsylvania, where a hospital had been located, hearing of Dr. Shippen's difficulties, wrote him:

"Respected Sir:

"As by your direction in the winter before last, a large hospital was established at Ephrata, indebted to bear a to which we submitted without reluctance, being proportionate share in the calamities of the present war, I should sooner have acknowledged the past favor of your protection, without which we should not have been in the condition to weather that storm. Indeed, all circumstances would then join to make the situation of the sick comfortable; such as your vigilance in visiting us as often as necessity called; a constant supply of medicines and refreshments, sent by your order from Manheim, which your deputies, the senior doctors, supplied with a peculiar care; a plentiful market, constantly kept up by the neighbors, furnishing veal, milk and other articles necessary to recruit the strength of the poor soldiers; a good government kept by the senior doctors, Messrs. Scott and E. Smith, in which vices attending a soldier's life were suppressed. I must say in praise of the Senior Surgeons and your person, that they merit your approbation.

"Should your labor not turn out to general satisfaction, remember that every critical circumstance commonly attends such officers who often traverse even the most sanguine hope of success, of which the public cannot be sufficiently acquainted; so satisfaction is conscience, etc.

"I conclude by recommending you to the wings of Divine protection. "July 15th, 1779."

Though Dr. Morgan wrote that he would discuss the fifth charge and the evidence submitted in his next article, he hardly mentioned the subject. The only interesting exhibit he offered was a letter that Morgan claims Shippen had written to a member of Congress, saying:

"I cannot with propriety, say all I know [regarding Dr. Morgan] lest it look like finding fault with a man with whom I have never had a good understanding."

Shippen claimed:

"That he [Morgan] stopped at nothing ever so mean, to gain testimony against me; as proof, read the following declaration made on oath by Robert Jewell, a friend of his country and a respectable citizen. "I hereby certify and declare that Dr. Morgan offered me a certificate to sign which he had ready, containing a reflection on the character of Dr. Shippen, which was not true. He importuned me much to sign but I refused; he then begged I draw one myself, as near to his as I would. I told him I knew nothing against Dr. Shippen and would not sign any. thing. He urged and persuaded me much to do something, saying: You know, Mr. Jewell, you are under obligations to me and ought to oblige. At length he obtained deposition from me before Justice a Adcock, in which I did not mean to reflect on Dr. Shippen's character as Director General or as an honest man.

"Mr. Jewell also deposed that Dr. Morgan appraised him that he was informed of the subject matter contained in his original certificate by Dr. Rush."

Two other examples of improperly obtained and used documents offered by the prosecution were submitted by Dr.

Morgan; one referred to Dr. Hinan, and the other to Dr. Bodo Otto. The first stated that:

"Dr. Hinan swore that prior to his giving a certificate to Dr. Morgan, Dr. Rush had asked him in what manner he would answer certain questions if he were called upon; he also declared that the form of his signed certificate was drawn by Dr. Rush."

Of Dr. Otto, Shippen wrote:

"Dr. Bodo Otto, a Senior Surgeon, when shown a paper drawn up by Dr. Rush, was asked after it had been distinctly read to him, whether he had signed it and if the facts contained therein were true? Answered thus on oath:

"I signed my name to one part of it but not to the other, according to the best of my recollection, but the statement in that paper I do not acknowledge to be true, or to have been assented to by me; I must have been imposed upon, to have signed it.

"Dr. Bodo Otto is an excellent officer and a very polite man but is not a master of English."

Frequent references by Shippen to Rush, with insinuations that he had resorted to clever arrangements of wording in the certificates he had composed, was apparently too much for Dr. Rush to ignore, so in the next edition of the paper, Rush joined in the altercation with:

"To Dr. William Shippen, Jr.

"It is with reluctance that I am obliged to appear in a newspaper controversy with a man of your unworthy character. I am well aware of the advantages you have over me in point of leisure. While every hour of my time is employed in discharging the duties of my profession, you have nothing to do from the manner in which you execute or rather hold your present office but to transcribe depositions of your stewards and commissaries.

"The regard I bear your worthy connections obliges me to lament that you have forced me to contribute my mite toward exposing your crime and awakening the resentment of your plundered country.

"Had you been well advised, you would have avoided a public scrutiny of your conduct, by resigning your commission and retiring with your blushing honors thick upon you. But you were permitted by Heaven, to continue in office that public infamy (the worst of all punishment) might supply the place of public justice.

"I am much obliged to you for the extract you have published from my letters written to you in the summer of 1776. They prove that I entered into the Hospital Department with a prejudice in your favor and that the rupture between us was only occasioned by your gross negligence of duty and your consuming and selling those stores that were proper and necessary for the hospitals.

"It is to no purpose for you to attempt to persuade the public that I used indirect measures with witnesses, to induce them to appear against you. You know I had no sinecure of rations, coffee, sugar, wine, spirits and forage to lavish upon them. How far a plentiful allowance of those articles has influenced your friends, the following extract of a letter from Dr. Otto, the most respectable of your witnesses, will sufficiently show. It was received three weeks before he subscribed to a certificate, reciting the wants of his hospital at Trenton and your neglect to supply them:

(the letter)

"'I beg I may be supplied with the articles on the enclosed list, of which things I stand in every necessity.'

"'I shall take the greatest care to do my duty in this important office here, to which you were pleased to appoint me, and all your orders shall be punctually obeyed, Respected Sir, by

"Your obedient and humble servant,"

"Bodo Otto, Surgeon."

"The articles mentioned in Dr. Otto's list, were the same he declared in his certificate to be wanting in his hospital. His application to me is a proof that he had applied to you to no purpose, for he well knew it was no more my business to furnish those articles, than to provide beef and flour to the Army. I take it for granted that the Attorney General of this State will take proper notice of this man's disposition. He knows the name and punishment of his crime.

"November 18th, 1780."

"Benjamin Rush."

The paper Morgan offered at the court-martial that Shippen had cited as being repudiated by Dr. Otto was a letter addressed to Dr. Shippen three years before (1777) under circumstances that have already been told. It had been composed and penned by Dr. Rush but signed by Dr. Otto for delivery to Dr. Shippen after a discussion of the needs of the Trenton Hospital. Rush had so composed the text that it could be interpreted either as an urgent request for necessities for the sick and wounded soldiers or as a charge of negligence, and these finer differences in English, Dr. Otto, with limited knowledge of the language, did not perceive.

For Dr. Rush to designate the communication "a deposition" was a deliberate and unwarranted misrepresentation and intended to support his following insinuation that by signing the paper and later giving favorable testimony for Dr. Shippen, Dr. Otto had committed perjury. Everyone knew that the term "deposition," as used in this controversy, was a statement for presentation to the court as evidence and made under oath, though few knew that they were not authorized until November 1779, two years after the letter had been written.

Dr. Otto's communication to Dr. Rush, quoted in the newspaper, was alleged to have been sent even before the Trenton conference three years before. It supplied Rush with ammunition to support a plausible argument for his position. The writing of such an epistle to Dr. Rush, Physician General, located only ten miles away, was quite characteristic of Dr. Otto. Military procedure and routine never stood in his way during six years of hospital service when he sought something he thought necessary for his patients. Many letters found among Government Revolutionary records bear testimony to the fact that he frequently recited grievances and sent lists of his needs directly to Congress or the source of supplies. So, according to Dr. Otto's method of reasoning, it seemed perfectly regular and natural to request Dr. Rush to send things he required at Trenton from the Princeton commissary, pending receipt of requisitioned supplies from the distant hospital warehouse. But now the prosecution was attempting to use this combination of letters to break down and discredit the man Dr. Rush had described as "the most respectable of Shippen's witnesses.

Surprised as Dr. Otto must have been to have this ancient, long-forgotten letter offered as evidence, the venerable physician promptly repudiated the interpretation put upon one part of it and denied all recollection of another section of the document. Dr. Morgan, who may have been quite ignorant of the circumstances related above, was greatly disturbed by Dr. Otto's testimony, and that night (May 27th, 1780) he wrote to Dr. Rush:

"It will doubtless surprise you to hear that after Dr. Otto's examination, the Judge Advocate produced a certificate signed by himself, by young doctors Frederick and John Otto, and Dr. Stockton, on one side of the paper, and Bodo Otto alone on the other. The certificate is in your handwriting. He [Dr. Otto] had given testimony in direct opposition to the facts therein set forth. He acknowledges the signature at the bottom of the first page to be his, but would not admit the facts contained to be true, or to have been assented to by him; nor would he acknowledge his name [signature] on the second page as his, and states he must have been imposed upon to have signed.

"On this declaration I found Shippen prepared to triumph. He intimates he shall in the course of examining other witnesses, show more of this [kind of] work. I think it my duty to inform you of these particulars."

Several days later, Dr. Morgan again wrote to Dr. Rush, repeating the subject matter of his previous letter, and saying he was sending it by Major Claybourne, that he might be sure it would be delivered. In this communication, he added:

"Dr. Shippen is making great use of Dr. Otto's statements, in his harangues and frequent references to you. He asserts he shall show more forgery, etc., which, in his language, 'must ever bless your character.'"

Dr. Otto did not tamely submit to Dr. Rush's reflection upon his honor, and quickly replied in print. The response must have been first written in German and by someone translated, for the English composition is much better than could have come direct from Dr. Otto's pen.

"To Dr. Rush:

"When an honest man feels himself injured in his honor and reputation, nature and reason point out the propriety of defending himself and resenting the abuse. The injury is much heightened and its effects more sensibly felt, when the person sustaining it is engaged in the service of his country as a public character, and of course accountable to it for his conduct.

"These considerations, more than any dread of incurring censure or suffering in character, where I am personally known, induced me to appear in this manner in defense of my reputation, unjustly attacked; to refute your groundless and base insinuations, lest a silence on my part should be accounted a tacit acknowledgment of your ungenerous charge you bring against me in the Pennsylvania 'Packet,' where after inserting an extract of a letter said to be received from me, you have the following paragraph:

"I take it for granted that the Attorney General of this State will take proper notice of this man's deposition; he knows the name and punishment of his crime.

"The plain and obvious design and intent of which is; (as far as your power and influence extends) an endeavor to blast my character and credit, by representing me to the public as guilty of the most odious and disgraceful offense to society.

"A charge or accusation of this kind in such a public manner (however weak and ineffectual in itself), must naturally excite the most keen sensation in a feeling mind; and I can, with satisfaction say, that in the course of seventy years' journey through life with its various changes and vicissitudes, both in Europe and America, I have never experienced an instance of similar treatment.

"What I have related in my examination as a witness in the case of Dr. Shippen's trial, was what I knew to be the truth, and to what I shall always religiously and truthfully adhere. Uninfluenced by prejudice or party, my conduct throughout the whole of that affair was actuated by love of justice and humanity, and I feel a satisfaction in the honest and conscious discharge of my duty of which the envenomed fling of slander cannot deprive me.

"With regard to my public character, since I have had the honor to be entrusted with the post in the Hospital Department, I beg leave to lay before the public the following unsolicited certificate left at my house after Dr. Shippen's trial, as appears by the date:

(the letter)

"General Hospital,

"Yellow Springs, August 12th, 1780. "Being about to leave the department of the General Hospital in which I have served as Physician General for upwards of three years, I cannot do less than give my testimony before departure on behalf of such officers who, during that time, have served under me with distinction; among these, I beg leave to number Dr. Bodo Otto, whose assiduous attention to his charge, whose industry and ability, have uniformly manifested themselves and been productive of the most essential benefits to the service and the highest honor to himself.

"William Brown,

"Physician General, Medical Department."

"I shall now leave it to your own feelings, whether in this ungenerous treatment of a person who never intentionally did you an injury, you have acted upon the principles of a gentleman or man of honor.

"For my own conduct as a public officer, I am, and at all times expect, to be held accountable at a proper tribunal, and I rest assured that my character in private life will ever be proof against the darts of slander and efforts of malice.

"Bodo Otto."

Dr. Rush must have experienced some feeling of regret at his unjust attacks, for the explanation he published in answer is couched in milder and more considerate language than he generally used to answer opposition.

"In order to understand more fully the nature and contradiction of Dr. Otto's evidence in favor of Dr. Shippen, it will be proper to lay before the public, the following facts:

"In the latter end of August or beginning of September, 1777, I visited the hospital at Trenton, then under the care of Dr. Otto. I found the rooms clean and everything as far as it related to Dr. Otto, in good order. The Doctor complained that his sick suffered only from want of medicines and stores. I examined the shop and found scarcely any medicine in it, of any use. Not an ounce of coffee, tea, rice, wine or sugar, could be obtained from the commissary stores. I asked Dr. Otto if he had applied to Dr. Shippen for the above articles and he told me that he had, but he received them in such small quantities and so out of time, that they did the sick but little good. I asked him if he would certify these facts that I might lay them before Dr. Shippen. He consented cheerfully for he then complained much of Dr. Shippen's negligence. The certificate was signed at the same time by a Junior Surgeon and two mates, who were witnesses of the readiness with which Dr. Otto subscribed his name; not only to a certificate which declared the suffering of the sick from want of medicines and stores, but to another which declared he had applied to Dr. Shippen for them, to no purpose. When I showed these certificates to Dr. Shippen at York Town, he looked at them with a sneer and said in the presence of a Committee of Congress, that he could prevail upon the old fellow to sign a counter certificate. At that time I thought it impossible, for I had the highest opinion of Dr. Otto's probity as well as his industry and humanity, in his profession. In the course of his evidence before the court, he showed that Dr. Shippen was better acquainted with him than myself. He acquitted the doctor of neglecting his duties; said the hospital at Trenton was, in general, plentifully supplied with stores and medicines; and added that one of the certificates he had signed, was obtained by persuasion, and the other he did not remember to have signed at all; unfortunately for him, his own original letter to me, written three weeks before I saw him, sets forth the wants of the Trenton hospital; the evidence of the gentleman who saw him subscribe both certificates in his own handwriting all concur to prove that the certificate he gave, contained what he then believed and knew to be the truth, the whole truth and nothing but the truth.

"It may not be improper in this place, to inform the public that by the hospital system imposed by Dr. Shippen and afterwards adopted by Congress, he possessed the power of dismissing any officer in the department, not appointed by Congress. He possessed likewise the power of disposing of hospital stores, and of creating as many officers and sinecures as he pleased. This will account for the many eulogies upon his industry and humanity with which he has lately filled the papers.

"If Dr. Otto's venerable age and habits of virtue could not secure him from yielding to the terrors and charms of Dr. Shippen's power, what then could be expected from men who had been so long steeped in vice that they were incapable of receiving a deeper hue, even from Dr. Shippen's company?

"B. RUSH."

Another of Dr. Shippen's articles included Dr. Barnabas Binney's testimony, in which he recited that:

"Dr. Binney when on oath, was asked whether he had not heard Dr Morgan express a desire to avenge an injury that he said he had received from Dr. Shippen, answered: "I have heard Dr. Morgan observe that Dr. Shippen had attempted to ruin him, and he added strong expressions of resentment."

Morgan's retort to this publication was:

"How ridiculous a figure do you make, by reproducing the testimony of Dr. Binney. Anger often extorts disagreeable truth and I do not exactly recollect what expressions I used to him, but perhaps I said, 'you were treacherous and cowardly, for treachery always acts with cowardice'; an unprincipled calumniator and secret assassin of my character. What I have said of you at any time to any man, I never have and never mean to unsay, and what I have said, I will undertake to prove to the conviction of the public. Dr. Binney has concurred with me in my sentiments concerning you, and I believe that without ever having altered his opinion."

Just what did Dr. Binney think about Doctors Rush, Morgan, and Shippen? Private opinions expressed to his intimate friend, Dr. Solomon Drowne, might properly be accepted as his real sentiments on the subject. In any event, his letters to his absent chum always spoke sympathetically of Shippen but contained many expressions of disapproval and dislike of both Morgan and Rush and their methods; once, he frankly said he would prefer to go without an M.D. degree rather than ask and obtain it from these men he so thoroughly despised.

In one of Shippen's articles, he wrote:

"I am pleased to find that my implacable enemies, stung to the quick at my having exposed their iniquity and finding all of their wicked practices and low arts to injure my reputation ineffectual, have betaken themselves to scurrility with pathetic declarations and assertions as wild and extravagant as they are false and unjust. This will make them more despicable, if possible, than before and they may be assured I shall not take up the time of the public with any remarks on such impertinences, nor shall it interrupt my great object of proving myself an honest and faithful officer."

Dr. Thomas Bond, Jr., an Assistant Director General, drew down Dr. Rush's wrath upon him by reason of Bond's testimony in support of Shippen. Rush quickly addressed another article to Shippen, saying:

"I will proceed to take notice of the evidence of Dr. Thomas Bond, Jr. I wish this good-tempered man had not lessened the reputation he acquired in office, by the evidence he has given in your favor. Too much praise cannot be given him for his humanity and even charity to the sick, but duty to my country and regard for my own testimony, oblige me to declare in this public manner, that I have repeatedly heard Dr. Bond complain of your manner of doing business; of your neglect to consult him upon those mercantile transactions relating to supplies for the hospitals. I have moreover, often heard him say that you would never settle your accounts and that you would be ruined when they were called for, and lastly I have heard him declare, that by his exertions at putting your hospital in Bethlehem in order and supplying it plentifully with hecessities, he had saved you from perdition. He meant by this that he had obviated the force of my complaints against your maladministration, to the Committee at York Town."

Dr. Bond replied to this Rush attack in the newspaper:

"To detect impositions on the public is the duty of every honest man, especially when the impositions are intended to gratify private malice and traduce the character of gentlemen who are now serving their country in very important places. This is my sole reason for taking notice of an article in the Pennsylvania 'Packet,"

"signed 'Benjamin Rush."

"In any other view, both the writer and his performance are too contemptible to deserve a moment's attention. That the reader may see of what impositions Dr. Rush is capable, when they are likely to serve the purpose of his malice against Dr. Shippen, the Court Martial, many worthy witnesses adducted to the trial, as well as two or three respectable members of Congress would not contribute to Dr. Rush's malevolent designs, I shall contrast what this same Dr. Rush wrote me on February 1st, 1778, what he has now imposed on the public, from which he will appear in his true light."

Dr. Bond then quoted the two different reasons given by Rush for resigning his commission in the Medical Department, both of which are reproduced in the preceding chapters. Dr. Bond then continued:

"Having thus shown that Dr. Rush is capable of lying in the worst sense of that approbation, it is unworthy of me to take any notice of the pretended private conversation concerning Dr. Shippen which he has imputed to me, other than to observe that his mention of it was prompted by the same malignant spirit which has so shamefully actuated Dr. Rush throughout the whole of his disgraceful writings, and carries in it the strongest mark of an unprincipled man. It also confirms me that Horace, who well knew the world, was right when he delineated such as character, thus:

"He who malignant, tears an absent friend,
or when attacked by others don't defend;
who trivial bursts of laughter strive to cease,
And courts of prating petulance the praise;
Or things he never saw, who tells his tale,
And friendship's secrets knows not to conceal,
This man is vile! Here, Roman, fix your mark;
His soul is black, as his complexion dark."

"Thomas Bond, Jr."

In a long article, Dr. Shippen reviews Morgan's five charges, the Court's action on each, and then continues:

"Am I not here acquitted of every charge, by a disinterested Court Martial? Ho How false then then the insinuation that I was convicted of speculating in stores belonging to the hospital, when the Court, lest such a construction might be put on their words, added: "That is, stores proper for hospitals.'

"It is also as falsely asserted that Congress did not approve the acquittal of the Court Martial, and a vote of that honorable body was published by Morgan to prove it; [and a statement made] that on a motion made by Mr. Adams, and seconded by Mr. Scott, that the words in the first motion on the subject, 'the acquittal be confirmed be struck out, was carried in the affirmative by nine States and therefore Congress did not approve the acquittal. The facts are otherwise; the gentlemen who made and seconded that motion, have assured me that they proposed it, lest Congress, by confirming the acquittal as it stood in the sentence, might be supposed to also approve their [the Court Martial's] opinion of reprehensibility for speculation, and that they [Congress] did not appear very plain [clear] from the next motion and the vote. A motion was therefore made by Mr. Clark and seconded by Mr. Folsom, to amend the motion by inserting after 'Dr. Shippen' the words: 'except that part of the second charge relating to speculation in hospital stores in which the Court judged him highly reprehensible."

"The yeas and nays were then taken, with a negative result. Hence it appears that eight States, and Maryland as far as represented, did approve the acquittal of the Court Martial but not their opinion that I was reprehensible because I happened to purchase and sell on my own account, articles similar to those used in hospitals. This seeming censure could only be considered as an opinion of the Court on a matter which was not properly before it; my trading in any article was not prohibited, and consequently not punishable.

"Although I ought to stand acquitted in the eyes of the sensible and candid, because the Court Martial have declared there was no evidence to prove they [articles bought and sold] were public [hospital] stores, or that the sick suffered for want of them, yet lest the smallest suspicion of fraud should remain, I have shown the Court that the articles were my own property by the following declaration.

"The public should first be informed that, exclusive of the Boston adventure [transaction] I am accused of selling [a total of] four and a half pipes of wine and three tierces of sugar. Two of them were sold to Mr. Denney of Lancaster, one to Mr. Hartmann at Reading, one to Mr. Haffa, near Reading, and one half of a pipe to Mr. Bennett; also one tierce of sugar to Mr. Bennett and two to Mr. James Biddle. These are the mighty speculations that you are told have caused the depreciation of our money and endangered the independence of North America."

Dr. Shippen produced two special witnesses from outside the Medical Department to give testimony on Morgan's charge of speculation. One was Thomas Smith, Commissioner of the United States Loan Office, who told of a conversation in which Shippen said he had just laid in the necessary supply of stores for the hospital and had an opportunity to purchase some wine for his own account; that he was inclined to take advantage of it, for he believed that a profit would result. Smith further stated that Shippen asked his opinion of the propriety of such a speculation and that he had replied that while there was nothing wrong in such a transaction, that it would be better for Shippen to choose some article outside the list of hospital purchases for an opportunity to make money; that Dr. Shippen had answered he had no time to give to business and that this opportunity was immediately available. Colonel Moylan, the other witness, testified to being present at the conversation related by Mr. Smith and concurring in his opinion. He also told that he personally had inspected the available wine and had made the selection that Dr. Shippen purchased. Many others told of knowing that Dr. Shippen had bought wine and sugar to sell for profit. Dr. Craik, Assistant Director, and Dr. William Brown, the Physician General, were among those who testified that the transaction was common knowledge. Shippen admitted the purchase of six pipes of wine, some of which he consumed, some he sold to friends, and the balance to tavern-keepers. Dr. Bond and Mr. Eames, who had examined the books, swore that the purchase of the six pipes specified did not appear on the hospital books; neither did the transportation charge for delivery to the different tavern-keepers, so Rush's and Morgan's charge that this specific wine was taken from Government stores and delivered in hospital wagons, was unfounded. In the article in which the foregoing was told, Shippen continued:

"That the sugar was also purchased with my own money and for my own use, will appear from the following declaration: Dr. Cutting, late Apothecary General of the Hospitals, was asked whether I had not sent him to Boston in the Fall of 1777, to look for medicines, instruments, and such stores as could be purchased cheaply, and at the same time, if I had given him a sum of my own money to lay out in sugar or any other article that would be worth bringing to Philadelphia. He answered, 'You did.' I then asked whether he did not purchase sugar for me and transport it to Bethlehem at my expense? His reply was, I did; I cannot collect the exact quantity but believe it was 2800 weight, contained in 3 tierces.' I next asked; instead of laying out all my money for my din vantage, did you not use the greater part of it to purchase and pay for medicine for the hospital? Things that you could not get and transport into Pennsylvania without cash? Dr. Cutting answered, 'I did; the public {Government} wanted many medicines which at that time could not be obtained without a prompt payment.' Hence it appears that my money not only purchased and transported 3 tierces of sugar for me, but a majority of it was laid out for public use."

It was unfortunate that a fictitious name was used in billing the sugar and wine that Shippen sold, for Morgan made much ado about it, though it appears from sworn testimony by the person responsible that this action was taken without Dr. Shippen's knowledge. In this situation, the Doctor wrote:

"But a bill was made out in the name of Thomas Brown, a man never heard of in or about Bethlehem, nor did I ever hear the name until nearly two years after the sale was made. Mr. Hugh James, late Commissary of the Hospitals, testified, he received my five pipes of Madeira wine for safekeeping and these were never entered on the hospital books; that my household furniture [sent from Philadelphia] and other private goods, as well as the hospital stores, were all stored in the cellar of Mr. Horsefield's house in Bethlehem; that I did desire [direct] him to send a tierce of my sugar and one-quarter cask of my wine, to Mr. Bennett by a careful driver but I did not direct him to employ a public wagon to transport them. He also deposed that I did not desire [order] him to make out a bill in the name of Thomas Brown, but that he did so of his own accord; not to cover a fraud but for fear lest the letter [bill] might fall into the hands of some person who might be officious and become suspicious at seeing the Director's name on a bill of sale for sugar and wine, both of which were regular Government supplies. Mr. James also testified, that I had not been in Bethlehem for ten days previous to the delivery of the wine and sugar and was ignorant of all the detailed arrangements."

When the University of Pennsylvania was organized, and the Medical School of the College of Philadelphia absorbed, all instructors of the old institution were invited to accept reappointments. Rush and Morgan then conceived a plan of conditional acceptance, depending upon Dr. Shippen's being excluded from the faculty, for they firmly believed that the Trustees would agree to the loss of one rather than two professors. To their great surprise, no notice was taken of their letter, and Dr. Shippen was reinstated. Rush, becoming worried over the silence of the Trustees, finally appealed to Dr. John Ewing, the University Provost, for his interest and influence in obtaining the former position, and it was only after withdrawing or repudiating the objectionable dictatorial condition that Rush was re-elected to his old professorship. This effort of Rush and Morgan to humiliate Shippen was told by Dr. Ewing when carrying on a Pennsylvania Packet newspaper controversy with Dr. Rush regarding Dickinson College in the late winter of 1785. Looking back on this long-drawn-out controversy, it may be stated that the most favorable testimony that could have been cited in favor of Dr. Shippen never appeared on the record.

First, no letters, petitions, depositions, complaints or witnesses from the rank and file of the Army were presented to support any of the charges made by Dr. Morgan.

Second, with all the available facts and court-martial records before it, Congress re-elected him to the position of Director General of the Continental Hospitals.

Third, General Washington apparently never seriously entertained the charges, commended him highly for his services when he resigned from the Army, remained a good personal friend throughout life and engaged him as a family physician during the Philadelphia administration.

During the four months' exchange of evidence to support both sides of the controversy, Rush's and Morgan's contributions in number greatly exceeded Shippen's, and this seems to support Rush's psychology, which he expressed in a letter dated September 4, 1781, to General Greene:

"Cardinal De Ritz remarked that in the civil wars of France, the party that wrote most and wrote best always prevailed."

That the prosecution wrote most there is no question, and it may be that this fact has contributed to the prevailing traditions regarding Dr. Shippen.

After four months of continual newspaper abuse between Morgan, Rush, Shippen and many witnesses who testified at the court-martial, the public became tired of the subject and disgusted with having it always present. On December 23, 1780, an article appeared in The Pennsylvania Packet signed "Calamas," which suggested a method of relief from a repetition of the offense. In part, it said:

"Having observed with real concern, that our newspapers for a long time past have been filled with private contests and calumny to the great abuse of the liberty of the press and dishonor of the city, I, who have ever been ambitious of devising something never before conceived for the public good, have set my wits to work to remedy this growing evil and restore your Gazette's Advertisers, Packets, etc. to their original design, viz., to make them vehicles of intelligence and not a common server of scandal.

"Let there be a new Court of Justice established, by the name and title of the 'High Court of Honor, to consist of twelve impartial and judicious persons, to be elected by the Free men of the State.....

"The Court shall have jurisdiction in all matters of controversy between man and man of whatever kind, provided no property, real or personal, comes in question. They shall determine on differences of opinion, points of honor, rank and precedence; in all cases of affronts, slights, abuse, scandal, slander, calumny, and in all matters of contest save as before excepted.

"The Clerk of the Court shall keep a large book to be called a 'Rascal Record,' in which shall be fairly entered the name, occupation and place of residence of any person on whom the judgment of the Court shall fall, which book shall be at all times open to the inspection of any person, by the payment of a fee.

"The process of the Court shall be as follows: if any man has cause of offense against another, he shall apply to the Court for a form of 'Declaration.'

"No counsel shall be admitted to the Court, but the parties must personally appear and plead their own case. If the judgment goes against the accused, his name, etc., shall be registered in the 'Rascal Record,' but if the accuser shall fail to make good, his name shall be duly entered."

The edition of The Pennsylvania Packet, in which this suggestion for a Court of Honor appeared, contained an unusual amount of Rush, Morgan, and Shippen controversial matters, but not one article was printed after that date. The cessation was so abrupt that it seemed as though the proprietor of the paper had taken action to exclude further argument. Morgan's life was greatly influenced by the disappointments of his Revolutionary Army experience. He continued lecturing at the University and attending his private practice but withdrew from public activities and died on October 15, 1789.

Rush, the greatest physician of his day, outlived both Morgan and Shippen, expiring on April 19, 1813. In his last illness, among others who attended him, was a favorite pupil, Dr. J. Conrad Otto, a grandson of Dr. Bodo Otto, his venerable revolutionary hospital associate. Shippen, grieved by the death of his son, gradually retired to a quiet life in Germantown and here he expired on July 11, 1806, among his family and friends. Dr. Rush's diary of that date contains this record:

"Shippen died today. I attended him in his last illness."

Let us hope that time and old age had softened their hearts and made them forget the bitter quarrels of many years' duration.

CHAPTER TWENTY

LEGISLATION AFFECTING OFFICERS • Revision of Department Otto's • Correspondence Reimbursement

THE CONTINENTAL CONGRESS seem to have had a habit of passing resolutions, which, if adopted by a private corporation, might have been regarded as contractual obligations, but not so by the Government, for they frequently changed them and even entirely repealed laws containing inducements that had enabled many men to enter the Continental service.

On October 27, 1779, Congress resolved that the Director General, each of his Deputy Directors, the Physicians and Surgeons General, every Senior Physician, Senior and Junior Surgeons, etc., should be entitled to draw clothing from the Clothier General's Department, in the same manner as had been established for officers of the line, on November 26, 1777. Just what this allotment included was not specified. If the State's allowance of clothing to their own Regimental officers followed Government rulings, then each Hospital officer would draw yearly: one hat, a coat, and waistcoat, two pairs of breeches, three pairs of stockings, three pairs of shoes, three shirts and three stocks, for this was the Pennsylvania law. Members of the Medical Department, during the Revolutionary War, did not wear a uniform or display any insignia to indicate their rank or corps.

It was also decreed that the various members of the hospital staff should be entitled to a subsistence allowance, but on the following day, both these resolutions, already passed and in the minutes, were reconsidered and returned to the Medical Committee. On November 20, 1779, the Committee again reported, and it was "Resolved, that the Director General, Deputy Directors General, the Physicians and Surgeons General, the Senior Surgeons, Junior Surgeons, Mates, etc., shall be entitled to clothing allowance as previously passed and in addition, shall be paid subsistence money in the same manner as had been granted to officers of the line, on August 17th, 1777. This amounted to 500 dollars a month to the Director General and to each of the Physicians and Surgeons General. The Assistant Deputy Director and the Senior Surgeons were allowed monthly, 400 dollars; Junior Surgeons, 300 dollars; and Surgeons' Mates, 100 dollars."

The sums mentioned here seem most generous in terms of money, but they only reflected the depreciated value of the Continental currency at that date.

Congress also resolved that all the said officers of the Continental Hospitals should be granted land under the same conditions as had been allowed to the officers of the Army. The provision for gifts of land to officers and men in the ranks had been passed as early as September 16, 1776, and directed that a Colonel should be entitled to 500 acres; a Lieutenant Colonel, 450; a Major, 400; a Captain, 300; a Lieutenant, 200; an Ensign, 150; and each noncommissioned officer and private soldier, 100 acres.

Under a later resolution, the land allotment to the hospital staff was more specifically set forth, providing that the Director should receive the same quantity as a Brigadier General and the Chief Physicians and Surgeons the amount granted a Colonel. Hospital Physicians and Surgeons were to be treated the same as Lieutenant Colonel, while Regimental Surgeons were placed on an equality with Majors, and Surgeons' Mates with Captains.

On October 8, 1794, Margaret and John Otto, Executors of the Estate of Bodo Otto, received military bounty land warrant #1621 for 450 acres in consideration of Dr. Bodo Otto's Revolutionary War service. This allotment was then sold to John Wright, who, combining it with other warrants he had purchased, took title to 4,000 acres in Section 4 to 7, R. 14, in the U. S. Military District, now included in Knox County, Ohio.

On January 3, 1780, a resolution was introduced in Congress:

"That each and every officer hereinafter mentioned, belonging to the Hospital Department, shall receive annually for the term of seven years if they live that long, viz.: Physicians and Surgeons General, and Deputy Director, a sum equal to one-half the pay granted a Colonel of the Army, by resolution of Congress dated May 15th, 1778; Senior Surgeons and Physicians, Asst. Deputy Directors and Apothecary Generals, each a sum equal to one-half the pay of a Lieutenant Colonel; Junior Surgeons, each, one-half that paid a Major; and Surgeon Mates, one-half that of a Lieutenant."

The proposed legislation, when put to vote, was defeated by the members of the House. No further effort was made to remove discriminations that existed in the treatment of the Hospital Corps until January 17, 1781, when Congress again took them under consideration, the result of a memorial filed by members of the Medical Department and endorsed by General Washington.

"And thereupon came to the following resolution: Whereas, by the plan for conducting the hospital department passed on September 30th last, no proper establishment is provided for the officers of the Medical staff, after their dismission from public service, which, considering the custom of other nations, and the late provisions made for the officers of the Army after the conclusion of the war, they appear to have a just claim to; for remedy whereof, it is resolved:

"That all the officers in the hospital department and medical staff hereinafter mentioned, who shall continue in service until the end of the war or be reduced before that time, as supernumeraries, shall be entitled to and receive during life, in lieu of half-pay, the following allowance, viz:

"Director, one-half the pay of a Lieutenant Colonel; Chief Physicians and Surgeons, one-half that of a Major; Hospital Surgeons, Purveyors, etc., one-half the pay of a Captain; and to a Mate, one-half the pay of a Lieutenant."

On March 22, 1783, Congress amended this legislation, providing for half-pay during life by giving those entitled to its benefit an option to accept a lump sum in the form of certificates of indebtedness, amounting to five years' pay based on their retiring rank. On October 31, 1783, the Secretary of War reported to Congress that among those who had accepted the alternative were Dr. Bodo Otto and his son, Dr. Frederick. At seventy-one years of age, when he resigned, Dr. Bodo Otto's decision was undoubtedly a wise choice, but the irony of it is that the amount then due was never paid. Shortly before he died, Dr. Otto addressed Congress on the subject:

"To the Honorable Congress of the United States of America.

"The Humble Petition of Bodo Otto Showeth:

"That your Petitioner, before the last war, lived in Reading Town, in the State of Pennsylvania, in good circumstances. But, at the beginning of the War, was chosen Doctor for a Battalion of the Flying Camp from Berks, by the Committee of said County. In an unexpected attack of the Enemy on Long Island, our troops retired with great haste and your Petitioner lost all his medicines and other useful utensils.

"After that, the Honorable Congress was pleased to give your Petitioner a Commission to act as Senior Surgeon in the Hospital of the United States, and in April, 1777, he was continued in that station (and thus he served) until the subsequent arrangement, September, 1780, when he was appointed 'Hospital Physician and Surgeon,' in which capacity he officiated until the reduction was made of a number of Officers of said Department, in January, 1782, at which period he was deranged [discharged].

"Your Petitioner's accounts were settled and certificates received, but on account of necessity, your Petitioner was obliged to sell them to speculators for a mere trifle; merely to relieve him of his present wants, and he has ever since been obliged to shift for necessities for himself and family.

"But, as the Honorable Congress, in January, 1782, resolved to pay all Officers in the Line, and Medical Department, half pay during life, as soon as the war was over, but was afterwards pleased to alter it, and resolve to pay all Officers five years' full pay instead of half pay during life; therefore, your Petitioner has yet some hope of receiving something for his great toil and service, and humbly prays the Honorable Congress would be pleased to relieve him in his distress, and inform him when he could have any hope of obtaining anything.

"And your Petitioner will forever pray.

"Bodo Otto, "Late Physician and Surgeon to the Middle Division."

This document lies among the Colonial archives in Washington and bears this endorsement:

"This appears to be a request for information as to when money due, will be paid. Ordered filed."

Dr. Otto, in his reference to the loss of a medicine chest and surgical instruments at Long Island, was registering a personal misfortune, for he, with many other regimental surgeons, had taken his own private stock with him, that the men under his care might be sure of proper treatment. The Rev. Henry Melchior Mühlenburg wrote in his diary of the great scarcity of medicines in Berks County, for, he said, Dr. Otto had taken all that was locally obtainable.

When Bodo Otto retired from the Army, he was due his pay and sustenance allowance for eighteen months of service. No money was available to discharge this obligation, so an acknowledgment of the Government's indebtedness was issued in the following form:

"By virtue of a warrant from the Superintendent of the Finances of the United States unto me directed, bearing the date of April 19th, 1782, I do certify that there is due Dr. Bodo Otto, late of the General Hospital, the sum of $2,138, bearing interest at 6%, as appears of record in my office.

"Joseph Nourse, Registrar."

Necessity evidently compelled Dr. Otto to exchange this admission of money due for cash, for on the same day it was received, the certificate was either sold outright or used as collateral for a loan, as evidenced by a power of attorney executed by him.

"Know all men by these presents, that I, Dr. Bodo Otto, late of the General Hospital, make and appoint .. my trusty and loving friend, Haym Salomon, Broker, of the City of Phila., my true and lawful attorney, for me and in my name and stead and to his use, to ask, demand and receive all such sums... due me, agreeable to a certificate issued by the Registrar's office, bearing date of April 19th, 1782...

Thus did Haym Salomon, one of the financiers of the War, extend personal assistance to one who had just given six of his declining years to the effort for independence. When Salomon died, his private papers revealed many similar kindnesses, besides gifts of large sums to various prominent public men, that they might be able to meet their immediate needs while engaged in the work of the Revolution. Among the recipients of his generosity were James Madison, Edmund Randolph, Joseph Reed, Arthur Lee, James Wilson, Joseph Jones, and Baron von Steuben. Salomon's purse was always open to any hard-pressed Government official for his necessities, and many of them afterward gratefully acknowledged their benefactor.

Financial help to worthy individuals was only a small part of the service Haym Salomon extended to the cause of the infant republic. Without his knowledge, experience, and active assistance in the world of finance and trade, Robert Morris's task of providing funds and credit for the Government would have been even more difficult. Salomon not only marketed the bills of exchange that the Treasurer issued but, at many critical times, pledged personal credit and gave from his own capital to meet emergencies. He died before a Government accounting and settlement of amounts due him had even been discussed, and many of the important papers involved were unfortunately destroyed when the British burned Washington in the War of 1812.

Salomon's executors presented a partial tabulation of their claims in 1848, which totaled $353,000, and in 1860, additional documents were found that increased the amount to $800,000 without figuring interest. Papers submitted to substantiate the items of this total carried the signatures of many important Revolutionary men, and autograph collectors within the Government departments so mutilated the documents that their legal value as proof of claim was destroyed.

Haym Salomon's son and heir, when seventy-eight years of age, offered to make a settlement with the Government for $100,000 cash and some members of Congress strongly urged acceptance of the proposal, but no action was taken.

In 1893, more than one hundred years after the war, descendants of Haym Salomon requested Congress to give recognition to the great service rendered by their illustrious forefathers in the form of some suitable resolution and the minting of a medal in his honor. They agreed, if this were done, to withdraw all claims for financial reimbursement, and though a Committee of the House approved this generous offer, Congress neglected to authorize the small sum of $250 necessary to cover the cost.

A national movement was inaugurated in 1911 to persuade Congress to establish Washington University, to be dedicated to Haym Salomon, a hitherto unrecognized American patriot of Jewish faith. Woodrow Wilson was one of many prominent Americans who served on the Committee, and the idea received the approval of President Taft, but Congress could not be persuaded to do its part.

Congress did, in 1925, introduce and debate a bill appropriating $50,000 to erect a statue to Robert Morris's able assistant, but again, the proposal failed to win legislative approval.

Finally, in 1926, the Congress of the United States decided and resolved that some recognition should be given to Haym Salomon's memory, so it was decreed that a Government document containing a biographical sketch of his life should be authorized and published at public expense.

Ten times, between 1846 and 1920, efforts were made in Congress by fair-minded members to in some way make a belated acknowledgment of the gratitude and debt due Haym Salomon, and six different Congressional Committees appointed to investigate and report recommended favorable action, but without any success.

In view of all these facts, and in the absence of any doubts regarding them, it would seem that the recognition of Haym Salomon's great Revolutionary War service and personal contributions, in the form of a Resolution to publish a story of his life, had better been left undone.

Truly might it be written:

"The mountain labored, and brought forth a mouse."

The court-martial evidence developed in the trial of Dr. William Shippen brought a realization of some weaknesses in the existing organization plan of the hospitals, besides certain abuses that were possible and within the law. Congress, therefore, began considering a revision, early in September, 1781, and, after much discussion, it declared on September 30th:

"Whereas, the late regulations for conducting the affairs of the general hospital are in many respects defective, and it is necessary that the same be revised and amended, in order that the sick and wounded may be properly provided for and attended, and the business of the hospital conducted with regularity and economy; it is, therefore, resolved:

"That there be one director of the Military hospital,... three chief hospital physicians, who shall be surgeons, fifteen hospital physicians, who shall also be surgeons.

"That the hospital physicians shall take charge of such particular hospitals as may be assigned them by the director; they shall obey the orders of the director, or, in his absence, of the chief hospital physician; they shall have power to suspend officers under them and to confine other persons serving in the hospital under their charge, for negligence or ill-behavior, until the matter be regularly inquired into. They shall dili. gently attend to the cases of the sick and wounded of the hospital under their care, administering at all times proper relief as far as may be in their power. They shall respectively give orders under their hands, to the assistant purveyor or steward at the hospital, for the issuing of stores and provisions, as well as for procuring any other articles that the exigencies of the hospital may require, and which the store is not provided with; having always a strict regard to economy, as well as the welfare of the sick, then to be provided for. They shall make a weekly return to the nearest hospital physician, of the state of the hospital under their care. "That no person concerned in trade on his own account shall be suffered to act as an officer in the hospital or medical department of the Army. "That no officer or other person in the hospital department, except the sick and wounded, be permitted to use any of the stores provided for the sick.

"That the Director, Chief Hospital Physicians, Physicians and Surgeons... be appointed and commissioned by Congress...

"That the pay and establishment of the officers of the hospital department and medical staff, be as follows:

"Director-$150 per month plus two rations for himself, and forage for two horses. "Chief Physician and Surgeon of the Hospitals $140 per month, two rations per day, and forage for two horses.

"Physicians and Surgeons of the Hospitals each $120 per month, one ration per day, and forage for one horse.

"That the several officers above mentioned shall receive their pay in the new currency, emitted pursuant to a resolution of

Congress of the 18th day of March last, and that they be allowed and paid at the rate of five dollars of said currency per month, for every retained ration.

"That the former arrangement of the hospital department, and all resolutions heretofore passed touching the same, as far as they are inconsistent with the foregoing, be repealed.

In the earlier days of the War, a pretense was made of keeping the wounded separated from the sick by putting them in different departments, under the care of either surgeons or physicians, but the records of hospital assignment indicate that most of the medical men chosen to take charge of a hospital were selected because of experience in both branches of service. The first hospital reorganization law of April 1777 provided that the Physician General and the Surgeon General should have different duties and responsibilities, but these prescribed distinctions apparently developed complications, for Congress later resolved:

"That the Surgeon General and the Physician General of the Hospitals shall each of them regulate the practice of both physics and surgery...."

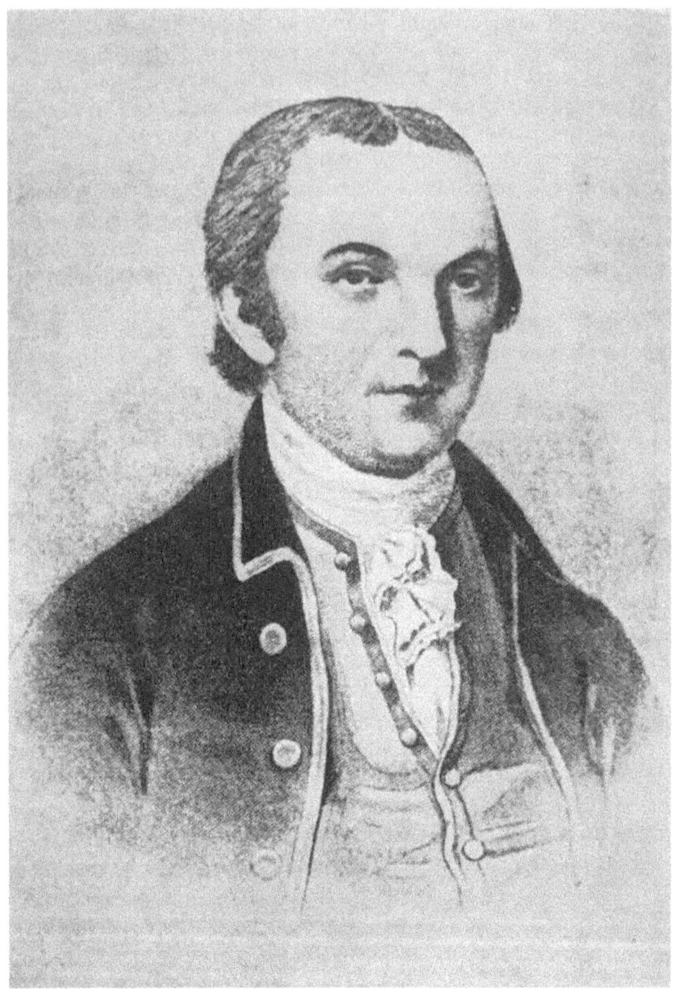

JOHN COCHRAN

Director General of the Military Hospitals of the Continental Army, 1781-1783.

This authority here shared in executive departments was then unofficially extended to those hospital surgeons and hospital physicians who could qualify on the two branches of the profession. Many medical men of the Revolution have been erroneously rated as "hospital physicians and surgeons" in existing rosters. It is true that quite a few had functioned as physicians and surgeons just as Bodo Otto did from the year 1776, in hospitals at Philadelphia, Trenton, Bethlehem, and Yellow Springs, but their commissions enrolled them as either "senior surgeons" or "senior physicians." In some of his letters, written before October 1780, when the rating of "hospital physicians and surgeons" was created, General Washington wrongly referred to several men of the profession by the combined title. The wording of the 1777 Act of Congress, relating to the subject and making a clear distinction, is:

"That the sick are to be taken care of by the physicians, and the wounded by the surgeons, in different departments. That the sick and wounded in the hospitals must be kept separate from each other, when circumstances will admit thereof; and that the sick shall be always placed at such a distance from those in health, as to prevent the spread of infection in the Army."

It might be inferred that General Washington was not consulted regarding the proposed hospital changes of October 1780, before the discussion by Congress, for on September 9th, 1780, he wrote to John Mathews, a member of the House:

"I have heard that a new arrangement is about to take place in the Medical Department, and that it is likely to be a good deal curtailed, in respect to many of its present appointments. Who will be the persons generally employed, do I wish to know? However, I do not know, nor do I I will mention to you that I think Dr. Cochran and Dr. Craik, for their services, abilities, experience and close attention, have the greatest claim to their country's notice, and are among the first officers in the establishment. The several gentlemen I have mentioned, as I have observed, appear to me to have the greatest pretensions to the public es teem and if they are honored with proper places, I am satisfied the public will be greatly benefited by their services. The reason of my mentioning these particularly proceeds from a hint given me that the new arrangement might be influenced by a spirit of party out of doors, which would not operate in their favor."

John Mathews answered General Washington's letter on September 15, 1780, and said:

"I had the pleasure of receiving your favor of the 9th, by Dr. Craig, two days ago.

"There is a new arrangement for the Medical Department now before Congress, and nearly completed, by which there will be a great reduction of officers.

"By the new system, there will be fifteen principal officers to be elected by Congress, which I apprehend will not be too much influenced by that spirit which has given a well-grounded alarm to the gentlemen concerned."

George Washington's communication to John Mathews was turned over to Congress, and James Duane, in an official capacity, replied on September 19, 1780: "I am to acknowledge the honor of your Excellency's favor of the 9th inst. on the subject of the Hospital Department.

"Your solicitude that gentlemen of distinguished merit should be employed, is a continual proof of your attention to the public good, and those you particularize, will not fail of being supported."

On October 2, 1780, the House resolved:

"That on Thursday next, Congress will proceed to the election of the Director, Chief Physician... and the Physicians of the Military Hospital.

So on October 6, 1780, they authorized the issuance of commissions to Dr. Wm. Shippen, Jr., as Director General; Dr. John Cochran as Chief Physician and Surgeon of the Army (attached to General Washington's staff); and to Doctors James Craik, Malachi Treat and Charles McKnight as Chief Hospital Physicians.

On the following day, Congress continued their election of officers for the reorganized hospital, and the ballots being taken were elected to fill the newly created positions of "Hospital Physicians and Surgeons."

Bodo Otto	
James Tilton	Barnabas Binney
John Warren	David Townshend
Samuel Adams	Francis Hagan
Henry Latimer	Wm. Burnet
Philip Turner	Moses Scott
David Jackson	Moses Bloomfield
Wm. Eustis	George Draper

Many men who had previously been prominent in the hospital organization were dropped from the service at this time.

The legislation of October 1780 was but the beginning of many Congressional changes in the Hospital Department regulations for the Army. A number of these might naturally have been expected, with the altered conditions in the Middle Division resulting from shifting battlegrounds and lesser Army activity. But the reduction in personnel and discharge of officers whose pay was generally in arrears left many of them stranded, far away from their homes.

The Medical Department of the Continental Army entered a period of Congressional neglect and parsimony with its reorganization of 1780. From that date until the end of the War, its history was indeed sad. One appeal sent to Congress for consideration of the sick and wounded stated:

"The poor fellows suffer for want of necessary supplies, which I hope soon will be afforded them; otherwise, there will be little encouragement for the physicians and surgeons."

Dr. Cochran wrote the Board of War, which had been substituted for the Medical Committee, and begged it to consider legislation for the relief of the hospitals, for many resignations were resulting from Congressional neglect, and only eight of the fifteen "hospital physicians and surgeons" selected by Congress, remained in the service. Again, he wrote:

"I hope some pay is ordered to be advanced to the officers of this department, without which it cannot much longer exist. Many of us have not received a shilling in near two years, nor can we procure public clothing from the Army supply."

Another seemingly ridiculous shortage was in writing material, and in one report, it was said:

"Several of the hospital physicians have not sufficient paper to make out their hospital returns; therefore, they are obliged to omit them."

It was also written:

"We are so squeezed for paper that I cannot afford you half a sheet, for cover and all."

One method adopted by Congress to reduce Medical Department expenses, was an arbitrary closing of hospitals regardless of their importance, and often without even consulting the proper authorities, or the Commander-in-Chief.

In October 1781, many hospitals were ordered discontinued, and Dr. Barnabas Binney, the Senior Officer in charge of the Philadelphia Hospital, fearing that he would be superseded by Dr. Bodo Otto, who outranked him, wrote the Director General asking how his status would be affected by the transfer of Yellow Springs Hospital patients and staff, to Philadelphia, Dr. John Cochran replied:

"Dear Sir:

I received your favor of the 16th instant and am at a loss to conceive on what principles the Board of War mean to break up the Hospitals at Yellow Springs, Boston and Albany, for, by their instructions to me, it is impossible to effect the two latter, unless at a most enormous expense, for if board cannot be promised at Boston, which it certainly cannot without money to pay for it, which they have not got, then the patients must be sent to another hospital, the nearest being upwards of two hundred miles. Ridiculous as this may appear, I have ordered Warren to put it into execution, as I am determined to obey my superiors. I have given no direction about the Albany Hospital, have assigned my reason to the Board of War, and shall await their further instructions. If economy is the object these gentry have in view, it will appear evident to any person with half an eye that they are saving on the small and expending on the large scale; a fault but too prevalent among the Great Ones; proceeding from a want of better information, and a too great proneness to listen to the idle whims of those who have their own interest more in view than the honor of Congress, the good of the service, or the Country they pretend to serve. I know not who is at the bottom of all these evolutions, for be assured they are new to me. If we take a view of the different metamorphoses of our poor Medical Department, it will give out the most genuine picture of the instability of all things here below. I have written my sentiments to the Board of War very fully on this subject, but fear to little purpose. I know no reason why you should be removed from Philadelphia to make way for another, for suppose the Board of War had taken it into their heads to break up the Hospital at Philadelphia and send the patients to Yellow Springs as they have done before, and which may be the case again tomorrow, surely it could not be supposed that you would take the place of Dr. Otto; besides I have written him to hold himself in readiness to join any other Hospital where his services may be most wanted. I fear we have some evil counsellors who are endeavoring to lead us astray, for astray we are going as fast as the Devil can drive us. I proposed seeing my friends in Philadelphia in a fortnight, but the indisposition of Mrs. Cochran will, I fear, deprive me of this pleasure. Compliments to Mrs. Binney, and believe me,

"Dear Sir, your most obedient and very humble servant,

"J. Cochran, M.D."

"To Dr. Binney, Phila."

On April 10th, 1780, the House

"Resolved, That when Congress shall be furnished with proper documents to liquidate the depreciation of the Continental bills of credit, they will as soon thereafter as the state of the Public Finance will admit, make good to the Line of the Army, and the independent Corps thereof, the deficiency of their original pay, occasioned by such depreciation, and that the money and articles heretofore paid or furnished, or hereafter to be paid or furnished by Congress or the States, or any of them, for pay, subsistence, or to compensate for deficiencies, shall be deemed as advances..., it being the determination of Congress that all troops serving in the

Continental Army, shall be placed on an equal footing; provided that no person shall have the benefit of this resolution, except such as were engaged during the year or for three years, and are now in service, or shall hereafter engage during the war.

"Resolved that a committee of three be appointed to report a proper compensation to the Staff of the Army, in consequence of the depreciation of the currency."

The Pennsylvania Assembly, acting under this authority, then passed a law providing for an adjustment of the pay to Officers of the Line, but it did not include all departments in this resolution, so on February 17, 1781, a second proposal was introduced and "A bill for admitting the Surgeons of the Pennsylvania Line to the advantages and emoluments of the commissioned officers thereof, was read and debated....."

The amendment here cited immediately called attention to discrimination being made against many Pennsylvanians who were serving on Continental Army Staffs and in independent corps, so Bodo Otto and Thomas Bond became their spokesmen through a communication addressed to the President of the Pennsylvania Assembly. On February 21, 1781, the minutes of the day record that:

"A letter from Bodo Otto, a Physician and Surgeon, and Thomas Bond, Purveyor of the General Hospitals of the United States, was read, requesting that the officers of the said hospitals, who are citizens of this State, may be admitted to the benefits and advantages of the Officers of the Pennsylvania Line, in the same manner as is proposed with respect to Regimental Surgeons. Ordered to be on the table."

It was further recorded in the Journal on March 13, 1781:

"On motion and by order, the letter of Bodo Otto and Thomas Bond received on the 21st ult., consideration it was read a second time, and on

"Ordered, That the said letter be committed to Mr. Boyd and Mr. Wynkoop, who are hereby instructed to make inquiry what provision has been made by Congress and the other States, for Chaplains, Brevet Officers and Hospital Surgeons, and report thereon to the House, and in the meantime, consideration of the Bill be postponed."

The Pennsylvania Committee's inquiry to Congress brought a realization to them that their own recommendation of April 10, 1780, had ignored all officers serving in the Continental Hospitals, so on June 13, 1781, a resolution was passed to correct the omission.

"Resolved, That it be, and hereby is recommended to the several States to which the officers of the Hospitals and Medical Departments now in service, respectively belong, to settle the accounts of the said officers for depreciation on the principle established by the Act of Congress of the 10th of April, 1780; and to make provision for paying the balance that may be found due, in the same manner with Officers of the Line."

It was not until October 1, 1781, that the Pennsylvania Assembly finally passed the necessary redrafted legislation, thus:

"Whereas, the United States, in Congress assembled, by their Act of the 13th of June, 1781, resolved and recommended to the several States, in the following words [then was inserted the wording of already quoted]. The Resolution

"Therefore, be it enacted that the officers of the Hospital and Medical Department now in the service of the United States, who are citizens of this State, be, and they are to all intents and purposes [on the same basis] as the Military Commissioned Officers, Chaplains and Regimental Surgeons of the Pennsylvania Line; all are entitled [to the benefit] under the Act ssed December 18, 1780, and April 10, 1781, and shall be entitled to half pay during life.

"And whereas, it may be difficult for the Auditors appointed by the Supreme Executive Council, to ascertain the rights of the Hospital Officers, who shall claim the benefits, be it enacted that the Supreme Executive Council are authorized to hear and determine the respective claims."

One month after the quoted legislation became effective both Dr. Bodo Otto and his son, Frederick, presented their applications to the designated authority. The first read:

"The Honorable, the Supreme Executive Council of the State of Pennsylvania:

"Gentlemen:

On the 1st ult. the Honorable House of Representatives of this State enacted a law to put the Officers of the Continental Hospital, who are citizens of this State, on the same footing with the Line, and in the 5th Clause of said Act, I find the Honorable, the Executive Council, are authorized and empowered to hear the claims of such persons as may apply for their benefits, and to direct the Auditors to settle and adjust their accounts without delay.

"Presuming that my service with the General Hospital since the year 1777 to this time, constantly employed in Active Duty with my residence in this State, and having paid rent, taxes, etc., has entitled me to the privileges of a freeman and consequently to these benefits.

"I pray your Honorable Body to give such orders therein as they shall think proper, and am with great respect

"Your most obedient and humble servant,

"Bodo Otto, "Hospital Physician and Surgeon.'

The action taken on Bodo Otto's communication, as recorded in the minutes, was:

"In Council, Phila., Nov. 2nd, 1781.

"A Petition from Thomas Bond, Jr., Purveyor of the Hospital of the United States, in behalf of himself and Dr. Goodwin Wilson, a Physician and Surgeon in the said hospital, praying the Board to direct the Auditors to settle the depreciation of their pay agreeable to the Act, was read; ..
Whereupon.. the said petition was granted, as far as respects the said Thomas Bond, Jr. Like petitions from Bodo Otto, Physician and Surgeon in the said Hospital, and Reading Beatty, Surgeon to the Regiment of Artillery, late Col. Proctor's, were read, and upon consideration the said petitions were granted."

Dr. Frederick Otto also filed a claim to the benefit of the Pennsylvania Act, but the Supreme Council recorded:

"Friday, November 2, 1781. "A Petition from Frederick Otto, Junior Surgeon of the Continental Hospital at the Yellow Springs, praying a settlement of the depreciation of his pay, was read; and thereupon it was Resolved by Council, that it is the opinion of the Board that the said Frederick Otto is a subject of the State of New Jersey, and therefore the prayer of said petitioner cannot be granted."

Frederick Otto indeed entered the Hospital Department on May 1, 1777, as a resident of New Jersey, but meanwhile, he had been recommissioned in October 1780 as a citizen of Pennsylvania because he had purchased and continuously occupied a property near his station at Yellow Springs. That he sincerely believed himself a Pennsylvanian is proved by the fact that he did not afterward make an application in New Jersey, as suggested by the Supreme Council's opinion.

The Continental Government was not in financial condition to promptly reimburse the States for any outlay required to adjust depreciated pay, nor were the States able to finance themselves. The Pennsylvania Assembly, therefore, appointed a committee of three members to determine a basis for the adjustment, with the authority to issue Certificates of Indebtedness in the proper amounts. It was found by the committee that the scale of depreciation for the year 1777 varied from 11/2 to 4, with a monthly average of 2.5. The 1778 variation was from 4 to 6, with an average of 5, while 1779 varied from 8 to 411/½ and averaged 22. The first seven months of 1780 had a low 401/2, a high 641/2, and an average of 57.

Pennsylvania had purchased a large area of land located in the Northwestern part of the State, and this section became known as "Donation Lands," the "Struck District," and the "Certificate Lands." The origin of these different names is interesting; when it became evident that the redemption of certificates issued to adjust depreciated pay could not be financed by either Congress or the States, an Act was passed by the Pennsylvania Assembly, declaring that the certificates should be accepted at the Land Office, in payment of land, as the equivalent of coin. To exchange the certificates for land, a vast stretch of this country was set apart, and the section was known as "Certificate Land."

Pennsylvania had also pledged itself to give to each of its citizens who served in the Continental Army, a specified quantity of land, varying with the rank of the recipient. A Major General was allotted 4,000 acres; a Brigadier General, 1,500; a Colonel, 1,000; a Lieutenant Colonel, 750; each Surgeon, Major and Chaplain, 600 acres; a Captain, 500; a Lieutenant, 400; every Ensign and Surgeon's Mate, 300; while a Sergeant received 250, and each Private, 200.

To fulfill this obligation, a second area was selected, located north of the "Certificate Land," and the section was called "Donation Lands."

When these areas were explored, one part was found to be totally unfit for farming and apparently of no value, so it was withdrawn and became known as the "Struck District."

There is no record or tradition of Bodo Otto taking title to any Pennsylvania Certificate or Donation land, and it is probable that the documents representing these rights were the certificates he wrote Congress he had been compelled to sacrifice. Speculation in both certificates and land was a popular business in the latter part of the eighteenth and beginning of the nineteenth century and resulted in the ruination of many men of means and prominence in public life. It was Robert Morris of Pennsylvania, who sold millions of acres of New York State land to the Holland Land Company, for resale to settlers, and in about 1824, Bodo Otto's grandson, Jacob S. Otto, became their agent. Thus was established a real estate business that has been continued by that branch of the family, into the present generation.

CHAPTER TWENTY ONE

POST-WAR DAYS • Removal to Baltimore Return to Reading • Otto's Illness and Death Otto's Monument

BODO ODO OTTO'S SEPARATION from the Continental service followed soon after an order from Congress to close the Yellow Springs hospital and was dated February 1, 1782. The last four months on duty were spent in Philadelphia, for he accompanied his patients when they were transferred to the Bettering House Hospital. Here, after rendering the necessary financial accounting and delivering all unused medicines and supplies, he received an official discharge from the Medical Department of the Army, accompanied by a letter expressing appreciation of his services.

Despite the absence of Bodo Otto and his son, the Reading apothecary shop had remained open throughout the entire war, as is evidenced by an old account book that recorded frequent purchases of drugs and other necessities. An attack of typhus fever caused the resignation of Dr. John A. Otto from the Hospital Department in 1780, and he then returned to his home, where he resumed private practice and acquired many of his father's old patients. A realization of the probable effect of his own return to

Reading and a desire to have his son well-established without any interference probably influenced Bodo Otto's decision to reopen an office in Philadelphia. The German newspaper of February 13, 1782, therefore, contained the announcement:

"DR. BODO OTTO who, for some years has served as Physician and Surgeon in the Continental Hospitals, herewith announces, by request of good friends, that he is again residing in Philadelphia on 5th Street opposite the old Lutheran Church, where he may be consulted in all cases of illness. Those who care to entrust themselves to his treatment, may depend upon his diligence and faithfulness."

"The following letter of commendation will satisfy everyone of his scientific and medical knowledge:

"This is to certify that Dr. Bodo Otto served in the capacity of a Senior Surgeon in the Hospital of the United States, in the year 1776, and when the new arrangement took place in April, 1777, he was continued in that position until the subsequent reorganization of October, 1780. He was then elected a 'Hospital Physician and Surgeon,' in which capacity he officiated until January, 1782, when a reduction occurred in the number of officers, and he was deranged.

"During the whole of the time Dr. Bodo Otto acted in the above stations, he discharged his duty with great faithfulness, care and attention. The humanity for which he was distinguished towards the brave American soldiers, claims the thanks of every lover of his country, and the success attending his practice will be a sufficient recommendation of ability in his profession. "Given under my hand, the 26th day of January, 1782.

"John Cochran, "Director of the Hospitals."

Many other retiring hospital physicians had likewise decided to locate in the Continental capital, and a list of medical men practicing in Philadelphia in 1783 contained the names of twenty-three who had served in the Army.

Whether Bodo Otto was disappointed in the amount of practice he developed in Philadelphia or was induced to make another start in the fast-growing town of Baltimore will probably never be known. Undoubtedly, many of his old patients had died during nine years of absence, and his seventy-one years may have handicapped him in attracting a younger generation. In any event, just eight months after he reopened his old office, a newspaper notice appeared that

"Dr. Bodo Otto, who has practiced medicine for many years, has settled in Baltimore and is now living in the house of the Widow Tripolet. He will treat patients, either in his own home or outside, and in his Apothecary Shop will be found everything necessary to a physician. Those who may become his patients or customers, will be served with the greatest diligence and care."

No record exists, among Baltimore archives, of Dr. Otto's stay in that city, but his landlady's memory is perpetuated in the name of an alley located in the old part of town. A local newspaper, dated November 30, 1791, contained a notice of:

"The death of Mrs. Mary Tripolet, an old inhabitant."

Baltimore had greatly increased in population and commercial importance during the period of the Revolution, and the condemnation of much Tory property, with resulting sales, brought ample funds for municipal improvements. The laying of sidewalks and paving of streets were then commenced, and in 1782 a considerable area was added to the city limits. General Greene commented on its growth after a visit in 1782, saying that no less than 300 houses had been erected each year. Communication with other sections of the country had been made more easily possible by the inauguration of a stage-coach service between Baltimore and Philadelphia, and shortly afterward, it was extended to Alexandria, Virginia.

It was in the summer of 1782 that 5,000 French troops, en route to the North to embark for home, encamped for a month's stay in Baltimore. The officers were extensively entertained by both the men and women of the city, and before leaving, they showed their appreciation by giving a large ball. One of the French nobles, Baron de Closen, wrote in his diary that the Baltimore women had more charm and style than any others of the fair sex he had met in America. It was also noted that the local citizens boasted of their "Market Street," claiming it could not be matched in Philadelphia or New York for its length, beauty or gayety.

Bodo Otto had been an inhabitant of Baltimore one year when the Continental Army passed through the city, returning from the Southern campaign. General Greene, who commanded, was tendered a large banquet, and undoubtedly, Dr. Otto saw something of his old associate of the Valley Forge encampment. It is also likely that he paid his respects to his beloved General Washington when the Commander-in-Chief stopped in Baltimore on his way to Annapolis to surrender his commission.

Urged by his son, whose practice now absorbed most of his attention, Bodo Otto returned to Reading in 1784 and spent the three remaining years of his life among grandchildren and old friends. He was physically active, mentally fit and apparently still able to operate, for two years later, he was sent to Germany for a new set of surgical instruments. His continued interest in the Reading Apothecary is disclosed in an advertisement that appeared in a Philadelphia newspaper:

"DR. BODO OTTO

and his son

announce to the public and to their good city and country friends, who have honored them with their patronage, that the Apothecary shop is now well supplied with a fresh stock of good medicines and other necessities.

"They ask their patrons to visit them and give an assurance that all will be served at the lowest possible prices and with the greatest care. "Reading, July 3rd, 1784."

The town of Reading did not publish a newspaper until 1796, so no local obituary notice is available to tell the details of Dr. Otto's last illness and death. The only record found was written in the Parish book:

"Buried: June 15th, 1787-The esteemed Dr. Bodo Otto, who was born in the City of Hanover, Electorate of Hanover, Germany. He was well known in his native land, as well as in America. Aged 78 years, 4 months."*

His remains were interred in the Trinity Lutheran Church grounds at the western end of the building, and his monument is now adorned with a bronze tablet dedicated by the local chapter of the Daughters of the American Revolution.

While no outstanding achievement appears in the life of Bodo Otto, his history has been well worth recording, for it includes the experiences of many unsung patriots of the late Colonial period and the early days of the republic. Conscientious and thorough, Dr. Otto met and solved the problems of his times to the best of his understanding and ability; unafraid and with self-confidence, he frequently changed his plans when proved wrong or he thought better opportunities presented themselves. He was the father of three sons, of whom he might well have been proud, grandfather

*Dr. Otto's correct age was 76+ of two physicians who left enviable reputations in their profession; besides the ancestor of a member of Abraham Lincoln's Cabinet and a number of creditable

descendants now living, it may be claimed that some of the characteristics of this venerable man have been carried through the blood of five generations.

Many years ago, the distinguished Pennsylvania historian Morton L. Montgomery wrote:

"Next to Washington, Gates, Mifflin, Wayne, and other leading Generals, Dr. Bodo Otto, of Reading, Pa., occupied a prominence and rendered useful service equal to any other man who was engaged in the great cause of the Revolution, not on the field of battle, leading his fellowmen into danger and death, but amongst the Hospitals, as a Senior Surgeon, caring for, and administering to the sick, wounded and dying soldiers. And yet his name is not mentioned in history."

ADDENDUM

EXTRACTS FROM THE JOURNAL OF REV. DR. JAMES SPROAT

The Rev. Dr. Sproat was appointed Chaplain to the hospitals of the Middle Department of the Revolutionary Army and rode the circuit every two weeks. His diary covering this period began March 9, 1778, and the original book was found among the documents in the Pennsylvania Historical Society Library. These records are of special interest because they not only list the hospitals but also give the names of the medical officers in charge.

Genealogy

April 2nd, 1778.

Rode to Bethlehem (from Easton)-travelling exceedingly bad - dined with Drs. Finley and Hall. In the afternoon, discoursed and prayed with all the sick, in their different departments, that were unable to attend the sermon. Drank tea with Dr. (Bodo) Otto-lodged at the tavern. The company of Mr. Caldwell and Dr. Laton rendered the evening agreeable.

April 3rd, 1778.

Preached to the convalescents-upward to one hundred-dined with the doctors. After dinner, rode to Allen Town-roads exceeding bad. Went to see Dr. Smith-met with Mr. and Mrs. Bryan and Miss Looky Smith-this was very agreeable. This night the doctor's wife was delivered of a son.

April 4th, 1778.

Visited, discoursed and prayed with the sick (Allen Town). In the afternoon rode up to the Settlement, seven miles, in company with Mr. Cowell.

April 6th, 1778.

Preached at 10:00 o'clock in the Settlement. A little more freedom, blessed be God. First part of this week spent among the people at the Forks the latter part rode to the hospital-preached in the Duch [Dutch] Church. Baptized Dr. Smith's son by the name of Thomas Graham. Went to old Mrs. Smith's kindly received-it is desirable to see old friends, citizens and neighbors. Saturday, rode up to the Settlement and preached twice on the Sabbath-on Monday, preached again and rode to Allen Town.

April 14th, 1778.

Rode to Reading.

April 15th, 1778.

Visited the hospitals-discoursed with all the confined preached in the afternoon-Easter sermon; visited the sick and saw a good many Philadelphia friends. Took leave.

April 16th, 1778.

Lodged the night in Mr. McIllhanie's. This day rode to Rheims Town where I supposed there was a hospital-very wet and poor entertainment. Met with Capt. Collens from Rhode Island.

April 17th, 1778.

Rode five miles to Dunkers Town, visited and prayed with all the sick-preached in the hospital. Dr. Scott is the Senior (Physician and Surgeon).

April 18th, 1778.

Rode to Shaffers Town. Visited the hospital and preached in the Duch [Dutch] Church where all that were able to attend were paraded, and attended in good order-lodged with Dr. (George)

Glentworth - genteely treated - here met with General McIntosh. Lord's Day. Rode from Shaffers Town to Lititz, twelve miles. Dined with Dr. [Francis] Allison, who is the Senior here. Visited the hospitals conversed with the sick at 3:00 o'clock preached to the convalescents Monday, rode to Lancaster in company with Mr. Mackey, one of the and father to Dr. Allison Spouse. Dined at Dr. Jackson's and visited the hospital. Prayed in five or six different departments very much fatigued.

April 21st, 1778.

Preached in ye Barracks to all the convalescents that were able to attend. Lodged at J. D. Smith's-Dined at Mr. Harbinson's drank tea at Mrs. Rhea's saw many of my Philadelphia friends.

April 23rd, 1778.

Rode to Mr. Woodhull's lodged there very kindly treated.

April 24th, 1778.

Rode to Mr. Whitehill's and Mr. Smith's at Pequga-neither of the gentlemen at home this day rode to Mr. Carmichael's lodged there but he was not at home.

April 25th, 1778.

Rose early got my horse fed hope to set off soon. Bless the Lord for all His goodness, oh my soul, and forget not all His benefits. This day rode to Yellow Springs-visited the hospitals-conversed and prayed with the sick that were not able to attend the sermon. Lodged at Dr. [Samuel] Kennedy's.

April 26th, 1778.

Lord's Day morning-had some time alone-found that in the midst of tumult, 'tis sweet to have a little retirement. This hospital seems to be very neat and the sick comfortably provided for, though wickedness, I understand, prevails among the convalescents. I endeavored, in my sermon as well as in my private discourses in their department, to show them the obligations they were under to love God to live to Him and for Him. This evening rode about three miles to Mr. Ralston's where I found my old friend William Ralston and his family-lodged there - kindly treated.

April 27th, 1778.

Mr. Ralston rode with me to French Creek. Mr. William Smith and G. Tennent, doctors here. The Senior doctor is abroad [away]. The hospital very neat and clean and the sick seem well attended. Here I again met with General McIntosh, who is visiting the hospitals in an official capacity. According to my usual methods, I first visited and conversed with the sick and wounded in the departments, in the forenoonin the afternoon I preached to all of them in the church. Rode this evening to Charles Town-lodged at Mrs. Pritchard's kindly entertained-discoursed and prayed with her. In the afternoon I applied to General Greene and to Col. Cox to transport my goods from Friends Ford to the Forks of the Delaware, which the Colonel, granted. Crossed the Schoolkill to lodge at Mr. Arthur McFarling's.

May 1st, 1778.

The wagons loaded and set out, when I followed-had great difficulty in finding them they and I both missed the way-met about noon and had a good passage. Lodged at a tavern-tolerably comfortable that night.

May 2nd, 1778.

Rode to Bethlehem-the hospital removed from this place, except for a few invalids. Called to see Capt. Balding, who has had his leg dissected [amputated] since I was here last. Conversed and prayed with him and then rode on to the Forks.

May 3rd, 1778.

Preached at the Settlement will spend the week here.

May 11th, 1778

Went to the Muster. The report of Borden Town and Trenton being destroyed by the enemy gave me great concern for my family.

May 12th, 1778.

Rode to Allen Town and returned before noon. Got wagon to go to Maiden Head for my family-heard the enemy had left Trenton and Borden Town, which gave me some encouragement and hope that my family was safe. Rode to Greenwich and lodged at the tavern.

May 13th, 1778.

Rode to Maiden Head*-stopped at Wilson Stunk kindly treated. Found my family all safe at this place, to my great comfort. Bless the Lord, oh my soul, for His goodness to me and mine in this day of trouble.

May 14th, 1778.

Thursday. Spent this day in getting my family to the Settlement where we arrived late Friday evening, much fatigued.

May 16th, 1778.

Arrived at the Parsonage with all our goods.

June 9th, 1778.

Set out [from the Settlement] for the hospital at York Town-dined at Mr. Tatem's at Allen Town-rode to Camp-saw my son rode to Graham's and dined. Saw Dr. Shippen, Dr. J. B. Smith, and received $60.00 rode to French Creek and lodged at the Commissaries.

June 11th, 1778.

Came up to the hospital-found Drs. Smith, Rodgers and Linwentin the afternoon, preached to one of the hospitals where Dr. Smith accompanied me. The hospital very airy and clean about sixty-six sick in this place returned to the other hospital and met my son, Billy. He and I dined with the Doctor. In the afternoon preached to the other hospital, a Duch [Dutch] Church-very clean and airy-ninety-six sick in it. Dr. Binney, the Senior, came in time for service drank tea with the doctors and my son after tea parted with my son and rode a mile with Dr. Binney-lodged at his house kindly treated he is genteel, learned and hospitable much pleased with his Lady from the City, the daughter of one Mr. Woodrom-very kind.

June 12th, 1778.

Rode long miles to the Yellow Springs-lit [alighted] at Dr. Kennedy's poor gentleman, very sick-visited Dr. [Bodo] Otto-dined at Dr. Kennedy's. After dinner, preached in the hospital-'tis airy and new-but not yet finished-smoked a pipe and then preached to a number in adjacent barn. Many sick here, though clean and airy. Drank tea with the matron and the doctors in the evening returned to Dr. Kennedy's, very much exhausted the poor doctor is no better, encouraged him in the things of God-prayed again with him retired to bed and slept comfortably.

Maiden Head was near Princeton, N.J.-now Lawrenceville.

June 13th, 1778.

Understand that the doctor [Kennedy] is no better after breakfast preached in the upper gallery of the hospital, where the gentleman is treated by Des. Otto went to a barn [nearby] and preached before dinner. Dined with Dr. Craig-rested a little after dinner, and then went to another barn and preached again-took little spirits and rode to a barn and preached again-much fatigued. In the barns are one hundred and eighty-two patients the barns are clean and airy and in good order. Dr. [James] Fallon is the Senior [Solomon] Halling and [John] Cowell, JuniorsWhite and Marshall, mates.

The number of patients at the Yellow Springs hospital and adjacent barns are about 125 or 130. Drs. Otto and sons are the Senior, Junior and mates-I have forgot their [first] names.

Dr. Kennedy, whose department is the three barns, is sick. After this tedious day's work, rode four or five miles to the Red Lion Tavern, where Dr. [John H.] Latimer is the Senior-lodged at the tavern.

June 14th, 1778.

Preached in the forenoon to the hospital in the Quaker Meeting127 patients. Dr. [John H.] Latimer, Senior, Garrison and... Juniors, [Ezekiel] Bull and Tobin, mates. Dined with the doctors and in the afternoon, preached in the barns. Drank tea at the lodgings of Latimer and Garrison-some dispute with Dr. [James] Fallon and others, concerning the liberty of human will.

June 15th, 1778.

After breakfast, set out in company with G. Tennent for Lancaster.

June 18th, 1778

Rode to Manheim-dined with Mrs. Shippen and old Dr. Shippenelegantly treated. Mrs. Shippen paid me $240.00 but could not settle with respect to rations. Rode to Lititz-put up with Dr. [Francis] Allison-spent the evening at Dr. William Brown's, the Physician General-lodged with Dr. [Francis] Allison.

June 19th, 1778.

Preached in the afternoon to the hospital. Dined with Dr. [William] Brown. Dr. [Francis] Allison and his wife were very kind and generously kept me and my horse.

This evening Mr. Malky, one of the Council of Safety, came to Mrs. Allison's and brought the second confirmation of the evacuation of the city by the enemy.

June 21st, 1778.

Rode to Dunker Town-no hospital here now-had some hesitation whether to put up or ride on to Reading thought duty to go to Reading—arrived there about 2:00 o'clock-obtained some refreshments at my good friend's, Mr. McIllhanie-his poor wife is very gloomy-preached at 6:00 o'clock, in the German School House.

July 29th, 1778.

Set out from the Forks toward the hospitals-stopped at Bethlehem.

July 30th, 1778.

Rode to Philadelphia.

August 3rd, 1778.

[Leaving Philadelphia] stopped by the gust [rain] at Robins Hood and at the Falls-reached Mr. Conford's.

August 4th, 1778.

Proceeded to Dr. [George] Glentworth's-much rain could not preach to the hospitals-lodged at the doctor's about seventy in this hospital-thirty of them expected to be sent away very soon. [NOTE-The identity and location of this hospital are unknown. Apparently, it lay somewhere between Philadelphia and Valley Forge and probably was but a temporary one used to break the transfer from some of the hospitals adjacent to the Yellow Springs, to Philadelphia, where a hospital was established in the Bettering House in charge of the same Dr. Glentworth.]

August 5th, 1778.

Preached at the hospital-the hearers seemed very attentive. Dr. [George] Glentworth rode with me to Camp-stopped at Col. Craig's quarters; then to Yellow Springs; the Doctor accompanied me. I lodged at Mrs. Kennedy's and endeavored to administer some consolation to her, in her mournful circumstances-Mrs. Kennedy kept my horse in

her pasture I obtained some feed from the Commissary. Preached at Yellow Springs to about seventy-odd patients. Rode to Yewklin (Uhlan). Dined with Dr. [William] Brown and Dr.

[James] Fallon very genteelly treated-Rode to East Coln, alias for Downing Town. Lodged with Dr. Smith-horse kept by the Commissary.

August 7th, 1778.

About seventy-one patients at Downing Town. After service, set out for Philadelphia.

August 13th, 1778.

Set out [from Philadelphia] on my journey-rode to Dr. [Malachi] Treat's-lodged there.

August 14th, 1778.

Dr. [Malachi] Treat rode with me to Craig's Tavern-parted with the doctor-rode to a Quaker Tavern.

August 15th, 1778.

Rode to a tavern within five miles of Bethlehem then to Bethlehemdined at tavern and then rode to my family [settlement at the Fork].

Sept. 7th, 1778.

Set out for the hospital at Philadelphia.

Sept. 11th, 1778.

Visited the hospital at the Bettering House-preached to a considerable number.

Sept. 14th, 1778.

Rode twenty-eight miles to French Creek-preached to the hospitals, where there are 130 persons who seem to be well attended by the physicians.

In the afternoon rode to the Yellow Springs preached in the hospital old Dr. Otto behaved politely then rode to Mrs. Pritchard's and lodged there.

Sept. 18th, 1778.

Received $180.00 from Mr. Joseph Shippen; in the afternoon, preached in the hospital at the Bettering House.

Oct. 11th, 1778. (Tuesday)

Set out for the hospitals in the country-preached at Yellow Springs on Thursday, in the morning-115 sick here-16 guards-total 131.

Rode to French Creek-preached to the hospital in the afternoon-89 sick here-lodged with Drs. Smith and Tennent.

Oct. 23rd, 1778.

Visited the hospitals at the Bettering House and preached to them, in Dr. [George] Glentworth's side [ward].

Oct. 26th, 1778.

Preached to the hospitals at the Bettering House, in Dr. Jackson's ward the poor sick very attentive.

Nov. 16th, 1778.

Rode to Yellow Springs-preached in the hospital. People seemed serious and attentive.

Jan. 12th, 1779.

Set out for the hospital at Yellow Springs.

Jan. 13th, 1779.

Arrived at the Springs about half past three-cold and rainy-lodged with Dr. Otto-supper with the Commissary-baptized his child this evening-breakfasted with Dr. Otto-preached at the hospital; the people attentive - dined in the matron's room with Dr. Otto, Jr. and the Commissary, and rode to Mr. Siemetous, eight miles, after dinner. Lodged there. Stormy evening.

Jan. 15th, 1779.

Rode to Philadelphia. Preached at the hospital (Bettering House). A number of new patients came in to be inoculated.

Jan. 26th, 1779.

Baptized four children for the Commissary at the hospital.

Feb. 4th, 1779.

Visited the hospital (Bettering House). Prayed with the poor sick Captain, whose smallpox seems to be attended with fatal symptoms. I discoursed with him and recommended Jesus Christ. Discoursed and prayed with nine inoculated people, who seemed to be attentive-oh, that some good may be done!

Feb. 10th, 1779.

Visited the hospital and preached in Dr. [George] Glentworth's ward. The patients seemed to be considerably affected.

Feb. 17th, 1779.

Preached in the Bettering House Hospital, Dr. Jackson's ward. One poor creature afflicted with the smallpox, was past instruction.

Feb. 23rd, 1779.

Set out for the hospitals at Yellow Springs. Rode eleven miles to the "Sign of the Buck." Baptized a child of Mr. Fullerton and then rode to Yellow Springs and lodged with Dr. Otto.

Feb. 24th, 1779.

Preached at the hospital-the hearers very attentive.

Feb. 26th, 1779.

Rode home [Philadelphia].

March 17th, 1779.

I could not preach at the hospital today, being called upon to attend ye funeral of Senior Dr. Jackson's wife.

April 13th, 1779.

Set out for the hospital at Yellow Springs in company with Capt. Hardy-dined at the "Sign of the Buck"-lodged this evening at Drs. Otto.

April 14th, 1779.

Preached at the hospital, from "I beseech you not to receive the grace of God in vain" took some refreshments in the matron's room and then rode to Mr. Trabling's, where I lodged.

April 29th, 1779.

Preached in the forenoon at the hospital in the Bettering House. The patients did not behave as well as usual.

May 25th, 1779.

Set out for the hospital at Yellow Springs. Rode with Mr. Proctor to Mr. McFarling's, in a chair-then rode a horse to the Springs. Much trouble in crossing the Schoolkill expenses for crossing, three shillings -lodged at Mr. McIllhanie's preached at the hospital, on the 26th of May the patients, about seventy, attended well.

July 7th, 1779.

Set out for Yellow Springs to visit the hospital-the weather hot-rode to Col. -kindly treated and dined there. Stopped at Mr. McFarling's rode to Mr. Pritchard's his wife went with me to the Springs arrived at the Commissary, whose wife is Mrs. Pritchard's daughter.

July 8th, 1779.

Preached at the hospital, patients attended well. Dined with Dr. Otto and Col. Syrus and then rode on to Mr. McFarling's.

Aug. 18th, 1779.

Set out [from Philadelphia] for the hospital at Yellow Springs, in company with Mr. Merchant. Rode to Mrs. Pritchard's and took lodging.

Sept. 27th, 1779.

Rode to Yellow Springs-dined with Dr. Otto, Sr. - preached in the afternoon - hospitals well provided for, and the gentlemen take good care of the sick. After the sermon rode to Mr. Pritchard's, about three and a half miles from the hospital-lodged there treated kindly.

Oct. 16th, 1779.

Sent in an order to Mr. James [Commissary of the Hospital Warehouse] for one gallon of wine.

Oct. 30th, 1779.

Set out to attend Presbytery and the Yellow Springs.

Nov. 4th, 1779.

Rose early and continued journey to Yellow Springs, distance of ten miles-preached-rode fifteen miles in the afternoon.

Nov. 28th, 1779.

Visited and prayed with poor Dr. Allison after the sermon; he appears to be dying.

Nov. 30th, 1779.

Attended the funeral of my good friend, Dr. Allison-Dr. Ewing preached the funeral sermon.

Set out for the hospital at Yellow Springs. Stopped at the "Sign of the Buck" rode to the hospital-lodged at Dr. Otto's.

Jan. 11th, 1780.

Set out in the morning, for the hospital at Yellow Springs extremely cold riding against the wind-stopped at the "Sign of the Buck" expenses four dollars then rode to Mr. Todd's here lodged and kindly treated.

Jan. 12th, 1780.

This morning, there were snow squalls and extreme cold. Mr. Todd accompanied me to the Springs the lanes filled with snow-travelling bad indeed I preached from John 40-"Ye will not come to me that ye might have life." Returned with my good friend, Mr. Todd-the weather was thought to be colder than it has been for the past twenty years. Lodged this night with Mr. Todd and his kind family. May the Lord reward their kindness.

March 29th, 1780.

Rose early "Buck's Tavern"-rode to the hospital at Yellow Springs -dined with Dr. Otto. Then rode to Mr. Pritchard's-lodged there - kindly treated.

May 2nd, 1780.

Dined with Dr. Otto, Jr., who preached at the hospital in the afternoon to a very serious congregation. Lodged with old Dr. Otto.

May 3rd, 1780.

Rode to Charles Town.

June 12th, 1780.

Rode to Yellow Springs [from Philadelphia]. Mr. Kennedy accompanied me part of the way-dined with the young Doctors Otto-lodged with the old doctor.

June 13th, 1780.

Preached. Dined with the young Drs. Otto. A child of a soldier has been baptized, and lately, they returned from the backwoods. They belonged to Mr. Eakin's congregation.

June 14th, 1780.

Rode to Philadelphia. Studied most all this day. Baptized the President's [Mr. Reed's] son, in the evening, by the name of George Washington. The French Ambassador and Mrs. Washington, the President of Congress and his Lady, were present.

July 3rd, 1780.

After dinner I went to the hospital to see some patients with the smallpox, who had sent for me. One died before I arrived three more are exceedingly bad. I discoursed and prayed with them, with some affection and acceptance.

July 10th, 1780.

Set out for Yellow Springs on half after four P.M. Weather exceedingly hot-stopped at Levering's.

July 11th, 1780.

Rose early and rode to McCallas. Crossed the Schoolkill, which was very high, to the Springs. Preached from Act 8th, "Repent of this, thy wickedness, and pray God." Though much fatigued, yet hope I had some assistance bless the Lord. Dined with Dr. Otto and the Commissary. Left the Springs about four o'clock and rode with Col. Corneys, where I lodged the season very hot, but rested pretty comfortably.

July 12th, 1780.

Rose rode early to Col. Basqard's, took breakfast with him, then on to the Leverings, took little refreshments there, and rode to the city, which was very dusty and hot.

July 31st, 1780.

Set out for the hospitals at the Yellow Springs-weather very hot-lodged at Dr. Otto's.

Aug. 1st, 1780.

A rainy morning-rode to the hospital-preached with some freedom -dined with Mr. Riley and several of the officers of the hospital. After dinner, set out and rode seven or eight miles to Major Bradley's, who is a consumptive-prayed and comforted him about his affliction.

Sept. 4th, 1780.

Set out for the Yellow Springs. Stopped at the "Buck" expenses only four dollars. Rode to Major Bradley's, who was still in a very low condition endeavored to impress on his mind a sense of Christ's all sufficiency rode to the hospital-lodged with Dr. Otto.

Sept. 5th, 1780.

Preached at the hospital and seemed, in some measure, to be favored.

Dined with the young Dr. Otto. After dinner, rode eight miles and lodged at Mr. John Lloyd's hospitably entertained.

Sept. 6th, 1780.

Rode to Philadelphia.

Sept. 12th, 1780.

Rode to the hospital at the Bettering House-preached to about forty-five sick.

Oct. 6th, 1780.

Purposed by divine leave to set out for the Springs set out, accompanied by Mr. Hide, stopped at the "Buck"-expenses sixteen dollars.

Oct. 10th, 1780.

Rode on to the hospital-preached to an attentive congregation-dined with Dr. Otto, Jr. rode to "Red Lion."

Nov. 1st, 1780.

Had Dr. Otto to dine with me [Philadelphia].

March 1st, 1782.

Attended to some necessary business with Col. Bayard in the Auditor's Office, relating to my hospital affairs.

March 2nd, 1782.

Wrote a letter to the Executive Council, relating to my affairs in the hospitals.

INDEX

REPRINTING NOTES

This reprint of Mr. James Gibson's book about the life and contributions of Dr. Bodo Otto was made possible by the Dr. Bodo Otto Association. The Association is comprised of descendants of Dr. Otto and others who are interested in honoring and perpetuating the memory of Dr. Otto and others who provided medical service during the American Revolution.

Any person desiring to join the Association may contact us through our web page at https://www.drbodootto.org/. Membership is open to the public. As of 2024, individual membership is $20 annually, family/household membership is $30 annually, and Lifetime membership is $250 for an individual. Family/household membership is defined as those residing at one address. To join, please send your name and address along with a check made out to the *'Dr. Bodo Otto Association 'to: Connie Barton, 2280 Vinson Road, Clayton, NC 27527-9145*

The Association sends a newsletter to members via email four times a year. In even numbered years, the bi-annual meeting / reunion is held at a site associated with Dr. Otto on the weekend following Father's Day. Information is shared in the spring issue of the newsletter and posted on the web page.

MARKERS RELATING TO DR. BODO OTTO

Several historical markers that pertain to the life and distinguished career of Dr. Bodo Otto can be found at the following locations:

- Behind the ruins of Washington Hall at Historic Yellow Springs in Chester Springs, PA. Dr. Otto attended the soldiers of the Valley Forge encampment at a hospital built at this location and named in honor of General George Washington. A plaque was installed by the Association in the garden area.
- In Penn Square in Reading, PA, between 5th and 6th streets marking the site of Dr. Otto's home in Reading until his death in 1787.
- There is a memorial grave marker on the grounds of Trinity Lutheran Church in Reading, PA. His actual grave is believed to be under a newer portion of the church along with many others.
- In Trenton, NJ at the Old Barracks Dr. Otto served during a yellow fever epidemic and provided inoculations for smallpox.
- In Emanuel Lutheran Church, 366 Cohansey Friesburg Rd, Elmer, NJ 08318 where Dr. Otto's wife Catherina Daechncken Otto and his daughter, Maria Elizabeth Otto Carman are buried.
- In Berks History Center, 940 Centre Avenue, Reading, PA 19601, there are portraits of Dr. Otto and his wife, his medical case and some tools and other archives. There is

also a diorama of Penn Square, which includes his home and apothecary shop.

- At Washington Memorial Chapel at Valley Forge, 2000 Valley Forge Park Rd., King of Prussia, PA 19406. Dr. Otto is honored on the Veterans' Wall of Honor and with a memorial in the adjacent prayer garden.

FOUR GENERATIONS OF DESCENDANTS OF DR. BODO OTTO

+ Spouses • Children ◆ Grandchildren

Bodo Otto (1711-1787)

+ Anna Elisabeth Sauken (1713-1738)

Maria Elizabeth Otto (1737-1768)

+ Marcus Kurrman (1731-1785)

Catharina Maria Carman (1760-1850)

+ Henrich Saul (1760-1826)

Johann Adam Saul (1786-1798)

Fredrich Saul (1788-1867)

Margareta Saul (1793-dec.)

Johann Saul (1797-1875)

◆Frederick Marcus Carman Sr. (1761-1832)

+ Margaretta (1765-1788)

Bodo Carman (1786-1791)

Henry Carman (1788-1814)

+ Hanna (1770-1792)

John Carman (b. 1792)

+ Catherine Fox (1772-1865)

Elizabeth Carman (b. 1794)

- Margarethe Carman (1795-1891)

Frederick Marcus Carman Jr. (1798-1879)

David Carman (b. 1800)

Marcus David Carman (b. 1802)

Anna Carman (b. 1805)

George Carman (b. 1807-1878)

Daniel Carman (b. 1809-1849)

Anna Marie Carman (1813-1880)

Elizabeth Carman (b. 1763)

+ Davis

Catherine Carman (b. 1765)

+ Bender (b. 1765)

Sarah Carman (b. 1767)

+ Catharina Dorathea Dahnken (1710-1765)

Great Grandchildren

Frederick Christopher Otto (1743-1795)

+ Mary Withers (1747-1794)

Sarah Otto (b. 1765)

Bodo Otto (b. 1767)

Margaret Otto (b. 1772)

+ Jonathan Morgan (1765-1840)

George Washington Morgan (b. 1798)

Bodo Morgan Sr. (b. 1799)

Maria Morgan (b. 1806-1902)

- Jonathon H. Morgan (1813-1888)

Peter Morgan (1817-1908)

Christopher Morgan (1829-1881)

Mary Otto (b. 1777)

+ Isaac Morgan

- Dorothea Sophia Otto (1744-1748)

Bodo Otto Jr. (1748-1782)

+ Catherine Schweighauser (1748-1782)

Jacob Schweighauser Otto (1768-1788)

+ Phoebe Whitehead

John Otto

Eliza Martin Otto

Catherine Margaretta Otto (1773-1815)

+ Dr. James Seargent Ewing (1770-1823)

- John Otto Ewing (1802-1810)
- Henry Ewing (1803-1826)
- Jacob Otto Ewing (1805-1863)
- William Davidson Ewing (1807-1831)
- Catherine Margaretta Ewing (1808-1871)
- Amelia Ewing (1813 - ?)

+ Tobias Hammer (1752-1815)

Francis Hammer (1786-1865)

John Conrad Otto (1774-1844)

+ Elizabeth Todd (1780-dec.)

William Todd Otto (1816-1905)

Bodo Otto (1776-1778)

John Augustus Otto (1751-1836)

+ Catharine Hitner (1758-1836)

Margaret Otto (1777-1838)

+ Benjamin Witman

Mary Otto (b. 1779)

+ Gabriel Heister

- Augustus Otto Heister (1799-1820)

Elizabeth Otto (1781-1788)

Bodo Otto (1783-11785)

John Bodo Otto (1785-1858)

+ Esther Green Witman (1785-dec.)

John Augustus Otto II

Bodo Otto II (1819-1904)

- Emma Otto

Maria Otto (b. 1820)

- Henry M. Otto
- Matilda Otto

Bodo Otto (1788-1793)

Elizabeth Otto (b. 1789)

+ Henry M. Richards

◆Daniel Hitner Otto (1792-1838)

+ Sarah Witman (1795-1840)

William Witman Otto (1815-1882)

Catherine Otto (1817-1840)

- Daniel Henry Otto (1819-1875)

John Bodo Otto (1821-1840)

Charles Witman Otto (1823-1901)

Mary Witman Otto (1825-1840)

◆Catharine Maria Otto (1794-1816)

+ Joseph Wood (1794-1816)

Catharine Elizabeth Otto Wood (1816-1840)

Henreiaty Otto (1797-1801)

Sarah Otto (b. 1799)

+ Jonathan Hiester, Esq.

+ Margaretha Paris (1719-1801)

www.ingramcontent.com/pod-product-compliance
Lightning Source LLC
Chambersburg PA
CBHW051129120626
46547CB00012B/726

9781968296599